AORTIC ANEURYSM - RECENT ADVANCES

Edited by **Cornelia Amalinei**

Aortic Aneurysm - Recent Advances
http://dx.doi.org/10.5772/45988
Edited by Cornelia Amalinei

Contributors

Gioachino Coppi, Valentina Cataldi, Guido Regina, Tetsuo Fujimoto, Petar Popov, Reidar Brekken, Toril A N Hernes, Geir Arne Tangen, Frode Manstad-Hulaas, Satoshi Yamashiro, Edward McFalls, Santiago Garcia, Cemşit Karakurt, Koichi Yoshimura, Cornelia Amalinei, Irina-Draga Caruntu, Futoshi Mori, Hiroshi Ohtake, Go Watanabe, Teruo Matsuzawa, Jiaxuan Feng, Zaiping Jing, Qingsheng Lu, Jian Zhou

Published by InTech

Janeza Trdine 9, 51000 Rijeka, Croatia

Publishing Process Manager Iva Lipovic
Technical Editor InTech DTP team
Cover InTech Design team

Additional hard copies can be obtained from orders@intechopen.com

Aortic Aneurysm - Recent Advances, Edited by Cornelia Amalinei
p. cm.
ISBN 978-953-51-1081-1

For EU product safety concerns:
IN TECH d.o.o., Prolaz Marije Krucifikse Kozulić 3, 51000 Rijeka, Croatia,
info@intechopen.com or visit our website at intechopen.com.

Meet the editor

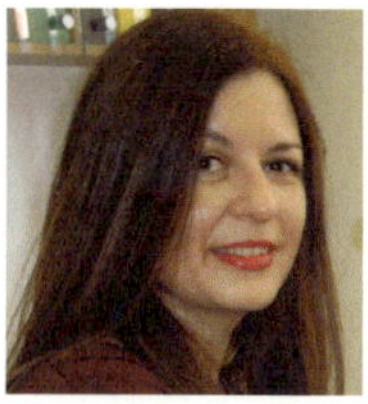

Associate-Professor Cornelia Amalinei, M.D., Ph.D., Histopathologist, of the "Grigore T. Popa" University of Medicine and Pharmacy, Iasi, Romania, is the author of 10 books and 110 articles, being also involved in international research projects. She is an editorial advisory board member of The Open Reconstructive and Cosmetic Surgery Journal. Based on her publications, she was invited as a member of the scientific committee and speaker in the first International Congress of the Kosova Association of Oncology, in 2004. The "Oxford Colleges Hospitality Scheme" selected her for a grant, in 2005. She was the beneficiary of a travel grant offered by the International Academy of Pathology, in 2006. The Adriatic Society of Pathology awarded her the Prize Pio Sodalizio Dei Piceni, in 2007.

Contents

Preface

The invitation to contribute to the editorial process of a book regarding the aortic aneurysm may seem for a histopathologist as an unchallenging project, considering that its morphological characteristics have been well-recognized and verified in individual practical diagnostic activity. Firstly described in the second century AD, by Antyllus, the complexity of the disease has been progressively evolving to a spectrum of anomalies based on genetic predisposition, stresses within the aortic wall, proteolytic degradation of the structural components, and/or inflammation and autoimmune response, factors that may be combined in a variable proportion.

Nevertheless, the increasing involvement of genetics, molecular biology and immunology, relatively recent findings in understanding the complex pathogenic mechanisms of a wide spectrum of diseases, including aortic aneurysm, provides an interesting and challenging research domain. The deep insight into these molecular cascades may facilitate not only the understanding of aortic aneurysm pathogenesis but also provide a fundament for an early diagnosis and further development of complex therapeutic modalities.

The amplitude of aortic aneurysm morbidity and mortality is constantly increasing, despite considerable advances in surgical or endovascular intervention which is still considered as the only successful form of therapy.

Furthermore, as a contribution to numerous studies currently conducted around the world aiming the improvement of patients' prognosis, mainly by the use of animal models, this book becomes a challenging project designed to gather the view of researchers with different background regarding fundamental notions and adding the updates resulted from world-wide scientific progress or from medical practice.

Consequently, the reader may find interesting data about etiology, risk factors and pathogenesis of aortic aneurysm, including an update of the genetic susceptibility and complex interactions of a wide panel of cytokines, growth factors and proteolytic enzymes, its characteristics in young age, and particularities of aneurysms affecting visceral arteries. Moreover, the chapters regarding the therapeutic management are preceded by a presentation of a complex algorithm of preoperative evaluation of the patients.

Several different perspectives regarding the surgical therapy, including the treatment of complications after prior surgery are completing the content of the book.

The authors' practical experience is added to an exhaustive and comparative review of the relevant scientific publications concerning the initiation mechanisms, clinical evaluation and complex therapeutic modalities. Furthermore, some original proposals regarding new therapeutic strategies are added, opening new and promising perspectives for the future management of the disease.

Last but not least, advanced imaging strategy contributions to the multidisciplinary management of the disease are offering the reader a wide picture of the current knowledge of aneurysmal disease.

The complex association of notions from fundamental sciences with practical therapeutic resources and original proposals for the management of the disease is providing an interesting lecture and an update of scientific literature.

Special consideration and thanks to all the authors for their efforts and to the publishing team which connected the authors from all over the world.

Associate-Professor Cornelia Amalinei
Department of Morphofunctional Sciences-Histology,
"Grigore T. Popa" University of Medicine and Pharmacy,
Iasi, Romania

Chapter 1

Etiology and Pathogenesis of Aortic Aneurysm

Cornelia Amalinei and Irina-Draga Căruntu

Additional information is available at the end of the chapter

http://dx.doi.org/10.5772/56093

1. Introduction

Aortic aneurysm is a multifactorial disease, with both genetic and environmental risk factors contributing to the underlying pathobiology.

Aortic aneurysms are atherosclerotic in origin, in older patients. Recognized predisposing factors are: hypertension, hypercholesterolemia, diabetes, and smoking.

Aneurysms are increased in frequency in patients with Marfan, Loeys-Dietz, Ehler-Danlos type IV, and Turner Syndrome, in Familial aortic disease (Hiratzka et al., 2010), and in repaired and nonrepaired congenital heart diseases (Hinton, 2012).

Less common causes, as Takayasu disease, giant cell arteritis, Behçet's disease, ankylosing spondylitis, rheumatoid arthritis, and infective aortitis should be considered (Hiratzka et al., 2010).

Histological examination demonstrates that the pathophysiological processes in aortic aneurysm involve all layers of the aortic wall in a variable proportion.

Although the aortic aneurysm morphological characteristics have been well- recognized, the mechanism which elicits its formation is incompletely understood. However, it is generally accepted that an aneurysm results from an association of genetic predisposition, stresses within the aortic wall, proteolytic degradation of the structural components, and/or inflammation and autoimmune response.

A review of the relevant scientific publications, concerning the etiology, pathogeny, histology, and molecular markers is presented in this chapter. These data provide valuable mechanistic insight into the pathogenesis of aortic aneurysm, reveal diagnostic markers, and identify new therapeutic targets.

2. Aortic anatomy

The thoracic aorta has four anatomical segments, as following: the aortic root, the ascending aorta, the aortic arch, and the descending aorta (Gray, Bannister, 1995; Hiratzka et al., 2010). The aortic diameter is influenced by age, gender, body mass index, location of measurements, and type of imaging technique (Hannuksela et al., 2006).

The aortic root contains the sinuses of Valsalva, the aortic valve annulus, and the aortic valve cusps measuring 3.50-3.72 ± 0.38 cm in female and 3.63-3.91 ± 0.38 cm in male (Hannuksela et al., 2006).

The ascending aorta contains the tubular portion extending from the sinotubular junction to the origin of the brachiocephalic artery measuring 2.82 cm (Hannuksela et al., 2006).

The aortic arch has a course in front of the trachea and to the left of the trachea and oesophagus, contains the origin of the brachiocephalic artery, and branches into the head and neck arteries (Hannuksela et al., 2006).

The descending aorta has a course anterior to the vertebral column, through the diaphragm to the abdomen, contains the isthmus between the origin of the left subclavian artery and the *ligamentum arteriosum* measuring, in mid-descending area, 2.45-2.64 ± 0.31 cm in female and 2.39-2.98 ± 0.31 cm in male and, in diaphragmatic region, 2.40-2.44 ± 0.32 cm in female and 2.43-2.69 ± 0.27-0.40 cm in male (Hannuksela et al., 2006).

The abdominal aorta is situated in front of the lower border of the last thoracic vertebra and descends in front of the vertebral column from the aortic hiatus of the diaphragm to the fourth lumber vertebra, to the left of the middle line and branches into the two common iliac arteries (Gray, Bannister, 1995). The lesser omentum and stomach, together with the branches of the celiac artery and the celiac plexus are anteriorly placed and below these, the inferior part of the duodenum, the mesentery, the splenic vein, the pancreas, the left renal vein, and aortic plexus are disposed (Gray, Bannister, 1995). The anterior longitudinal ligament and left lumbar veins are posteriorly disposed. The azygos vein, thoracic duct, cisterna chyli, and the right crus of the diaphragm are situated to the right side and the inferior vena cava is situated below (Gray, Bannister, 1995). The left crus of the diaphragm, the ascending part of the duodenum, the left celiac ganglion, and some coils of the small intestine are disposed to the left (Gray, Bannister, 1995).

The normal adult infrarenal aorta has a 12 cm length, a diameter of 2 cm, and a thickness of 2 mm (Humphrey, Taylor, 2008).

The abdominal aorta has the following branches: visceral (celiac, mesenteric, renals, middle suprarenals, internal spermatics, and ovarian), parietal (lumbars, middle sacral, and inferior phrenics), and terminal (common iliacs) (Gray, Bannister, 1995).

3. Aortic embryology

The development of the aorta and aortic valves includes aortopulmonary septation, followed by semilunar valve and two large arteries formation (Hinton et al., 2012). A process of endothelial-mesenchymal transition is responsible for the development of endocardial cushions. Cell proliferation and extracellular matrix development results in valve cusps layer formation (Hinton, Yutzey, 2011). Consequently, while cells from the semilunar valve cusps are endothelial-derived, the smooth muscle cells of the proximal aorta originate from neural crest (Majesky, 2007), with reciprocal influences of both types of cells on the development of both cell populations (Jain et al., 2011). In aorta and valve development several signalling pathways are involved, such as TGF-beta and Notch (Garg et al., 2005), and Wnt (Hinton et al., 2012).

4. Aortic histology

The histological structure of the human adult aortic wall comprises three layers. Intima is composed of a monolayer of endothelial cells supported by a special type of connective tissue (subintima), with a basement membrane between the two types of tissues (Hannuksela et al., 2006). The endothelium is continuous with endocardium and represents the interface between the vascular wall and blood (Saito et al., 2013). The endothelium is actively involved in production and reaction to inflammation mediators, such as growth factors, adhesion molecules, and a wide panel of cytokines (Saito et al., 2013). The basement membrane is composed of type IV collagen and laminin. The subendothelial layer contains collagen type I and II, elastic fibers, and abundant extracellular matrix rich in proteoglycans. Supplementary, dual phenotypic myocytes, myointimal cells, and macrophages are also components of the subendothelial layer.

The internal limiting membrane is composed of condensed elastic fibers forming a crenelated structure delimiting the intima from media. Media is composed of fenestrated concentrically disposed elastic lamellae with interposed smooth muscle cells (abundant in abdominal aorta), multiple types of collagen, and proteoglycans (Humphrey, Taylor, 2008), and external elastic lamina (Hannuksela et al., 2006). Media occupies approximately 80% of the wall thickness and contains up to 70 elastic lamellae.

Adventitia is composed of connective tissue rich in type I collagen fibers admixed with elastin and fibroblasts (Humphrey, Taylor, 2008), containing *vasa vasorum* and *nervi vasorum*. Periadventiteal tissue facilitates the aortic fixation in mediastinum and abdomen.

The aortic valve is semilunar and is composed of connective tissue forming three components: a fibrosa of fibrillar collagen, a spongiosa with proteoglycans, and a ventricularis layer made up of elastic fibers (Hinton, Yutzey, 2011). The aortic root has a different morphology compared to the aorta, consisting of the fibrous valve annulus region, situated at the cusp and aortic wall junction and of arterial tissue within the sinuses of Valsalva (Nesi et al., 2009), without elastic lamellae (Hinton, 2012).

5. Aortic aneurysm gross findings

According to the location, aortic aneurysms may be thoracic (25.9%), abdominal (62.7 %), thoracoabdominal (8.3%), and unspecified (3.0%) (Hiratzka et al., 2010).

Aortic aneurysm may exhibit two patterns, as following (Waller et al., 1997):

1. The most common type is cylindrical or fusiform pattern involving the entire aortic circumference and being diagnosed in almost all abdominal aortic aneurysms, distal to the renal arteries.
2. The saccular type is involving a limited portion of the circumference of the aorta and is diagnosed in the arch and in the descending aorta, associated to atherosclerosis, or in the abdominal aorta, mostly proximal to the renal arteries. The saccular type may be further subdivided into two subtypes, as following (Edwards, 1979):

- True type is a bulge of aorta located in an area of medial weakness, exhibiting a mouth of a similar diameter as the size of the aortic bulge.
- False type contains adventitia and a portion of media and an intra-aneurysmal thrombus, with a mouth diameter smaller than the diameter of the aortic bulge.

As chronic aneurysms are frequently associated in their evolution with atherosclerosis, the traumatic saccular aneurysm which may develop is wrongly considered as atherosclerotic in origin (Waller et al., 1997).

Within aneurysms, thrombi develop serving as a protective mean against the intra-aortic pressure (Waller et al., 1997). Due to progressive development, the outermost layers of the thrombus become organized with the consequent development of a "tree trunk" appearance (Waller et al., 1997). If it is dislodged, thromboembolic complications may occur (Waller et al., 1997).

6. Aortic aneurysm histopathology

The thoracic aortic aneurysm has been termed cystic medial necrosis which is currently considered as a misnomer because the histopathology of the disease is not characterized by necrosis or cysts (Hiratzka et al., 2010). The term medial degeneration is more accurate as the process involves disruption of elastic fibers and accumulation of proteoglycans (Hiratzka et al., 2010). Although degenerative changes, not related to hypertension, are identified in approximately two thirds of ageing population, variably associated to fibrosis and atherosclerosis (Klima et al., 1983), there are quantitative differences comparative to aortic aneurysm (Savunen, Aho, 1985).

6.1. Light microscopy

Histological examination demonstrates that pathophysiological processes in aortic aneurysm involve all layers of the aortic wall, contrasting to those observed in occlusive atherosclerosis.

http://dx.doi.org/10.5772/56093

From our experience, the biopsies demonstrate significant degradation of extracellular elastin (Fig. 1) and collagen fibers, cystic medial change (Fig. 2) (Amalinei et al., 2009) and fibrosis, reduction in the number of vascular smooth muscle cells, medial and adventitial infiltration by mononuclear lymphocytes and macrophages forming vascular associated lymphoid tissue, and thickening of the *vasa vasorum* (Fig. 3). An increase in medial neovascularisation has also been reported in aneurysmal tissue biopsies. Moreover, medial splitting by haemorrhage associated to elastic fragmentation and fibrosis was observed in dissecting aneurysms from our files (Fig. 4).

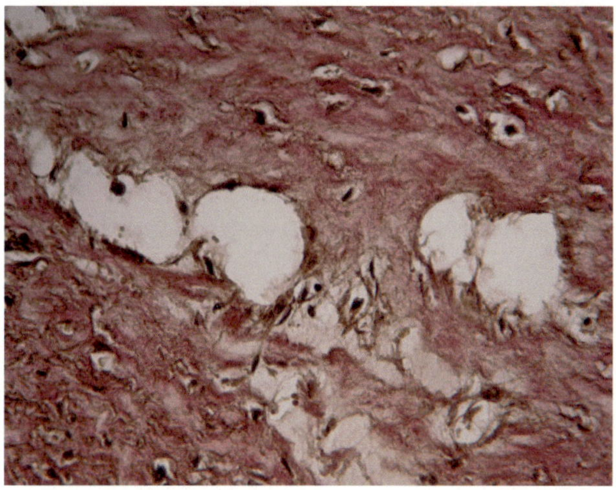

Figure 1. Elastic fibers fragmentation (Elastic-van Gieson staining)

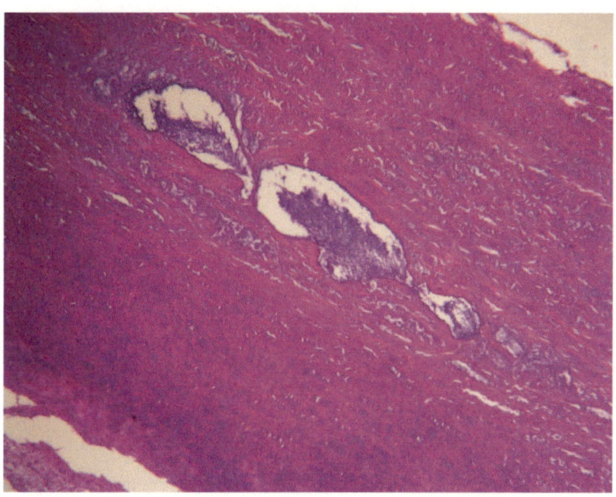

Figure 2. Cystic medial degeneration (HE staining)

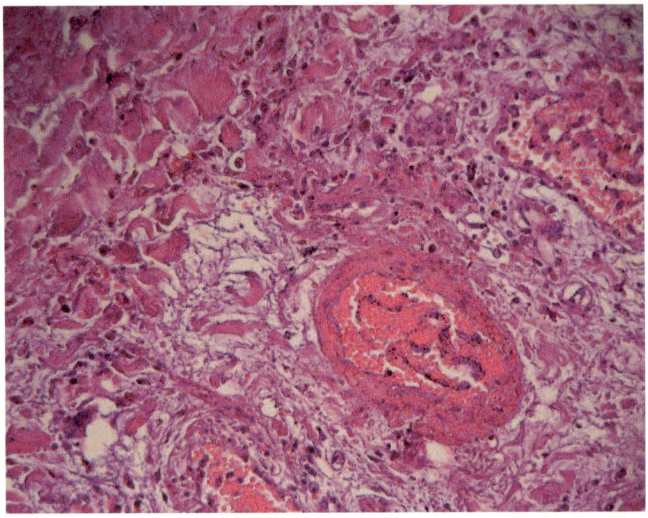

Figure 3. Adventitial inflammatory infiltrate and thickening of the *vasa vasorum* (HE staining)

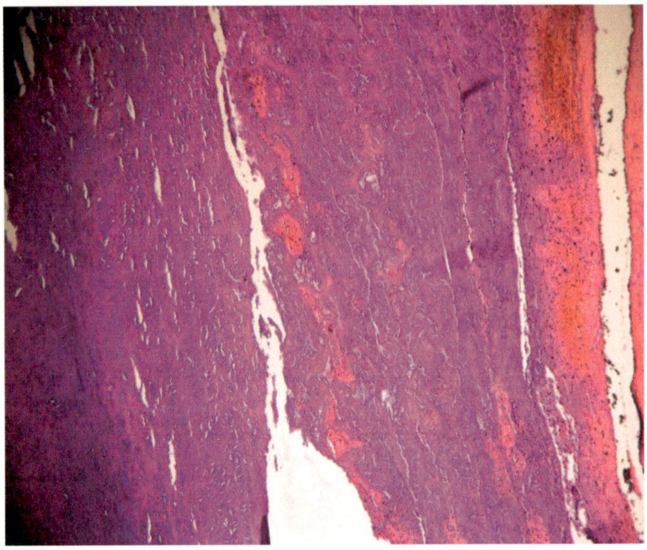

Figure 4. Dissecting aneurysm (HE staining)

Cystic changes are characterized by accumulation of basophilic material (in haematoxylin-eosin staining), showing Alcian blue positivity and metachromatic characteristics (in toluidine blue staining) between the elastic lamellae of the aortic media (Savunen, Aho, 1985). Occasional elastin deposits are identified in areas with fibers disruption or severe fragmentation when associated to atherosclerotic lesions, in orcein (Savunen, Aho, 1985) or in Elastic-van Gieson staining.

http://dx.doi.org/10.5772/56093

According to the amount of material accumulated, the lesions may be classified into three degrees, as following (Savunen, Aho, 1985):

- Grade I shows minute cysts, involving up to five foci of elastic fibers degeneration extended to two to four lamellae within the total width of the media.
- Grade II involves maximum the width of one lamellar unit, being extended to more than five foci.
- Grade III is extended more than the width of a lamellar unit and it is also involving the smooth muscular tissue.

There are two types of degeneration, according to the location of the aortic damage, as following (Doerr, 1974):

- microcystic (Gsell-type);
- disseminated cystic (Erdheim-type).

The elastic fiber degeneration is positively correlated to an increase in collagen content, less severe in Marfan-related disease and more advanced in atherosclerotic aorta (Savunen, Aho, 1985). The fibrosis may be also graded, as following (Savunen, Aho, 1985):

- Grade I fibrosis involves less than one third of the medial thickness.
- Grade II fibrosis is extended to more than one third until maximum two thirds of the media.
- Grade III fibrosis involves more than two thirds of the aortic media.

The smooth muscle is progressively lost corresponding to the structurally ineffective reparative elastogenesis, as normal elastin inhibits smooth muscle apoptosis (Humphrey, Taylor, 2008).

The medial degeneration is variable associated to atherosclerosis and inflammation (Hiratzka et al., 2010).

6.2. Electron microscopy

Normal elastin comprises 3-4 nm diameter filaments showing a parallel disposition of the fibers and a periodicity of about 4 nm (Gotte et al., 1974). Although the filamentous component is not observed in elastic lamellae, the normal aorta shows elastin streaks attached to the elastic lamellae (Dingemans et al., 1981).

In aortic aneurysms, the elastic lamellae show irregular surfaces, granulofilamentous densities, and amorphous centre holes or a normal appearance exhibiting only a variable width (range 1.2- 1.5 μm) (Savunen, Aho, 1985). New elastin formation is indicated by bundles composed of non-banded microfibrils (Savunen, Aho, 1985).

The electron microscopy shows a network of proteoglycan matrix associated to a variable amount of collagen tissue (Savunen, Aho, 1985). The collagen bundles are disposed both between elastic lamellae and in areas of elastic fibers degeneration and normal 64 nm periodicity of individual fibers has been identified (Savunen, Aho, 1985).

The smooth muscle shows degenerated cells, fragments of organelles, debris, with focal nuclei loss in Grade I, extended to less than one third in Grade II, and more than two thirds in Grade III medial necrosis (Savunen, Aho, 1985). Although smooth muscle cells are focally lost, there is no indication of a reduced total amount of muscular tissue (Hiratzka et al., 2010). Moreover, an initial hyperplastic smooth muscle cell remodelling of the aortic wall has been suggested by morphometry (Dong et al., 2002; Pannu et al., 2005; Guo et al., 2007).

6.3. Ascending aortic aneurysms particularities

The aneurysms of the ascending aorta are usually fusiform, being associated to degenerative or inflammatory processes, and occasionally calcified (Tazelaar, 2004).

The most common histopathological feature noticed in ascending aorta aneurysm is cystic medial degeneration. The patients' age ranges from 6 to 89 years, with a male dominance (M:F, 1.7:1) (Tazelaar, 2004).

The medial degenerative changes are variably associated with wall thinning, elastic lamellae disruption, and consecutive glycosaminoglycans deposition. Another finding is coagulative necrosis or laminar medial necrosis, exhibiting nuclei loss and elastic lamellae degeneration, in elderly or hypertensive patients (Tazelaar, 2004).

The consequence is the wall expansion, resulting in aortic root dilatation, anuloaortic ectasia, or ascending aortic aneurysm (type A).

According to the risk factors, patients with inherited connective tissue diseases are younger (mean age 42 years) and the lesions are more severe than those diagnosed with bicuspid aortic valve (56 years) or hypertension (65 years) (Tazelaar, 2004).

If disruption occur adjacent to small intramedial *vasa vasora*, either scant lymphoplasmacytic infiltrates or microfocal medial hemorrhage may occur, without active aortitis features.

Intima may be normal or unrelated co-existent atherosclerosis may be identified.

From our experience, during the aortic aneurysms evolution, descending aorta dilation is commonly progressive, and is accompanied by the formation of a non-occlusive, intraluminal, laminated thrombus, continuously remodelled and increasing in size. Localised hypoxia has been demonstrated in regions of the aorta covered by the thrombus and this has been suggested to contribute to physiological stresses within the arterial wall (Tazelaar, 2004).

Intramedial dissection is another manifestation of ascending aortic aneurysm most commonly diagnosed in men (63 %) with a mean age of 63 years (range 22–87 years) (Tazelaar, 2004). A higher susceptibility is registered in patients with hypertension (70% of cases), inherited connective tissue diseases, bicuspid aortic valve, cystic medial degeneration, and arteritis (Tazelaar, 2004).

The false channel developed in the outer third of the media results in hematoma with fresh platelet fibrin thrombus, sometimes with the detachment of the adventitial layer, and occasional intimal tear (Tazelaar, 2004), added to the background process of cystic degeneration, being rarely associated to laminar medial necrosis or giant cell aortitis (Tazelaar, 2004).

Variable degrees of healing may result in development of a thick, new intima possibly associated to atherosclerosis, mimicking the natural lumen or of obliterative dense linear fibrosis, or of an acute process developed against a background of chronic dissection (Tazelaar, 2004).

Despite extensive sampling, normal histological media is also reported in ascending aortic aneurysm, although associated with bicuspid valve, hypertension, or atherosclerosis (Tazelaar, 2004).

Isolated aortitis with foci of medial necrosis and no evidence of a temporal arteritis or other systemic inflammatory disease may be associated to ascending aorta aneurysm without dissection (Tazelaar, 2004). The histopathological findings reported are the following: 0.4 cm mean aortic thickness, laminar medial necrosis (50% of cases), and cystic medial degeneration (30%) (Tazelaar, 2004). Variable giant cells aortitis (44 to 75% of cases) and granulomas formation (20% of cases) have also been reported (Tazelaar, 2004).

6.4. Abdominal aortic aneurysms particularities

Abdominal aortic aneurysms are usually atherosclerotic in origin, being found in up to 3% of patients older than 50 years. Beside age, other predisposing factors are: hypertension, hypercholesterolemia, diabetes, and smoking (Heuser, Lopez, 1998).

As the abdominal aorta shows a wider pulse pressure, a thinner wall thickness, a different elastic/muscular tissue ratio, with only 28-30 concentric elastic lamellae (Humphrey, Taylor, 2008), there is a higher predisposition both for atherosclerosis and aneurysm (Heuser, Lopez, 1998).

The infrarenal segment is involved in 80-90% of cases and approximately 50% of cases show extension to the iliac arteries (Heuser, Lopez, 1998), with aneurysm being defined by a diameter greater than 3 cm and a tendency toward diffuse involvement (Humphrey, Taylor, 2008).

The histopathology of abdominal aortic aneurysm reveals a dilated lumen, a degenerated media containing disorganized collagen fibers, proliferation of fibroblasts and extracellular matrix production or external media and adventitia containing chronic inflammation (Tsuruda et al., 2006), and the development of an intraluminal thrombus (Humphrey, Taylor, 2008). The initial event is debated, either inflammation and early loss of elastin, or either a ruptured atherosclerotic plaque (Humphrey, Taylor, 2008).

Approximately 5% of patients develop a dense lymphocytic adventitial inflammation and adhesion to the duodenum or inferior vena cava, being called inflammatory aneurysms.

Numerous evidences support the significant role of Renin-angiotensin system in abdominal aortic aneurism (Blanchard et al., 2000; Lu et al., 2008). Angiotensinogen and Angiotensin II type I receptor (AT1) are overexpressed in aneurysms in comparison to healthy or atherosclerotic aorta (Kaschina et al., 2009).

In animal experiments, exogenous Angiotensin II stimulates aneurysm development (Daugherty, Cassis, 1999; Daugherty et al., 2000), while AT1a deletion inhibits its progression

(Cassis et al., 2007). Consequently, Angiotensin converting enzyme (ACE) inhibitors is preventing the aneurysmal disease progression and the AT1 blockers are currently under testing (Thompson et al., 2010; Iida et al., 2012).

7. Natural history

Aortic aneurysms are usually asymptomatic, as they initially have a slow expansion. Due to a complex association of pathogenic factors the process becomes faster, the aneurysm may continue to enlarge, and the diagnosis may be frequently be given by autopsy, due to lethal complications (Hiratzka et al., 2010).

Aortic dissection is an acute aortic syndrome caused by the disruption of the medial layer of the aortic wall with hemorrhage causing the separation of the layers (Hiratzka et al., 2010).

From our experience, an intimal lesion is found in most of the patients, resulting in tracking of the blood in a dissection plane inside medial layer (Hiratzka et al., 2010); it may rupture externally through the adventitia or back, through the intimal layer causing a septum or flap between the two lumens. The false lumen may be obstructed by a thrombus. The intimal disruption is visible on autopsy in 96% of cases (Roberts, Roberts, 1991). Atheromatosis may lead to dissection, intramural hematoma, or penetrating atherosclerotic ulcer (Hiratzka et al., 2010).

The DeBakey classification is based on the location of the intimal tear and its extension, into the following three types (Hiratzka et al., 2010):

Type I dissection is originating in the ascending aorta and extends to the aortic arch and the descending aorta.

Type II dissection is originating in the ascending aorta and it is limited to its territory.

Type III dissection is originating in the descending aorta and it is limited to its territory (Type IIIa), or it extends below the diaphragm (Type IIb).

The Stanford classification has two types: Type A involves the ascending aorta and Type B does not involve the ascending aorta (Hiratzka et al., 2010).

The risk factors of the aortic dissection comprise situations associated to medial degeneration, such as: inflammatory vasculitides, genetic conditions, pregnancy, polycystic kidney disease, chronic corticosteroid or immunosuppression, infections, or extreme stress of the aortic wall (hypertension, coarctation of the aorta, cocaine use, pheochromocytoma, weight lifting, deceleration, or torsional injury (Hiratzka et al., 2010).

Rupture of aorta may result in extravasation of blood into the pericardial sac, mediastinum, pleural sac, pulmonary trunk, main pulmonary arteries, cardiovascular defects, lung, esophagus (in thoracic aneurysms), inferior vena cava, retroperitoneum, duodenum (in abdominal aneurysms) (Roberts, 1981; Waller et al., 1997). The risk of rupture is correlated to the size of the dilated segment, to the type of aneurysm, as fusiform aneurysms are correlated to a higher pressure directed against the wall of the bulge (Roberts, 1979; Waller et al., 1997), to the possible compression against a rigid adjacent structure, such as vertebra, and infection (Bless et al., 1968).

Intramural hematoma is identified in 10-20% of patients, most commonly in descending aorta, in older patients, without a false lumen or intimal tears, possibly originating from *vasa vasorum* hemorrhage (Nienaber, Sievers, 2002) or from microscopic lesions within intima. The evolution is variable: resolution (in 10% of cases), dissection (in 11-88% of cases of ascending segment involvement and in 3-14% of cases of descending aorta involvement), or aortic dilatation and rupture (Hiratzka et al., 2010).

Obstruction by hematoma of the aortic lumen may lead to true aortic stenosis and intussusception or an obstruction of the lumen of aortic branches may result in: acute myocardial infarction and sudden death (in coronary obstruction), oliguria and renal infarction (in renal artery obstruction), bowel ischemia and infarction (in mesenteric obstruction), syncope and stroke (in innominate and/or common carotid obstruction), upper limb gangrene, paralysis, and paraplegia (in innominate and/or subclavian obstruction), leg gangrene and paralysis (in common iliac obstruction) (Roberts, 1981; Waller et al., 1997).

Aortic regurgitation and **separation of a branch of aorta from aorta** are other complications which may occur (Roberts, 1981; Waller et al., 1997).

Penetrating atherosclerotic ulcer is diagnosed mostly in the descending thoracic aorta with atherosclerotic lesions associated to ulcerations penetrating the internal elastic lamina resulting in hematoma formation within the media (Stanson et al., 1986).

Pseudoaneurysms of the thoracic aorta are associated to deceleration or torsion aortic trauma, following aortic surgery, or in infectious aortitis and penetrating ulcers (Hiratzka et al., 2010).

8. Etiologic factors and pathogenesis

8.1. Genetic susceptibility

Several genetic anomalies are known to be associated to aortic aneurysm, such as: Marfan, Loeys-Dietz, Ehlers-Danlos, Turner, and familial aortic aneurysm and dissection. Recently, a panel of genes has been involved in the development of the disease. Supplementary, inherited cardiovascular conditions are also considered as risk factors of aortic aneurysms.

8.1.1. Genetic syndromes associated to aortic aneurysm

Marfan syndrome is a high penetrance heritable disease of the connective tissue or may appear due to sporadic mutations in 25% of patients (Hiratzaka et al., 2010).

Mutations of the *FBN1* gene encoding the fibrillin-1 glycoprotein of the microfibrils from the periphery of the elastic fibers are causing the disorder (Dietz, Pyeritz, 1995).

MFS2 represents a second locus recently identified in Marfan syndrome. This is caused by mutations of the transforming growth factor-beta type II receptor (TGFBR2) showing a locus which may be common to that identified in Loeys-Dietz syndrome (Mizuguki et al., 2004).

The diagnosis criteria of Marfan syndrome are cardiovascular, ocular, and skeletal clinical findings along with family history, and *FBN1* mutations (De Paepe et al., 1996).

The cardiovascular features are thoracic aortic aneurysm and/or dissection, valvular disease (mitral valve prolapse), and aortic regurgitation, as a consequence of an enlarged aortic root causing distortion of the aortic valve cusps.

The skeletal features result from the excessive growth of the long bones and are manifested as kyphoscoliosis, pectus deformities, dolichocephaly, dolichostenomelia, and arachnodactyly, associated to manifestations of the connective tissue disorders, such as dural ectasia, hernia, striae atrophica, and joint laxity (De Paepe et al., 1996).

The lens dislocation and ectopia lentis are specific ocular findings that are useful to differentiate Marfan from Loeys-Dietz syndrome (Loeys et al., 2006).

The common clinical presentation of Marfan syndrome is that with involvement of both sinuses of Valsalva and of the tubular aortic portion, resulting a pear-shaped or an inverted light bulb ascending aortic aneurysm, possible complicated with type A dissection and rupture (Tazelaar, 2004). The prognosis is better if the dilatation is limited to the sinuses of Valsalva (Roman et al., 1993).

Beside the histopathological findings commonly found in aortic aneurysm (severe cystic medial degeneration without an inflammatory infiltrate), prolapse of the mitral and aortic valves may be associated in non-complicated cases (Tazelaar, 2004).

Type B dissection necessitating early surgical repair (at a threshold of an external diameter of 5.0 cm) (Milewicz et al., 2005) and rarely abdominal aortic aneurysm may occur in some of the patients.

Loeys-Dietz syndrome results from mutations of *TGFBR1* or *TGFBR2* genes, has an autosomal dominant transmission mechanism (Loeys et al., 2006), and is clinically manifested with a characteristic clinical triad (Singh et al., 2006). The triad comprises hypertelorism, uvula anomalies, and head and neck arterial tortuosity and aneurysms. The patients may also show skeletal anomalies similar to Marfan syndrome, dural ectasia, cervical spine anomalies, joint laxity, craniosynostosis, malar hypoplasia, retrognathia, blue sclera, and translucent skin (Loeys et al., 2006).

The vascular abnormalities include patent *ductus arteriosus*, atrial septal defects, aortic root aneurysms complicated with aortic dissection even if the aortic diameter is less than 5.0 cm (Loeys et al., 2006).

Type IV Ehlers-Danlos syndrome (vascular form) is an autosomal dominant disease due to a defect of collagen type III encoded by *COL3A1* gene (Hiratzka et al., 2010) and the clinical findings are: thin skin, easy bruising, characteristic facial appearance, and rupture of gastro-

http://dx.doi.org/10.5772/56093

intestinal tract, uterus, and arteries, leading to death until 48 years-old with or without documented aneurysms (Pepin et al., 2000).

Turner syndrome is characterized by a 45, X karyotype, manifested with a short stature, webbed neck, low-set ears, low hairline, broad chest, ovarian failure, and cardiovascular disease with hypertension. The cardiovascular anomalies are: bicuspid aortic valve, aortic coarctation, aortic dilatation diagnosed as an ascending/descending aortic diameter ratio greater than 1.5 (Ostberg et al., 2004), and aortic dissection.

Aortic root dilatation may also occur in other types of Ehlers-Danlos syndrome (other than the vascular form), in **Beals syndrome** (congenital contractural arachnodactyly due to mutations of *FBN2*) (Gupta et al., 2004), in **Autosomal dominant polycystic kidney disease** (less common than cerebral aneurysm) (Lee et al., 2004), in **Noonan syndrome** (Purnell et al., 2005), in **Alagille syndrome** (McElhinney et al., 2002), and in Shprintzen-Goldberg syndrome (Doyle et al., 2012).

8.1.2. Nonsyndromic familial aortic aneurysm and dissection

Nonsyndromic familial aortic aneurysm and dissection is inherited in an autosomal dominant manner with decreased penetrance (Milewicz et al., 1998) and exhibits genetic heterogeneity (Guo et al., 2009).

The *TAAD4* defective gene located at the locus *10q23-24* is *ACTA2* (actin, alpha 2, smooth muscle aorta). *ACTA2* was identified in 14% of familial thoracic aneurysms Type A or Type B and dissections, being associated to the following features: patent *ductus arteriosus*, bicuspid aortic valve, *liveo reticularis*, and *iris flocculi* (Hiratzka et al., 2010).

The *TAAD2* locus defective gene is *TGFBR2*, being identified in 4% of familial thoracic aneurysms and dissections, showing the following features: arterial tortuosity, aneurysms, and thin, translucent skin (Pannu et al., 2005; Hiratzka et al., 2010).

The mutant gene at 16p is *MYH11* (smooth muscle cell-specific myosin heavy chain 11) gene, identified in 1% of familial thoracic aortic aneurysms and dissections, and associated to patent *ductus arteriosus* (Zhu et al., 2006). The mutant myosin molecules due to *MYH11* mutations inhibit the filament formation preventing the smooth muscle cells contraction mechanism (Zhu et al., 2006). As *Caenorhabditis elegans* studies have demonstrated that a proper folding and assembly of thick filaments require a distinct ratio β-myosin/UNC45 (its cellular chaperone), researchers have hypothesized that this imbalance might lead to the β-myosin degradation and contraction dysfunction due to *MYH11* overexpression (Kuang et al., 2011).

The 16p13.1 duplications are overlapping in thoracic aortic disease, schizophrenia, and attention-deficit hyperactivity disorder (Kuang et al., 2011). In familial thoracic aortic aneurysms and dissections, both inherited and *de novo* duplications of 16p13.1 were identified (Kuang et al., 2011), supporting the hypothesis of its influence in changing the age of onset and of dissection risk. In cases where familial single gene mutations have been identified (Kuang et al., 2011), other risk factors are required for the clinical phenotype expression (Girirajan et al., 2010).

8.1.3. Novel validated genes in aortic aneurysm

In the development of abdominal aortic aneurysms a panel of genes has been recently identified, as following: *FOSB, LYZ, MFGE8, ADCY7, SMTN, NTRK3, GATM, CSRP2, HSPB2, PTPRC, CD4, RAMP1,* and *NCF4* (Hinterseher et al., 2013).

FOSB belongs to FOS family and it is highly increased (both its mRNA and immunohistochemical staining of FOSB protein) in human abdominal aortic aneurysm (Hinterseher et al., 2012). Transcription factors associated to FOS are known to be involved in apoptosis, cell proliferation and differentiation (Ameyar et al., 2003). Vascular smooth muscle cells apoptosis may be related to transcription factors associated to FOS family proteins, such as AP1 (Hinterseher et al., 2013).

LYZ is encoding human lysozyme produced by macrophages, as a function of innate immunity. The enzyme acts on the bacterial wall, as the enzyme breaks down peptidoglycans (Levy et al., 1999). In the pathogenesis of abdominal aortic aneurysm, pathogens have been considered as initiators, so an increased *LYZ* mRNA and immunohistochemical staining of LYZ protein would be expected (Hinterseher et al., 2012). Two hypotheses have been launched to explain this finding, either the accumulation of microorganisms into the thrombus associated to the expanded aortic segment triggering a focal aortitis (Marques da Silva et al., 2003), or either phagocytic cells recruitment triggered by vascular smooth cells apoptosis, as an autoimmune reaction (Hinterseher et al., 2013).

MFGE8 represents the milk fat globule epidermal growth factor 8 which encodes lactahderin produced by macrophages (Hinterseher et al., 2013). This protein recognizes surface proteins of apoptotic cells, binds them to integrins, as a marker for their removal (Dasgupta et al., 2006). MFGE8 protein function is important, as the failure of apoptotic cells removal triggers inflammatory and autoimmune mechanisms (Hanayama et al., 2004). Both the gene expression and MFGE8 protein immunostaining are down regulated in abdominal aortic aneurysms, suggesting a failure of lactadherin function and a consecutive lack of appropriate marking of cells which need to be removed (Hinterseher et al., 2013).

ADCY7 is a gene encoding an enzyme which catalyzes the conversion of ATP to cAMP (Beeler et al., 2004) and the corresponding cell adhesion protein is represented in human platelets (Hellevuo et al., 1995). ADCY protein is involved in calcium and chemokine signaling pathways (Beeler et al., 2004). This membrane-bound adenylate cyclase activates vascular smooth muscle contraction (Akata, 2007) and it is significantly up regulated in human abdominal aortic aneurysms (Hinterseher et al., 2013).

SMTN is involved in the smooth muscle cells development, differentiation, structural maintenance, and contraction mechanism (Krämer at al., 2001). Mouse experiments have demonstrated the risk of cardiac hypertrophy and hypertension development (Rensen et al., 2008). SMTN is down regulated in abdominal aortic aneurysms and in intracranial aneurysms (Shi et al., 2009; Hinterseher et al., 2013).

NTRK3 represents a tyrosine kinase receptor involved in cellular development and differentiation (Hinterseher et al., 2013). Multiple cardiac malformations associated to a reduced amount of stem cells have been described in *Ntrk-3* deficient mouse (Youn et al., 2003) and in human abdominal aortic aneurysm, suggesting its involvement in the differentiation process of vascular smooth muscle cells (Hinterseher et al., 2013).

GATM is a gene involved in embryonic development, tissue regeneration, and metabolic activities, such as serine, threonine, proline, and arginine pathways (Hinterseher et al., 2013). GATM belongs to the amidinotransferase family, as a mitochondrial enzyme which is involved in creatine precursor (guanidinoacetic acid) synthesis (Humm et al., 1997). In heart failure, even post-therapy, a high GATM level has been demonstrated (Cullen et al., 2006). Similarly, in abdominal aortic aneurysms, a high expression of both the gene and its correspondent protein has been demonstrated, supporting its contribution to the high serum creatinine values (Nakamura et al., 2009).

CSRP2 is a gene involved in myoblast differentiation and development (Hinterseher et al., 2013). Both the gene and its corresponding protein are down regulated in injuries of the arterial walls, both in mouse and in human abdominal aortic aneurysms (Hinterseher et al., 2013).

HSPB2 is a gene encoding a stress protein of skeletal muscle cells with poorly delimited biological functions in humans although a cardio-protective role has been demonstrated in *ex vivo* experiments (Benjamin et al., 2007). HSPB2 is down regulated in human aortic aneurysms (Hinterseher et al., 2013).

PTPRC (CD45) codifies a membrane protein with multiple functions, including the regulation of cell cycle, focal adhesion (extracellular domains similar to those of cell adhesion molecules) (Bouyain, Watkins, 2010), and sequestered calcium releasing into the cytosol (Barell et al., 2009). PTPRC is up regulated in human aortic aneurysms (Hinterseher et al., 2013), with a concurrently low level in patients' peripheral blood (Giusti et al., 2009). In a genome-wide association study, the PTPRG subtype revealed interaction with contactin 3 (Bouyain, Watkins, 2010) harboring polymorphism associated to abdominal aortic aneurysms. As the PTPRC protein is strongly positive in inflammatory infiltrate of the abdominal aortic aneurysms but has been also observed in control aortas, it is considered as an unspecific marker of the aortic wall inflammation (Treska et al., 2002; Hinterseher et al., 2013).

CD4 is a gene which encodes a membrane protein involved in calcium signaling, cell adhesion, and immune reactions (Hinterseher et al., 2013). Several studies have demonstrated its up regulation in abdominal aortic aneurysms (Abdul-Hussien et al., 2010; Hinterseher et al., 2013), with a suggested involvement in an autoimmune mechanism.

RAMP1 belongs to the calcitonin receptor modifying proteins family and the corresponding protein encoded is involved in blood pressure regulation, by inducing vascular relaxation (Hinterseher et al., 2013). RAMP1 is down regulated in abdominal aortic aneurysms (Hinterseher et al., 2013).

NCF4 gene encodes a protein belonging to a multi-enzyme complex, as a cytosolic regulatory component of the superoxide-producing phagocyte NADPH-oxidase (NOX complex) (Hinterseher et al., 2013). NCF4 is up regulated in human abdominal aortic aneurysms (Hinterseher et al., 2013). As a gene variant has been identified in men diagnosed with rheumatoid arthritis (Olsson et al., 2007), its involvement in an autoimmune mechanism might influence the abdominal aortic aneurysm development (Hinterseher et al., 2013).

8.1.4. Aortic aneurysm and cardiovascular diseases

Different cardiovascular conditions are associated to an increased risk of aortic aneurysm, such as bicuspid aortic valve, aberrant right subclavian artery, coarctation of the aorta, and right aortic arch (Hiratzka et al., 2010).

Recently, the association of aortic aneurysm to several repaired and non-repaired congenital heart diseases has led to the term "aortopathy" (Zanjani, Niwa, 2012).

Bicuspid aortic valve is a congenital anomaly identified in 0.5-1.4% of population (Pisano et al., 2011).

According to the morphology, several types of bicuspid aortic valve have been identified, as follows: fusion of the right and left coronary cusps (approximately 70% of cases), fusion of the right and non-coronary cusps, and rare cases of fusion of the left and non-coronary cusps (Roberts, Ko, 2005). The valves are prone to regurgitation in young people or stenosis in older people, with concurrent ascending aortic aneurysm in 10- 35% of cases (Svensson, 2008), as a latent manifestation of the malformation (Hinton, 2012).

The patients diagnosed with bicuspid aortic valve have degenerative developmental changes, with elastolysis, smooth muscle cells anomalies in the media of the aorta and the pulmonary artery (De Sa et al., 1999). The matrix metalloproteinases (MMPs) activation followed by extracellular matrix abnormal remodeling might be initiated by deficiency of elastin, fibrillin, emilin, known as fibers proteins (Fedak et al., 2003; Fondard et al., 2005). Supplementary, asymmetric blood flow demonstrated by computational fluid dynamics is contributing to the aortic aneurysm formation (Hope et al., 2010; Viscardi et al., 2010).

As bicuspid aortic valve and aneurysm share the pathogenesis and show overlapping genetic causes, the supposition of a single disease has been proposed (Hinton et al., 2012). In order to examine the mechanism of the disease, specific mouse models have been used, as following: *ACTA2*-deficient mouse is a model of aorta malformation and *eNOS*-deficient mouse (Lee at al., 2000) is a model of bicuspid aortic valve. Further studies are needed to develop the hypothesis of an associated diseases model (Hinton et al., 2012). Family-based research has identified 10q23-24 locus as the genomic site of *ACTA2*, as already mentioned, and *NOTCH1* on 9q34 (Garg et al., 2005; Martin et al., 2007), with complex inheritance underlying bicuspid aortic valve and thoracic aortic aneurysm (Sans-Coma et al., 2012). Genetic heterogeneity, variable expressivity, combined to epigenetics result in different clinical risks (Hinton et al., 2012). The identification of the variable genetic and clinical patterns might facilitate prognosis evaluation and management of complex aortopathies.

Aberrant right subclavian artery may arise as the fourth branch of aorta causing dysphagia due to its course behind the esophagus and its enlargement forming the Kommerell diverticulum (Freed, Low, 1997). This congenital abnormality is associated to aortic aneurysms, dissection, and rupture.

Coarctation of the aorta may be associated to aortic aneurysms if untreated or after repair surgery (Ou et al., 2006).

Right aortic arch is identified in 0.5% of population and may be associated with two types of symptoms. An enlarged aorta or the vascular ring formed by the atretic *ductus arteriosus* result in esophagus or trachea compression in Type I anomaly or the aberrant left subclavian artery running posterior to the trachea and compressing it in Type II right aortic arch (Felson, Palayew, 1963).

Aortopathy

Aortic aneurysm is one of the late complications in repaired or non-repaired congenital heart diseases (Zanjani, Niwa, 2012), such as bicuspid aortic valve (Gurvitz et al., 2004), coarctation of the aorta (Istner et al., 1987), tetralogy of Fallot (Ramayya et al., 2011), *truncus arteriosus* (Carlo et al., 2011), double-outlet right ventricle (Taussig-Bing anomaly)- ventricular septal defect- pulmonary stenosis (Losay et al., 2006), hypoplastic left heart syndrome (Cohen et al., 2003), ventricular septal defect (Eisenmenger syndrome), and single ventricle- pulmonary stenosis (Niwa et al., 2001).

Genetic anomalies are associated to intrinsic aortic wall defects, aortic overflow resulting in aortic wall dilatation (Chowdhury et al., 2008).

The histopathological appearance is similar but milder than that observed in Marfan syndrome (Niwa et al., 2001). As the aortic dilatation is correlated to aortic regurgitation, and aortic and ventricular disfunctions, the result is a complex pathophysiological abnormality creating the new concept of "aortopathy" (Zanjani, Niwa, 2012).

8.2. Atherosclerosis role in the aortic aneurysm pathogenesis

The degenerative atherosclerotic disease results in hypoxia, as the diffusion of blood from the lumen is prevented by the plaques. The consequence is the onset of aortic wall structural anomalies which may lead to arterial dilatation, in a traditional view (Heuser, Lopez, 1998).

Higher coronary disease prevalence has been found in abdominal aortic aneurysm when compared to their thoracic counterpart (Agmon et al., 2003). Supplementary, a higher incidence of atherosclerosis in type B dissections compared to type A dissection has been identified, in autopsy studies (Nakashima et al., 1990). There is a statistical difference demonstrated in C-reactive protein (CRP)/Interleukin-6 (IL-6) ratio in cases of descending aortic aneurysms when compared to ascending aortic aneurysms (Artemiou et al., 2012). Moreover, CRP/IL-6 ratio shows a positive correlation to the size of aneurysms (in both ascending and descending aorta), with the cut-off value of 0.8 (Artemiou et al., 2012).

Although a variable degree of inflammation is seen in all atherosclerotic aneurysms (Rijbroek et al., 1994), rare cases of inflammatory abdominal aortic aneurysm have been diagnosed mainly in elderly patients with only few cases being diagnosed in young patients (Sharif et al., 2008). The characteristics of inflammatory abdominal aortic aneurysm are the following: thick aortic wall containing a variable mononuclear infiltrate, periaortitis, with possible association of perianeurysmal fibrosis or involvement of ureters and duodenum (Sharif et al., 2008). It is currently considered that inflammatory abdominal aortic aneurysm, associated with variable perianeurysmal fibrosis, and idiopathic retroperitoneal fibrosis are all components of the chronic periaortitis spectrum (Jois et al., 2004). In 19% of patients this process is part of a systemic autoimmune disorder but sometimes the autoimmune diseases cannot be identified (Sharif et al., 2008). A possible reaction to the antigens released from the atherosclerotic plaques has been also considered (Sharif et al., 2008).

The disturbed fibrinolytic balance in extracellular matrix remodelling has been demonstrated in atherosclerotic human aortic aneurysm (Hayashi et al., 2008). Two plasminogen activators, tissue-type and urokinase-type (both corresponding genes being enhanced in atherosclerotic human aortic aneurysms), transform plasminogen into plasmin. Consequently, plasmin, as a trypsin-like proteolytic enzyme, degrades the extracellular matrix and activates MMPs (Hayashi et al., 2008). Annexin II, a receptor for fibrinolytic proteins, binds plasminogen and tissue-type plasminogen activators, amplifying the catalytic effect of plasminogen activation. Recently, annexin II has been identified in pathophysiological intervention of macrophages in inflammatory process associated to human atherosclerotic aneurysms, suggesting a correlation between its expression and disease progression (Hayashi et al., 2008).

8.3. Inflammatory and autoimmune conditions in the aortic aneurysm pathogenesis

8.4. Infective thoracic aortic aneurysm (infected aneurysm or infectious aortitis)

Inflammatory diseases associated to aortic aneurysms are Takayasu arteritis, giant cell arteritis, Behçet disease, ankylosing spondylitis (Hiratzka et al., 2010), and rheumatoid arthritis (Tazelaar, 2004).

Takayasu arteritis involves elastic arteries (aorta and its branches) being more prevalent in women, in the third decade of life, exhibiting a moderate Asian overexpression (Kerr et al., 1994). The distribution of the aortic segments involved by Takayasu arteritis in Japanese population is: the descending aorta, followed by the abdominal, and then ascending aorta (Matsumura et al., 1991). The abdominal aorta and renal arteries are more commonly affected in Indian population (Kerr et al., 1994).

The American College of Rheumatology criteria may be used to diagnose Takayasu arteritis if three of the following criteria are found: age younger than 40 years, diminished brachial artery pulse, intermittent claudication, subclavian artery or aortic bruit, variation of blood pressure higher than 10 mm Hg between arms, and stenosis identified by angiography (Kerr et al., 1994). Supplementary, increased CRP and erythrocyte sedimentation rate are useful for diagnosis, mainly in acute phase (Kerr et al., 1994).

Several types have been described according to the extension of the disease (Tazelaar, 2004):

- Type I involves the aortic arch, the proximal brachiocephalic, and the common carotid, with IA subtype, involving the ascending aorta and associated with aortic valve regurgitation.
- Type II involves the descending thoracic and abdominal aorta.
- Type III involves the entire aorta.

- Type IV involves the pulmonary arteries, with the possible association of aorta and systemic vessels.

The histopathological findings in active arteritis have been described as: a thick wall (mean 0.7 cm, range 0.4-0.9 cm) mainly due to inflammation involving the media and adventitia, containing lymphocytes, macrophages, plasma cells, eosinophils, and neutrophils. Rare granulomas may be identified (14% of cases), showing central necrosis. Other findings are: laminar necrosis (40-50 %) and rare cystic degeneration (Tazelaar, 2004).

Obstruction of large arteries by a mural thrombus followed by its organization and association to medial and circumferential adventitial fibrosis, and intimal hyperplasia may occur in evolution (Tazelaar, 2004). Healing process may be associated with aneurysm formation (type IA) (Tazelaar, 2004).

The pathogenesis of Takayasu arteritis is attributed to a clonal T-cell-mediated panarteritis, initiated in adventitial *vasa vasorum* (Hiratzka et al., 2010). The destruction process leads to aneurysm, while fibrosis causes stenosis (Hiratzka et al., 2010).

Giant cell arteritis or temporal arteritis is a vasculitis of elastic vessels and its secondary and tertiary branches (Hiratzka et al., 2010), more prevalent in Scandinavian population, suggesting a genetic component (Nordborg et al., 1994).

The diagnosis is accomplished in case of positivity of three or more of the following criteria: localized headache, age more than 50 years, attenuation of the temporal artery pulse, increased erythrocyte sedimentation rate (greater than 50 mm/h), and positive biopsy (Achkar et al., 1994). The biopsy may be performed even during therapy, as it remains positive within 7 days of steroid therapy initiation (Achkar et al., 1994).

Isolated aortitis histopathological findings may be seen in systemic giant cells arteritis. Caucasians, over 50 years old, with women: men ratio of 4:1 may be diagnosed with systemic giant cells arteritis, being associated in 10-15% of patients with temporal arteritis and polymyalgia rheumatica (Tazelaar, 2004).

Giant cell arteritis and Takayasu arteritis share an inflammatory response with T-cell clonal expansion initiated in adventitia and amplified by cytokines and MMPs, resulting in granuloma formation and followed by vessel destruction (Salvarani et al., 1995). The granulomatous reaction protects the affected vessel from the inciting antigen but results in wall destruction (Hiratzka et al., 2010).

Behçet disease is another inflammatory vasculitis which may also result in thoracic aortic aneurysm (Hiratzka et al., 2010). The eponymous syndrome is most common in Turkey and diagnostic criteria comprise aphtous stomatitis, associated to another two of these three lesions: uveitis or retinal vasculitis, recurrent genital ulcers, or skin manifestations, such as pseudofolliculitis, pathergy, or erythema nodosum (Criteria for diagnosis of Behçet's disease, 1990; Sarica-Kucukoglu et al., 2006).

Variable arteries and veins involvement may occur in approximately one third of patients (Hiratzka et al., 2010), such as thrombosis and varices (Sarica-Kucukoglu et al., 2006).

Aortic inflammation of media and surrounding *vasa vasorum* is composed of lymphocytes, macrophages, eosinophils, and giant cells. The inflammation leads to multiple aneurysms, stenotic lesions, and brachiocephalic arteries occlusion (Tunaci et al., 1995).

Ankylosing spondylitis

There is strong association of major histocompatibility complex *HLA B-27* and the lack of rheumatoid factor in spondyloarthropaties, including Ankylosing spondylitis (Khan, Ball, 2002).

The diagnosis is set by finding four of the following five criteria: subtle onset, with morning stiffness, back pain prolonged more than three months, showing improvement with exercise, and diagnosis in young age (Roldan et al., 1998). Variable constitutional symptoms, acute anterior uveitis, aortic root involvement, nodular aortic valve, and aortic valvular regurgitation may also be associated (Roldan et al., 1998).

Rheumatoid arthritis

Rarely, a variable extension of inflammation of media and adventitia, composed of mononuclear cells, macrophages, and neutrophils, associated to granulomas (up to 50% of cases), laminar necrosis, and increased aortic wall thickness may occur in rheumatoid arthritis (Tazelaar, 2004).

Infective thoracic aortic aneurysm (infected aneurysm *or***infectious aortitis)** may be caused by fungal, bacterial, spirochetal, viral, or mycobacterium microorganisms (Hiratzka et al., 2010).

It was firstly described by Osler, as *mycotic endarteritis* (Osler, 1885). The disease may involve the ascending thoracic aorta, aortic arch, and descending aorta, usually in opposite sites to the great vessels in the aortic arch or to the abdominal visceral arteries, in the common shape of saccular or rare fusiform types, or pseudoaneurysms (Hiratzka et al., 2010).

The pathogenic mechanism involves contiguous spread from adjacent infected lymph nodes, pericarditis, mediastinitis, empyema, or abscesses, by septic emboli from a endocarditis, or by hematogenous spread in intravenous drug abuse or sepsis (Hiratzka et al., 2010).

Preexisting atherosclerotic plaque, trauma, or aneurysm may facilitate the onset of the infectious process (Hiratzka et al., 2010).

The organisms responsible for the aortitis are variable, such as bacteria of *Staphylococcus aureus, Salmonella, Pneumococcus,* and *Escherichia coli* species (Hiratzka et al., 2010), or fungi (in immunodeficient hosts) either *Candida* or *Aspergillus* (Byard et al., 1987).

Treponema species mainly affect ascending thoracic aorta, with the syphilitic aortitis onset 10-25 years after the initial infection (Hiratzka et al., 2010).

An increased thickness of the aortic wall associated to narrower or occluded lumina may occur in syphilitic aortitis, which mostly involves the aortic arch and descending thoracic aorta.

Histopathological findings consist of: variable elastic fibers degeneration, compensatory fibrosis, *vasa vasorum* with increased thickness, partial or complete lumen obliteration, and perivascular chronic inflammatory infiltrate (Tazelaar, 2004). Atherosclerosis is sometimes superimposed. Occasionally, gumas and diffuse secondary intimal fibrosis with linear folds creating the "tree bark" appearance may be identified (Tazelaar, 2004).

Tuberculous aortitis may spread by direct extension from lymph nodes, pericarditis or empyema, affecting the distal aortic arch and descending thoracic aorta (Allins et al., 1999).

Human immunodeficiency virus has been also associated to ascending thoracic aorta dilatations (Brawley, Clagett, 2005).

8.5. Matrix Metalloproteinases (MMPs) involvement in aortic aneurysm pathogenesis

Aortic aneurysms risk factors are currently correlated to initiation associated to elastin and collagen proteolytic degradation, altered expression of contractile proteins in smooth muscle cells, destruction of the extracellular matrix, and inflammation or progression and rupture, related to added angiogenesis.

The action of proteolytic enzymes, notably matrix metalloproteases and serine proteases, has been associated with the destruction of the extracellular matrix (Amalinei et al., 2007). Typically, protease activity is regulated by endogenous inhibitors (e.g. α2-macroglobulins, α 1-antitrypsin and tissue inhibitors of metalloproteinases) (Amalinei et al., 2010), and unbalanced proteolysis within the aortic media suggests that over-expression of proteinases, or deficiency in protease inhibitors may be involved in aortic aneurysm pathophysiology.

MMP-1, MMP-2, MMP-3, MMP-7, MMP-9, and MMP-12 have been associated to the aortic aneurysm pathogeny.

Gelatinase-A (MMP-2) and gelatinase-B (MMP-9) show a strong expression in media of aortic aneurysms, on the surface of disrupted elastic fibers (Ikonomidis et al., 2007; Lemaire et al., 2007).

MMP-2 results from an overexpression by the resident (mesenchymal) cells of the aortic wall, while MMP-9 is attributed to a strong expression of macrophages (Thompson et al., 1995), similar findings being also found in mouse models (Longo et al., 2002).

Gene expression analyses in animal models have demonstrated the up regulation of mRNA encoding MMP-1, MMP-3, and MMP-9, together with an enhanced cysteine protease cathepsin-D, -H, -K, and –S level, corresponding to an increased extracellular matrix degradation (Trollope et al., 2011).

Immunohistochemistry demonstrated the expression of MMP-1, MMP-2, MMP-3, MMP-7, MMP-9, and MMP-12 in macrophage-rich areas of abdominal aortic aneurysms (Curci et al., 1998).

Recent proteomics studies on tissue lysates have revealed increased levels of MMP-12 (macrophage metalloelastase) in abdominal aortic aneurysms. The MMP-12 overexpression was associated to enhanced levels of type XII collagen (correlated to exposure to high tensile forces), aortic carboxypeptidase-like protein (ACLP) (associated to collagen fibers and considered a possible regulator of fibrosis), fibronectin (accumulated in injured tissues), tenascin (correlated to the macrophage functions), thrombospondin 2 and periostin (related to cellular adhesion) (Didangelos et al., 2011). Furthermore, concomitant poor expression of glycoproteins which mediate the link between hyaluronic acid and proteoglycans, namely perlecan, aggrecan, and versican has been demonstrated (Didangelos et al., 2011).

8.6. ADAMs (a disintegrin and metalloproteases) involvement in aortic aneurysm pathogenesis

ADAMs are produced by smooth muscle cells in a healthy aorta (Lipp et al., 2012). Supplementary, ADAMs 10, 12, 15, and 17 expression are significantly correlated to the amount of smooth muscle tissue in the aortic wall (Lipp et al., 2012), without any influence on the expression of macrophages or other inflammatory cells or of the neovascularisation extent. Their complex biological roles have been demonstrated, including: proteolysis, cell adhesion, zymogen activation, cell migration, cell-matrix relation, angiogenesis (Oksala et al., 2009), and a possible role in the pathogenesis of atherosclerosis.

The experiments analysing the role of ADAM family of metalloproteases in aneurysm pathogenesis showed ADAMs 8, 9, 10, 12, 15, and 17 expressions in inflammatory cells and in neovessels of abdominal aortic aneurysm (Lipp et al., 2012).

As tissue inhibitors of metalloproteases, TIMP-1 and TIMP-3 counteract ADAMs activity, an increased TIMP-3 expression being found in abdominal aortic aneurysms (Lipp et al., 2012).

8.7. Angiogenesis in aortic aneurysm pathogenesis

An important pathway in the aortic aneurysm pathogenesis is attributed to angiogenesis.

Angiogenesis is regulated by ephrin-B1 and its cognate receptor, EphB2, members of a 21 gene family involved in morphogenesis by regulating cell adhesion and migration (Palmer, Klein, 2003; Sakamoto et al., 2008; Pasquale, 2010). In contrast to cytokines and chemokines that are soluble molecules, ephrins and Ephs are membrane-bound molecules that act locally by cell-to-cell interactions (Kepler, Chan, 2007; Janes et al., 2008). Thus, ephrins and Ephs modulate various types of cell interactions, conditioned by cytokines and chemokines, as macrophages-to-macrophages, macrophages-to-T-lymphocytes, and macrophages-to-endothelial cells (Sakamoto et al., 2012).

Human abdominal aortic aneurysm expresses high levels of ephrin-B1 and EphB2 in macrophages, T lymphocytes, and endothelial cells (Sakamoto et al., 2012).

Supplementary, ephrin-5 is up regulated in human abdominal aortic aneurysm (Armstrong et al., 2002).

8.8. Mast cells key role in aortic aneurysm pathogenesis

Mast cells, as cellular components of the media and adventitia are also important players in aortic aneurysm pathogenesis *via* several mechanisms, such as: activation of metalloproteinases and of the Renin-Angiotensin system, contribution to smooth muscle cells apoptosis, and release of proteolytic enzymes. Thus, drugs targeting the pathways of mast cell-derived mediators may be of value in future treatment of aortic aneurysm.

Two types of mast cells may be identified in human aorta (Kaartinen et al., 1994; Lindstedt et al., 2007): T type containing tryptase and TC type supplementary expressing chymase, carboxypeptidase A, and cathepsin G within cytoplasmic granules. The granules may also contain variable quantities of the following substances: tumor necrosis factor alpha (TNF-α), transforming growth factor beta (TGF-β), vascular endothelial growth factor (VEGF), basic fibroblast growth factor (bFGF), and chemokines (Swedenborg et al., 2012). Following mast cells activation, a prolonged synthesis and secretion of cytokines, chemokines, and eicosanoids takes place (Swedenborg et al., 2011).

As in normal human aorta, mast cells are located within intima and adventitia; their identification within media of abdominal aortic aneurysm in a higher amount in comparison to their expression in atherosclerosis demonstrates their involvement in the extracellular matrix degradation, smooth muscle cells apoptosis, renin-angiotensin system activity, and in neovascularization (Swedenborg et al., 2011). Moreover, their overall count increases along the aneurysm expansion, being associated to T cells and macrophages (Swedenborg et al., 2011).

Various types of cells are involved in producing chemotactic factors for mast cells, such as stem cell factor (SCF). Both the homing of the progenitor cells and their terminal differentiation are performed by SCF (Swedenborg et al., 2011).

Experimental studies on rats and mice which lack SCF or its receptor (c-kit) expression are used as mast cell deficient models (Swedenborg et al., 2011). In mast cell deficient rodents, elastase or $CaCl_2$ infusion cannot produce abdominal aortic aneurysm. Wild-type mast cells derived may restore the capacity of aneurysm formation. Alternatively, similar results have been obtained in experimental models in which mast cells degranulation has been pharmacologically prevented (Swedenborg et al., 2011).

Adrenomedullin, a 52-amino acid peptide firstly isolated from human pheochromocytoma, inhibits myofibroblastic differentiation and collagen synthesis and stimulates MMP-2 activity. In abdominal aortic aneurysms, an increased amount of adrenomedullin has been found in mast cells situated in the outer media and adventitia, showing a stronger expression in comparison to atherosclerotic aortas without aneurysmal changes (Tsuruda et al., 2006). This finding suggests anti-fibrotic function of adrenomedullin released from mast cells demonstrating its complex role in extracellular matrix modulation in the development of abdominal aortic aneurysms (Tsuruda et al., 2006).

8.9. Cytokines invovement in aortic aneurysms pathogenesis

Using comparative quantitative proteins profile within aortic aneurysm biopsies and aortic samples from cadaveric controls, significant differences in the expression of numerous proteins, including proinflammatory cytokines (IL-1α, IL-1β, TNF- α and TNF-β, oncostatin M, and IL-6), chemokines (ENA-78, GRO, IL-8, monocyte chemoattractant proteins [MCP-1, MCP-2], and regulated upon activation normal T cell expressed and secreted [RANTES]), anti-inflammatory cytokines (IL-10 and IL-13), and growth factors (VEGF, Angiogenin, GCSF [granulocyte colony stimulating factor], EGF [epidermal growth factor], SCF, leptin, IL-3, IL-7, and thrombopoietin) were reported (Quillard et al., 2011).

IL-6 has synergic effect as IL-1 in regulating the hepatic synthesis of CRP (Artemiou et al., 2012). There are both experimental and clinical evidences supporting the CRP involvement in stenotic atherogenesis and the significance of its increased level as a marker of cardiovascular diseases (Venugopal et al., 2005). IL-6 is involved in acute and chronic inflammation associated to aneurysm formation (Smallwood et al., 2008). Both thoracic and abdominal aortic aneurysms are positively correlated to IL-6 high circulating levels (Artemiou et al., 2012).

8.10. COX-2 involvement in aortic aneurysms pathogenesis

COX-2 (cyclooxygenase-2) is expressed in smooth muscle cells of the media, in mouse models of abdominal aortic aneurysm (Ghoshal, Loftin, 2012).

Chronic infusion of Angiotensin II induces abdominal aortic aneurysm but the process can be significantly reduced by pre-treatment with a COX-2 inhibitor or by targeted genetic inactivation of COX-2 (Gitlin et al., 2007). COX-2 inactivation is associated to significat decrease of macrophage-dependent inflammation (Gitlin et al., 2007).

A reduced progression of abdominal aortic aneurysm has been also obtained by inactivation of microsomal prostaglandin E synthase-1 (mPGES-1) (Wang et al., 2007), acting on COX-2-dependent mechanism and being correlated to a reduced activity of MMP-2 (Wang et al., 2007).

The experimental findings that COX-2 inhibition results in significantly reduced MMP-2 expression supports the hypothesis that COX-2 is involved in smooth muscle cell dedifferentiation during the abdominal aortic aneurysm progression (Ghoshal, Loftin, 2012).

During abdominal aortic aneurysm progression, smooth muscle cells produce hyaluronic acid and show a variable expression of α-actin, as characteristics of de-differentiation (Jain et al., 1996). Mouse experiments demonstrated that COX-2 inhibition results in α-actin mRNA expression and a hyaluronic acid synthase reduced expression (Ghoshal, Loftin, 2012). These findings suggest the COX-2 pathway involvement in smooth muscle cells de-differentiation is associated to abdominal aortic aneurysm development (Ghoshal, Loftin, 2012).

8.11. Macrophage role in aortic aneurysm pathogenesis

Experimental subcutaneous infusion of Angiotensin II into mice induces histopathological changes that result in proteolytic generation of elastin and collagen degradation products which can attract circulating inflammatory cells, such as macrophages and mononuclear lymphocytes (Daugherty et al., 2011). The cellular changes involve the early macrophage infiltration into media and adventitia, demonstrated by CD68 immunostaining in the suprarenal aortic region (Daugherty et al., 2011).

Once activated, inflammatory infiltrates produce (amongst others) leukotriens, proinflammatory cytokines, chemokines, prostaglandin derivatives, immunoglobulins, cysteine and serine proteases, thereby perpetuating the wall degradation and vascular smooth cell apoptosis (Daugherty et al., 2011). This infiltration of proinflammatory cells and the observation that IgG purified from aneurysm tissue is reactive to aortic extracellular matrix proteins suggest that its development may have an autoimmune component (Daugherty et al., 2011).

Macrophages along with smooth muscle cells produce elastolytic cathepsin L that results in elastic lamina fragmentation, muscle cell migration into neointima, and wall expansion (Liu et al., 2006). Cathepsin S produced by smooth muscle cells is amplifying the cathepsin L effect (Liu et al., 2006). Moreover, cathepsin L may process caspases and induce apoptosis in human abdominal aortic aneurysms and atherosclerosis. Both cathepsin L and VEGF-A (Kaneko et al., 2011), as macrophages products, are involved in neovascularization. The high expression of cathepsin L in atherosclerosis and abdominal aortic aneurysm, or its higher serum levels suggest a strong involvement in their pathogenesis (Liu et al., 2006).

There are several surface targets used for macrophage imaging, such as scavenger receptors (Tawakol et al., 2008), vascular cell adhesion protein-1 (VCAM-1) (Nahrendorf et al., 2006), inter-cellular adhesion molecule-1 (ICAM-1) (Choi et al., 2007), $\alpha_v\beta_3$ integrin (Chen et al., 2010), and chemokine (C-C motif) receptor 2 (CCR-2) (Hartung et al., 2007). Supplementary, phagocytosis may be useful for cell detection by internalization of probes (Quillard et al., 2011), such as nanoparticles (Christen et al., 2009). The possibility of developing therapies based on drugs marked with imaging moieties opens up the perspectives of "theranostic" approaches (Quillard et al., 2011). An illustrative example is the use of agents targeting macrophages scavenger receptor 1A which may detect MMP-9 activity (Suzuki et al., 2008). Reactive oxygen species and proteases, including MMPs and cysteinyl cathepsins (Lutgens et al., 2007), could also be used in macrophages detection (Quillard et al., 2011).

8.12. Utility of animal models in the study of aortic aneurysms pathogenesis

The study of the pathogenic mechanism operative in aortic aneurysm may be performed on experimental models, using normal transgenic animals or choosing one of the following methods: intra-aortic elastase infusion, topical aortic treatment with $CaCl_2$, or angiotension infusion (Swedenborg et al., 2011).

The advantage of animal research is that the study of the progressive stages of aneurysm is possible but the limits of this type of studies is that the results cannot be directly applied in interpreting human aortic aneurysm and interspecies biological and physiological variations must be considered (Trollope et al., 2010; Swedenborg et al., 2011).

The experiments on large animal models are helpful in development of new surgical techniques, being performed by turbulent flow method, vein patch, or xenografts (Trollope et al., 2010).

Another possibility of research is to study the plasma concentration of various markers or of the surgical specimens with the limitation that they represent just the end stage of the disease, as the intervention is recommended when the diameter is significantly increased (Daugherty et al., 2011; Swedenborg et al., 2011).

In experimental models, the initial disintegration of elastic fibers has been identified (Daugherty et al., 2011). The following stage is the medial rupture occurring several days after the progressive lumen expansion and followed by thrombi and adventitial dissection (Barisione et al., 2006; Daugherty et al., 2011). After thrombi resolving, abundant infiltration by macrophages, lymphocytes, disarrayed collagen deposition, and neovascularization follow (Saraff et al., 2003; Rateri et al., 2011; Daugherty et al., 2011). Supplementary, atherosclerotic lesions associated to hypercholesterolemia may be detected (Rateri et al., 2011; Daugherty et al., 2011).

The heterogeneity of angiotensin II induced abdominal aortic aneurysm is illustrated by their classification into four types, as following (Daugherty et al., 2011):

- type I- a small single dilation (x 1.5-2 times of a normal diameter);
- type II- a large single dilation (> 2 times of a normal diameter);
- type III- multiple dilations;
- type IV- aortic rupture.

The angiotensin II induced abdominal aortic aneurysm model may validate the therapeutic usage of renin angiotensin inhibitors (Daugherty et al., 2011).

Using mouse model with Angiotensin II-induced abdominal aortic aneurysm formation, the involvement of oxidative stress-induced changes in biomechanical and microstructural alterations characteristic for abdominal aortic aneurysm development have been investigated (Maiellaro-Rafferty et al., 2011). Although the aortic pressure-diameter mechanics has been preserved, an increased mean circumferential strain in the outer abdominal aortic wall has been registered (Maiellaro-Rafferty et al., 2011). Moreover, the strong expression of aortic smooth muscle cell-specific catalase might prevent the development of the mechanical alterations resulted from Angiotensin II perfusion (Maiellaro-Rafferty et al., 2011), suggesting reactive oxygen species production association to early remodelling process and mechanical adaptation (Maiellaro-Rafferty et al., 2011). As expected, up regulated reactive oxygen species have been found in abdominal aortic aneurysms (Gavrila et al., 2005) stimulating MMP action via the NADPH oxidase and thus promoting extracellular matrix degradation (Grote et al., 2003).

Numerous cellular abnormalities and ultrastructural alterations in extracellular matrix cross-linking might be added to the mentioned biomechanical events (Maiellaro-Rafferty et al., 2011). Enzymatically-related mechanisms have been identified in the genesis of abdominal aortic aneurysms both in animal models and in humans. These are related to the stimulator role of dysfunctional collagen and elastin cross-linking in aneurysmal progression in mice showing lysyl oxidase-deficiency (Maki et al., 2002). Moreover, cysteine protease inhibitor cystatin C human deficiency has been correlated to abdominal aortic aneurysms (Lindholt, Henneberg, 2001). Several other elements may complicate the aneurysm genesis, such as reduced proteoglycans (Tamarina et al., 1998), collagen microarchitecture anomalies (Lindeman et al., 2010), and inflammation (Freestone et al., 1995).

Additionally, the activation of endothelial NF-κB in transgenic mice results in an increased expression of adhesion molecules initiating macrophage infiltration and inflammation in adventitia and media, demonstrating the endothelium role in remodelling of the vascular wall and in aneurysm development (Saito et al., 2013).

9. Conclusion and perspectives

Aortic aneurysm is a multifactorial disease, with both genetic and environmental risk factors contributing in variable degrees to the underlying pathobiology, leading to proteolytic degradation of aortic wall components, stresses within the aortic wall, and variable intervention of inflammation and/or autoimmune response.

Although the aortic aneurysm morphological characteristics have been well-recognized, the mechanisms underpinning these changes are extremely complex and only partially discovered.

Numerous research data provide valuable mechanistic insight into the genetic, environmental, and mechanistic pathogenesis of aortic aneurysm, reveal diagnostic markers, and identifies new therapeutic targets, such as recently described "theranostic" approaches.

The translation of data resulted in animal models to human pathology may lead to the refinement of clinical risk categories and consequently to development of novel management strategies for the prevention and treatment of aortic aneurysms.

Author details

Cornelia Amalinei and Irina-Draga Căruntu

Department of Morphofunctional Sciences- Histology, „Grigore T. Popa" University of Medicine and Pharmacy, Iasi, Romania

References

[1] Abdul-hussien, H, Hanemaaijer, R, Kleemann, R, et al. The pathophysiology of abdominal aortic aneurysm growth: Corresponding and discordant inflammatory and proteolytic processes in abdominal aortic and popliteal artery aneurysms, J Vasc Surg, (2010)., 51, 1479-1487.

[2] Achkar, A. A, Lie, J. T, Hunder, G. G, et al. How does previous corticosteroid treatment affect the biopsy findings in giant cell (temporal) arteritis? Ann Intern Med, (1994)., 120(12), 987-992.

[3] Agmon, Y, Khandheria, B. K, Meissner, I, et al. Is aortic dilatation an atherosclerosis-related process? Clinical, laboratory and transesophageal echocardiographic correlates of thoracic aortic dimensions in the population with implications for thoracic aortic aneurysm formation, J Am Coll Cardiol, (2003)., 42, 1076-1083.

[4] Akata, T. Cellular and molecular mechanisms regulating vascular tone.2.Regulatory mechanisms modulating Ca^{2+} mobilization and/or myofilament Ca^{2+} sensitivity in vascular smooth muscle cells, J Anesth, (2007)., 21, 232-242.

[5] Allins, A. D, Wagner, W. H, Cossman, D. V, et al. Tuberculous infection of the descending thoracic and abdominal aorta: case report and literature review, Ann Vasc Surg, (1999)., 13(4), 439-444.

[6] Amalinei, C, Caruntu, I. D, & Balan, R. A. Biology of Metalloproteinases, Rom J Morphol Embryol, (2007)., 48(4), 316-320.

[7] Amalinei, C, Caruntu, I. D, Giusca, S. E, & Balan, R. Matrix metalloproteinases involvement in pathologic conditions, Rom J Morphol Embryol, (2010)., 51(2), 215-228.

[8] Amalinei, C, Manoilescu, I, & Hurduc, C. Cystic medial necrosis in Marfan and non-Marfan aortic dissection, Virchows Arch, (2009). suppl. 1): SS250., 249.

[9] Ameyar, M, Wisniewska, M, Weitzman, J. B, & Role, A. for AP-1 in apoptosis: the case for and against, Biochimie, (2003)., 85, 747-752.

[10] Armstrong, P. J, & Johanning, J. M. Calton Jr. WC, et al., Differential gene expression in human abdominal aorta: aneurysmal versus occlusive disease, Journal of Vascular Surgery, (2002)., 35(2), 346-355.

[11] Artemiou, P, Charokopos, E, Sabol, F, et al. C-Reactive protein/interleukin-6 ratio as marker of the size of the uncomplicated thoracic aortic aneurysms, Interactive CardioVascular and Thoracic Surgery, (2012)., 15, 871-877.

[12] Barell, D, Dimmer, E, Huntley, R. P, et al. The GOA data-base in an integrated gene ontology annotation resource, Nucleic Acids Res, (2009). D396-D403., 2009.

[13] Barisione, C, Charnigo, R, Howatt, D. A, et al. Rapid dilatation of the abdominal aorta during infusion of angiotensin II detected by noninvasive high-frequency ultrasonography, J Vasc Surg, (2006)., 44(2), 372-376.

[14] Beeler, J. A, Yan, S. Z, Bykov, S, et al. A soluble C1b protein and its regulation of soluble type 7 adenylyl cyclase, Biochemistry, (2004)., 43, 15463-15471.

[15] Benjamin, I. J, Guo, Y, Srinivasan, S, et al. CRYAB and HSPB2 deficiency alters cardiac metabolism and paradoxically confers protection against myocardial ischemia in aging mice, Am J Physiol Heart Circ Physiol, (2007). HH3209., 3201.

[16] Blanchard, J. F, Armenian, H. K, & Friesen, P. P. Risk factors for abdominal aortic aneurysm: results of a case-control study, Am J Epidemiol, (2000)., 151, 575-583.

[17] Bless, B. P, Maini, R. N, & Scott, J. T. Ruptured abdominal aorta infected with *Salmonella brandenbug*, Br Med J, (1968)., 4, 751-762.

[18] Bouyain, S, & Watkins, D. J. The protein tyrosine phosphatases PTPRZ and PTPRG bind to distinct members of the contactin family of neural recognition molecules, Proc Natl Acad Sci USA, (2010). , 107, 1433-2448.

[19] Brawley, J. G, & Clagett, G. P. Mycotic aortic aneurysm, J Vasc Surg, (2005).

[20] Byard, R. W, Jimenez, C. L, Carpenter, B. F, & Hsu, E. Aspergillus-related aortic thrombosis, CMAJ, (1987). , 136(2), 155-156.

[21] Carlo, W. F, Mckenkie, E. D, & Slesnick, T. C. Root dilatation in patients with truncus arteriosus, Congenit Heart Dis, (2011). , 6(3), 228-233.

[22] Cassis, L. A, Rateri, D. L, Lu, H, & Daugherty, A. Bone marrow transplantation reveals that recipient AT1a receptors are required to initiate angiotensin II-induced atherosclerosis and aneurysms, Arterioscler Thromb Vasc Biol, (2007). , 27, 380-386.

[23] Chen, W, Jarzyna, P. A, Van Tilborg, G. A, et al. RGD peptide functionalized and reconstituted high-density lipoprotein nanoparticles as a versatile and multimodal tumor targeting molecular imaging probe, FASEB J, (2010). , 24(6), 1689-1699.

[24] Choi, K. S, Kim, S. H, Cai, Q. Y, et al. Inflammation-specific T1 imaging using anti-intercellular adhesion molecule 1 antibody-conjugated gadolinium diethylenetriaminepentaacetic acid, Mol Imaging, (2007). , 6(2), 75-84.

[25] Chowdhury, U. K, Seth, S, Govindappa, R, et al. Congenital left atria; appendage aneurysm: a case report and brief review of literature, Heart Lung Circ, (2009). , 18(6), 412-416.

[26] Christen, T, Nahrendorf, M, Wildgruber, M, et al. Molecular imaging of innate immune cell function in transplant rejection, Circulation, (2009). , 119(14), 1925-1932.

[27] Cohen, M. S, Marino, B. S, Mcelhinney, D. B, et al. Neo-aortic root dilatation and valve regurgitation up to 21 years after staged reconstruction for hypoplastic left heart syndrome, J Am Coll Cardiol, (2003). , 42(3), 533-540.

[28] Criteria for diagnosis of Behçet's diseaseLancet, (1990). , 335, 1078-1780.

[29] Cullen, M. E, Yuen, A. H, Felkin, L. E, et al. Myocardial expression of the arginine: glycine amidinotransferase gene is elevated in heart failure and normalized after recovery. Potential implications for local creatine synthesis, Circulation, (2006). , 114, 116-120.

[30] Curci, J. A, Liao, S, Huffman, M. D, et al. Expression and localization of macrophage elastase (matrix metalloproteinase-12) in abdominal aortic aneurysms, J Clin Invest, (1998). , 102, 1900-1910.

[31] Dasgupta, S. K, Guchhait, P, & Thiagarajan, P. Lactadherin binding and phosphatidylserine expression on cell surface-comparison with annexin A5, Transl Res, (2006). , 148, 19-25.

[32] Daugherty, A, & Cassis, L. Chronic angiotensin II infusion promotes atherogenesis in low density lipoprotein receptor-/- mice, Ann N Y Sci, (1999).

[33] Daugherty, A, Cassis, L. A, & Lu, H. Complex pathologies of angiotensin II-induced abdominal aortic aneurysms, J Zheijiang Univ-Sci B (Biomed & Biotechnol), (2011). , 12(8), 624-628.

[34] Daugherty, A, Manning, M. W, & Cassis, L. A. Angiotensin II promotes atherosclerotic lesions and aneurysm in apolipoprotein E-deficient mice, J Clin Invest, (2000). , 105, 1605-1612.

[35] De Paepe, A, Devereux, R. B, Dietz, H. C, et al. Revised diagnostic criteria for the Marfan syndrome and related disorders, Ann J Med Genet, (1996). , 62, 417-426.

[36] De Sa, M, Moshkovitz, Y, Butany, J, et al. Histologic abnormalities of the ascending aorta and pulmonary trunk in patients with bicuspid aortic valve disease: clinical relevance to the Ross procedure, Journal of Thoracic and Cardiovascular Surgery, (1999). , 118(4), 588-596.

[37] Didangelos, A, Yin, X, Mandal, K, et al. Extracellular matrix composition and remodelling in human abdominal aortic aneurysms: a proteomics approach, Molecular & Cellular Proteomics, (2011). mcp.M111.008128-1-15.

[38] Dietz, H. C, & Pyeritz, R. E. Mutations in the human gene for fibrillin-1 (FBN1) in the Marfan syndrome and related disorders, Hum Mol Genet, (1995). spec (1799-1809), 1799-1809.

[39] Dingemans, K. P, Jansen, N, & Becker, A. E. Ultrastructure of the normal human aortic media, Virchows Arch [Pathol Anat], (1981). , 392, 199-216.

[40] Doerr, W. Herz und Gefäße. In: Doerr W (ed) Organpathologie. Band I. Georg Thieme Verlag, Stuttgart, (1974).

[41] Dong, C, Wu, Q. Y, & Tang, Y. Ruptured sinus of valsalva aneurysm: a Beijing experience, Ann Thorac Sirg, (2002). , 74, 1621-1624.

[42] Doyle, A. J, Doyle, J. J, Bessling, S. L, et al. Mutations in the TGF-β repressor SKI cause Shprintzen-Goldberg syndrome with aortic aneurysm, Nat Genet, (2012). , 44(11), 1249-1254.

[43] Edwards, J. E. Manifestations of acquired and congenital diseases of the aorta, Curr Probl Cardiol, (1979). , 3(1), 1-51.

[44] Fedak PWMDe Sa MPL, Verma S, et al., Vascular matrix remodelling in patients with bicuspid aortic valve malformations: implications for aortic dilatation, Journal of Thoracic and Cardiovascular Surgery, (2003). , 126(3), 797-806.

[45] Felson, B, & Palayew, M. J. The two types of right aortic arch, Radiology, (1963). , 81, 745-759.

[46] Fondard, O, Detaint, D, Iung, B, et al. Extracellular matrix remodelling in human aortic valve disease: the role of matrix metalloproteinases and their tissue inhibitors, European Heart Journal, (2005). , 26(13), 1333-1341.

[47] Freed, K, & Low, V. H. The aberrant subclavian artery, AJR Am J Roentgenol, (1997). , 168(2), 481-484.

[48] Freestone, T, Turner, R. J, Coady, A, et al. Inflammation and matrix metalloproteinases in the enlarging abdominal aortic aneurysm, Arterioscler Thromb Vasc Biol, (1995). , 15, 1145-1151.

[49] Garg, V, Muth, A. N, Ranson, J. F, et al. Mutations in NOTCH1 cause aortic valve disease, Nature, (2005). , 437(7056), 270-274.

[50] Gavrila, D, Li, W. G, Mccormick, M. L, et al. Vitamin E inhibits abdominal aortic aneurysm formation in angiotensin II-infused apolipoprotein E-deficient mice, Arterioscler Thromb Vasc Biol, (2005). , 25, 1671-1677.

[51] Ghosal, S, & Loftin, C. D. Cyclooxygenase-2 inhibition attenuates abdominal aortic aneurysm progression in hyperlipidemic mice, PLoS ONE, (2012). e44369.

[52] Girirajan, S, Rosenfeld, J. A, Cooper, G. M, et al. A recurrent 16microdeletion supports a two-hit model for severe developmental delay, Nat Gen, (2010). , 12.

[53] Gitlin, J. M, Trivedi, D. B, Langenbach, R, & Loftin, C. D. Genetic deficiency of cyclooxygenase-2 attenuates abdominal aortic aneurysm formation in mice, Cardiovasc Res, (2007). , 73, 227-236.

[54] Giusti, B, Rossi, L, Lapini, I, et al. Gene expression profiling of peripheral blood in patients with abdominal aortic aneurysm, Eur J Vasc Endovasc Surg, (2009). , 38, 104-112.

[55] Gotte, L, Giro, M. Y, Volpin, D, & Horne, R. W. The ultrastructural organization of elastin, J Ultrastruct Res, (1974). , 46, 23-33.

[56] Gray, H, & Bannister, L. H. Gray's Anatomy: The Anatomical Basis of Medicine and Surgery, Churchill Livingstone, (1995).

[57] Grote, K, Flach, I, Luchtefeld, M, et al. Mechanical stretch enhances mRNA expression and proenzyme release of matrix metalloproteinase-2 (MMP-2) via NADPH oxidase-derived reactive oxygen species, Circ Res, (2003). , 92, 80-86.

[58] Guo, D. C, Pannu, H, & Tran-fadulu, V. Mutations in smooth muscle alpha-actin (ACTA2) lead to thoracic aortic aneurysms and dissections, Nature Genetics, (2007). , 39, 1488-1493.

[59] Guo, D. C, Papke, C. L, Tran-fadulu, V, et al. Mutations in smooth muscle alpha-actin (ACTA2) cause coronary artery disease, stroke, and moya-moya disease, along with thoracic aortic disease, Am J Hum Genet, (2009). , 84, 617-627.

[60] Gupta, P. A, Wallis, D. D, Chin, T. O, et al. FBN2 mutation associated with manifestations of Marfan syndrome and congenital contractural arachnodactyly, J Med Genet, (2004). e56.

[61] Gurvitz, M, Chang, R. K, Drant, S, & Allada, V. Frequency of aortic root dilation in children with bicuspid aortic valve, Ann J Cardiol, (2004). , 94(10), 1337-1340.

[62] Hanayama, R, Tanaka, M, Miyasaka, K, et al. Autoimmune disease and impaired uptake of apoptotic cells in MFG-E8- deficient mice, Science, (2004). , 304, 1147-1150.

[63] Hannuksela, M, Lundqvist, S, & Carlberg, B. Thoracic aorta- dilated or not? Scand Cardiovasc J, (2006).

[64] Hartung, D, Petrov, A, Haider, N, et al. Radiolabeled monocyte chemotactic protein 1 for the detection of inflammation in experimental atherosclerosis, J Nucl Med, (2007). , 48(11), 1816-1821.

[65] Hayashi, T, Morishita, E, Ohtake, H, et al. Expression of annexin II in human atherosclerotic abdominal aortic aneurysms, Thrombosis Research, (2008). , 123, 274-280.

[66] Hellevuo, K, Berry, R, Sikela, J. M, & Tabakoff, B. Localization of the gene for a novel human adenylyl cyclase (ADCY7) to chromosome 16, Hum Genet, (1995). , 95, 197-200.

[67] Heuser, R. R, & Lopez, A. Abdominal aorta aneurysm and ELG: A review of a treatment in its infancy, Journal of Interventional Cardiology, (1998). , 11(6), 591-602.

[68] Hinterseher, I, Erdman, R, Elmore, J. R, et al. Novel pathways in the pathobiology of human abdominal aortic aneurysms, Pathobiology, (2013). , 80, 1-10.

[69] Hinterseher, I, Gäbel, G, Corvinus, F, et al. Presence of *borrelia burgdorferi sensu lato* antibodies in the serum of patients with abdominal aortic aneurysms, Eur J Clin Microbiol Infect Dis, (2012). , 31, 781-789.

[70] Hinton, R. B. Bicuspid aortic valve and thoracic aortic aneurysm: three patient populations, two disease phenotypes, and one shared genotype, Cardiology Research and Practice, (2012). ID 926975.

[71] Hinton, R. B, & Yutzey, K. E. Heart valve structure and function in development and disease, Annual Review of Physiology, (2011). , 73, 29-46.

[72] Hiratzka, L. F, Bakris, G. L, Beckman, J. A, et al. ACCF/ AHA/ AATS/ ACR/ ASA/ SCA/ SCAI/ SIR/ STS/ SVM guidelines for the diagnosis and management of patients with thoracic aortic disease: executive summary- a report of the American College of Cardiology Foundation/American Heart Association for Thoracic Surgery, American College of Radiology, Catheterization and Cardiovascular Interventions, (2010). EE86., 43.

[73] Hope, M. D, Hope, T. A, et al. Bicuspid aortic valve: four-dimensional MR evaluation of ascending aortic systolic flow patterns, Radiology, (2010). , 255(1), 53-61.

[74] Humm, A, Fritsche, E, Steinbacher, S, & Huber, R. Crystal structure and mechanism of human L-arginine: glycine amidinotransferase. A mitochondrial enzyme involved in creatine biosynthesis, EMBO J, (1997). , 16, 3373-3385.

[75] Humphrey, J. D, & Taylor, C. A. Intracranial and abdominal aortic aneurysms: similarities, differences, and need for a new class of computational models, Annu Rev Biomed Eng, (2008). , 10, 221-246.

[76] Iida, Y, Schultz, G. M, Chow, V, et al. Efficacy and mechanism of Angiotensin II Receptor blocker treatment in experimental abdominal aortic aneurysm, PLoS ONE, (2012). e49642.

[77] Ikonomidis, J. S, Jones, J. A, Barbour, J. R, et al. Expression of matrix metalloproteinases and endogenous inhibitors within ascending aortic aneurysms of patients with bicuspid or tricuspid aortic valves, J Thorac Cardiovasc Surg, (2007). , 133, 1028-1036.

[78] Istner, J. M, Donaldson, R. F, Fulton, D, et al. Cystic medial necrosis in coarctation of the aorta: a potential factor contributing to adverse consequences observed after percutaneous balloon angioplasty of coarctation sites, Circulation, (1987). , 75(4), 689-695.

[79] Jain, M. K, Fujita, K. P, Hsieh, C. M, et al. Molecular cloning and characterization of SMLIM, a developmentally regulated LIM protein preferentially expressed in aortic smooth muscle cells, J Biol Chem, (1996). , 271, 10194-10199.

[80] Jain, R, Engleka, K. A, Rentschler, S. L, et al. Cardiac neural crest orchestrates remodelling and functional maturation of mouse semilunar valves, Journal of Clinical Investigation, (2011). , 121(1), 422-430.

[81] Janes, P. W, Adikari, S, & Lackmann, M. Eph/ephrin signalling and function in oncogenesis: lessons from embryonic development, Current Cancer Drug Targets, (2008). , 8(6), 473-489.

[82] Jois, R. N, Gaffney, K, Marshall, T, & Scott, D. G. Chronic periaortitis, Rheumatology (Oxford), (2004). , 43(11), 1441-1446.

[83] Kaartinen, M, Penttila, A, & Kovanen, P. T. Mast cells of two types differing in neutral protease composition in the human aortic intima. Demonstration of tryptase- and tryptase/chymase-containing mast cells in normal intimas, fatty streaks, and the shoulder region of atheromas, Arterioscler Thromb, (1994). , 14, 966-972.

[84] Kaneko, H, Anzai, T, Takahashi, T, et al. Role of vascular endothelial growth factor-A in development of abdominal aortic aneurysm, Cardiovasc Res, (2011). , 91, 358-367.

[85] Kashina, E, Scholz, H, Steckelings, U. M, et al. Transition from atherosclerosis to aortic aneurysm in humans coincides with an increased expression of RAS components, Atherosclerosis, (2009). , 205, 396-403.

[86] Kepler, T. B, & Chan, C. Spatiotemporal programming of a simple inflammatory process, Immunological reviews, (2007). , 216(1), 153-163.

[87] Kerr, G. S, Hallahan, C. W, Giordano, J, et al. Takayasu arteritis, Ann Intern Med, (1994). , 120(11), 919-929.

[88] Khan, M. A, & Ball, E. J. Genetic aspects of ankylosing spondylitis, Best Pract Res Clin Rheumatol, (2002). , 16(4), 675-690.

[89] Klima, T, Spjut, H. J, Coelho, A, et al. The morphology of ascending aortic aneurysm, Hum Pathol, (1983). , 14, 810-817.

[90] Krämer, J, Quensel, C, Meding, J, et al. Identification and characterization of novel smoothelin isoforms in vascular smooth muscle, J Vasc Res, (2001). , 38, 120-132.

[91] Kuang, S. Q, Guo, D. C, Prakash, S. K, et al. Recurrent chromosome 16duplications are a risk factor for aortic disease, PLoS Genetics, (2011). e1002118., 13.

[92] Lee, C. C, Chang, W. T, Fang, C. C, et al. Sudden death caused by dissecting thoracic aortic aneurysm in a patient with autosomal dominant polycystic kidney disease, Resuscitation, (2004). , 63(1), 93-96.

[93] Lee, T. C, Zhao, Y. D, Courtman, D. W, & Stewart, D. J. Abnormal aortic valve development in mice lacking endothelial nitric oxide synthase, Circulation, (2000). , 101(20), 2345-2348.

[94] Lemaire, S. A, Pannu, H, Tran-faddulu, V, et al. Severe aortic and arterial aneurysms associated with a TGFBR2 mutation, Nat Clin Pract Cardiovasc Med, (2007). , 4, 167-171.

[95] Levy, O, Martin, S, Eichenwald, E, et al. Impaired innate immunity in the newborn: Newborn neutrophils are deficient in bactericidal/permeability-increasing protein, Pediatrics, (1999). , 104, 1327-1333.

[96] Lindeman JHNAshcroft BA, Beenakker JWM, et al., Distinct defects in collagen microarchitecture underlie vessel-wall failure in advanced abdominal aneurysms and aneurysms in Marfan syndrome, Proc Natl Acad Sci USA, (2010). , 107, 862-865.

[97] Lindholt JSEEHenneberg EW, Cystatin C deficiency is associated with the progression of small abdominal aortic aneurysms, Br J Surg, (2001). , 88, 1472-1475.

[98] Lindstedt, K. A, Mayranpaa, M. I, & Kovanen, P. T. Mast cells in vulnerable atherosclerotic plaques- a view to a kill, J Cell Mol Med, (2007). , 11, 739-758.

[99] Lipp, C, Lohoefer, F, Reeps, C, et al. Expression of a Disintegrin and Metalloprotease in Human Abdominal Aortic Aneurysms, J Vasc Res, (2011). , 49, 198-206.

[100] Liu, J, Sukhova, G. K, Yang, J. T, et al. Cathepsin L expression and regulation in human abdominal aortic aneurysm, atherosclerosis, and vascular cells, Atherosclerosis, (2006). , 184, 302-311.

[101] Loeys, B. L, Scwharze, U, Holm, T, et al. Aneurysm syndromes caused by mutations in the TGF-beta receptor, N Engl J Med, (2006). , 355, 788-798.

[102] Longo, G. M, Xiong, W, Greiner, T. C, et al. Matrix metalloproteinases 2 and 9 work in concert to produce aortic aneurysms, J Clin Invet, (2002). , 110(5), 625-632.

[103] Losay, J, Touchot, A, Capderou, A, et al. Aortic valve regurgitation after arterial switch operation for transposition of the great arteries: incidence, risk factors, and outcome, J Am Coll Cardiol, (2006). , 47(10), 2057-2062.

[104] Lu, H, Rateri, D. L, Cassis, L. A, & Daugherty, A. The role of the renin-angiotensin system in aortic aneurysmal diseases, Curr Hypertens Rep, (2008). , 10, 99-106.

[105] Lutgens, S. P, Cleutjens, K. B, Daemen, M. J, et al. Cathepsin cysteine proteases in cardiovascular disease, FASEB J, (2007). , 21(12), 3029-3041.

[106] Maiellaro-rafferty, K, Weiss, D, Joseph, G, et al. Catalase overexpression in aortic smooth muscle prevents pathological mechanical changes underlying abdominal aortic aneurysm formation, Am J Physiol Heart Circ Physiol, (2011). HH362., 355.

[107] Majesky, M. W. Developmental basis of vascular smooth muscle diversity, Arteriosclerosis, Thrombosis, and Vascular Biology, (2009). , 27(6), 1248-1258.

[108] Maki, J. M, Rasanen, J, Tikkanen, H, et al. Inactivation of the lysyl oxidase gene lox leads to aortic aneurysms, cardiovascular dysfunction, and perinatal death in mice, Circulation, (2002). , 106, 2503-2509.

[109] Marques da Silva RLingaas PS, Geiran O, et al., Multiple bacteria in aortic aneurysms, J Vasc Surg, (2003). , 38, 1384-1389.

[110] Martin, L. J, Ramachandran, V, Cripe, L. H, et al. Evidence in favour of linkage to human chromosomal regions 18q, 5q and 13q for bicuspid aortic valve and associated cardiovascular malformations, Human Genetics, (2007). , 121(2), 275-284.

[111] Matsumura, K, Hirano, T, Takeda, K, et al. Incidence of aneurysms in Takayasu's arteritis, Angiology, (1991). , 42(4), 308-315.

[112] Mcelhinney, D. B, Krantz, I. D, Bason, L, et al. Analysis of cardiovascular phenotype and genotype-phenotype correlation in individuals with a JAG1 mutation and/or Alagille syndrome, Circulation, (2002). , 106, 2567-2574.

[113] Milewicz, D. M, Dietz, H. C, & Miller, D. C. Treatment of aortic disease in patients with Marfan syndrome, Circulation, (2005). e, 150-157.

[114] Mizuguchi, T, Collod-beroud, G, Akiyama, T, et al. Heterozygous TGFBR mutations in Marfan syndrome, Nat Genet, (2004). , 36(8), 855-860.

[115] Nahrendorf, M, Jaffer, F. A, Kelly, K. A, et al. Noninvasive vascular cell adhesion molecule-1 imaging identifies inflammatory activation of cells in atherosclerosis, Circulation, (2006). , 114(4), 1504-1511.

[116] Nakamura, S, Ishibashi-ueda, H, Suzuki, C, et al. Renal artery stenosis and renal parenchymal damage in patients with abdominal aortic aneurysm proven by autopsy, Kidney Blood Press Res, (2009). , 32, 11-16.

[117] Nakashima, Y, Kurozumi, T, Sueishi, K, & Tanaka, K. Dissecting aneurysm: a clinicopathologic and histopathologic study of 111 autopsied cases, Hum Pathol, (1990). , 21, 291-296.

[118] Nesi, G, Anichini, C, Tozzini, S, et al. Pathology of the thoracic aorta: a morphologic review of 338 surgical specimens over a 7-year period, Cardiovascular Pathology, (2009). , 18(3), 134-139.

[119] Nienaber, C. A, & Sievers, H. H. Intramural hematoma in acute aortic syndrome: more than one variant of dissection? Circulation, (2002). , 106, 284-285.

[120] Niwa, K, Perloff, J. K, Bhuta, S. M, et al. Structural abnormalities of great arterial walls in congenital heart disease: light and electron microscopic analyses, Circulation, (2001). , 103(3), 393-400.

[121] Nordborg, E, Andersson, R, & Bengtsson, B. A. Giant cell arteritis, Epidemiology and treatment, Drugs Aging, (1994). , 4, 135-144.

[122] Oksala, N, Levula, M, Airla, N, et al. ADAM-9, ADAM-15, and ADAM-17 are up regulated in macrophages in advanced human atherosclerotic plaques in aorta and carotid and femoral arteries- Tampere vascular study, Ann Med, (2009). , 41, 279-290.

[123] Olsson, L. M, Lindqvist, A. K, Kallberg, H, et al. A case-control study of rheumatoid arthritis identifies an associated single nucleotide polymorphism in the NCF4 gene, supporting a role for the NADPH-oxidase complex in autoimmunity, Arthritis Res Ther, (2007). R98.

[124] Osler, W. The Gulstonian Lectures, on Malignant Endocarditis, Br Med J, (1885). , 1(1264), 577-579.

[125] Ostberg, J. E, Brookes, J. A, Mccarthy, C, et al. A comparison of echocardiography and magnetic resonance imaging in cardiovascular screening of adults with Turner syndrome, J Clin Endocrinol Metab, (2004). , 89(12), 5966-5971.

[126] Ou, P, Mousseaux, E, Celermajer, D. S, et al. Aortic arch shape deformation after coarctation surgery: effect on blood pressure response, J Thorac Cardiovasc Surg, (2006). , 132, 1105-1111.

[127] Palmer, A, & Klein, R. Multiple roles of ephrins in morphogenesis, neural networking, and brain function, Gens and Development, (2003). , 17(12), 1429-1450.

[128] Pannu, H, Fadulu, V. T, Chand, J, et al. Mutations in transforming growth factor-beta receptor type II cause familial thoracic aortic aneurysms and dissections, Circulation, (2005). , 112, 513-520.

[129] Pasquale, E. B. Eph receptors and ephrins in cancer: bidirectional signalling and beyond, Nature Reviews Cancer, (2010). , 10(3), 165-180.

[130] Pepin, M, Schwarze, U, Superti-furga, A, et al. Clinical and genetic features of Ehlers-Danlos syndrome type IV, the vascular type, N Engl J Med, (2000). , 342, 673-680.

[131] Pisano, C, Maresi, E, Balisteri, C. R, et al. Histological and genetic studies in patients with bicuspid aortic valve and ascending aorta complications, Interactive CardioVascular and Thoracic Surgery, (2012). , 14, 300-306.

[132] Purnell, R, Williams, I, Von Oppell, U, & Wood, A. Giant aneurysm of the sinuses of Valsalva and aortic regurgitation in a patient with Noonan's syndrome, Eur J Cardiothorac Surg, (2005). , 28(2), 346-348.

[133] Quillard, T, Croce, K, Jaffer, F. A, et al. Molecular imaging of macrophage protease activity in cardiovascular inflammation in vivo, Thromb Haemost, (2011). , 105(5), 828-836.

[134] Ramayya, A. S, Coelho, R, Sivakumar, K, & Radhakrishnan, S. Repair of tetralogy of Fallot with ascending and proximal aortic arch aneurysm: case report, J Card Surg, (2011). , 26(3), 328-330.

[135] Rateri, D. L, Howatt, D. A, Moorleghen, J. J, et al. Prolonged infusion of angiotensin II in apoE-/- mice promotes macrophage recruitment with continued expansion of abdominal aortic aneurysms, Am J Pathol, (2011). , 179(3), 1542-1548.

[136] Rensen, S. S, Niessen, P. M, Van Deursen, J. M, et al. Smoothelin-b deficiency results in reduced arterial contractility, hypertension, and cardiac hypertrophy in mice, Circulation, (2008). , 118, 828-836.

[137] Rijbroek, A, Moll, F. L, Von Dijk, H. A, et al. Inflammation of the abdominal aortic aneurysm wall, Eur J Vasc Surg, (1994). , 8(1), 41-46.

[138] Roberts, C. S, & Roberts, W. C. Dissection of the aorta associated with congenital malformations of the aortic valve, Journal of the American College of Cardiology, (1991). , 17(3), 712-716.

[139] Roberts, W. C. Aortic dissection: Anatomy, consequences, and causes, Am Heart J, (1981). , 101, 195-207.

[140] Roberts, W. C, & Ko, J. M. Frequency by decades of unicuspid, bicuspid, and tricuspid aortic valve replacement for aortic stenosis, with or without associated aortic regurgitation, Circulation, (2005). , 111(7), 920-925.

[141] Roberts, W. C. The aorta: Its acquired diseases and their consequences as viewed from a morphologic perspective. In The Aorta (eds. Lindsay J, Hurst JW), Orlando: Grune & Stratton, (1979). , 51.

[142] Roldan, C. A, Chavez, J, Wiest, P. W, et al. Aortic root disease and valve disease associated with ankylosing spondylitis, J Am Coll Cardiol, (1998). , 32, 1397-1404.

[143] Roman, M. J, Rosen, S. E, Kramer-fox, R, et al. Prognostic significance of the pattern of aortic root dilatation in the Marfan syndrome, J Am Coll Cardiol, (1993). , 22, 1470-1476.

[144] Saito, T, Hasegawa, Y, Ishigaki, Y, et al. Importance of endothelial NF-κB signalling in vascular remodelling and aortic aneurysm formation, Cardiovasc Res, (2013). , 97, 106-114.

[145] Sakamoto A Ishibashi-Ueda HSugamoto Y, et al., Expression and function of ephrin-B1 and its cognate receptor EphB2 in human atherosclerosis: from an aspect of chemotaxis, Clinical Science, (2008). , 114(10), 643-650.

[146] Sakamoto, A, Kawashiri, M, Ishibashi-ueda, H, et al. Expression and function of Ephrin-B1 and its cognate receptor EphB2 in human abdominal aortic aneurysm, International Journal of Vascular Medicine, (2012).

[147] Salvarani, C, Gabriel, S. E, & Fallon, O. WM, et al., The incidence of giant cell arteritis in Olmsted County, Minnesota: apparent fluctuations in a cyclic pattern, Ann Intern Med, (1995). , 123, 192-194.

[148] Sans-coma, V. Carmen Fernández M, Fernández B, et al., Genetically alike Syrian hamsters display both bifoliate and trifoliate aortic valves, Journal of Anatomy, (2012). , 47(7), 476-485.

[149] Saraff, K, Babamusta, F, Cassis, L. A, & Daugherty, A. Aortic dissection precedes formation of aneurysms and atherosclerosis in angiotensin II-infused, apolipoprotein E-deficient mice, Arterioscler Thromb Vasc Biol, (2003). , 23(9), 1621-1626.

[150] Sarica-kucukoglu, R, Akdaq-kose, A, Kayaball, M, et al. Vascular involvement in Behçet's disease: a retrospective analysis of 2319 cases, Int J Dermatol, (2006). , 45(8), 919-921.

[151] Savunen, T, & Aho, H. J. Annulo-aortc ectasia, Virchows Arch [Pathol Anat], (1985). , 407, 279-288.

[152] Sharif, M. A, Soong, C. V, Lee, B, et al. Inflammatory infrarenal abdominal aortic aneurysm in a young woman, J Emerg Med, (2008). , 34(2), 147-150.

[153] Shi, C, Awad, I. A, Jafari, N, et al. Genomics of human intracranial aneurysm wall, Stroke, (2009). , 40, 1252-1261.

[154] Singh, K. K, Rommel, K, Mishra, A, et al. TGFBR1 and TGFBR2 mutations in patients with features of Marfan syndrome and Loeys-Dietz syndrome, Hum Mutat, (2006). , 27, 770-777.

[155] Smallwood, L, Allcock, R, Van Bockxmeer, F, et al. Polymorphisms of the interleukin-6 gene promoter and abdominal aortic aneurysm, Eur J Vasc Endovasc Surg, (2008). , 35, 31-36.

[156] Stanson, A. W, Kazmier, F. J, Hollier, L. H, et al. Penetrating atherosclerotic ulcers of the thoracic aorta: natural history and clinicopathologic correlations, Am Vasc Surg, (1986). , 1, 15-23.

[157] Suzuki, H, Sato, M, & Umezawa, Y. Accurate targeting of activated macrophages based on synergistic activation of functional molecules uptake by scavenger receptor and matrix metalloproteinase, ACS Chem Biol, (2008). , 3(8), 471-479.

[158] Svensson, L. G. Acute aortic syndromes: time to talk of many things, Cleve Clin J Med, (2008). , 75(1), 25-29.

[159] Swedenborg, J, Mayranpaa, M. I, & Kovanen, P. T. Mast cells: important players in the orchestrated pathogenesis of abdominal aortic aneurysm, Arterioscler Thromb Vasc Biol, (2011). , 31, 734-740.

[160] Tamarina, N. A, Grassi, M. A, Johnson, D. A, & Pearce, W. H. Proteoglycan gene expression is decreased in abdominal aortic aneurysms, J Surg Res, (1998). , 74, 76-80.

[161] Tawakol, A, Castano, A. P, Gad, F, et al. Intravascular detection of inflamed atherosclerotic plaques using a fluorescent photosensitizer targeted to the scavenger receptor, Photochem Photobiol Sci, (2008). , 7(1), 33-39.

[162] Tazelaar, H. D. Diseases of aortic dilatation, Pathology International, (2004). suppl.1): SS56., 52.

[163] Thompson, A, Cooper, J. A, Fabricius, M, et al. An analysis of drug modulation of abdominal aortic aneurysm growth through 25 years of surveillance, J Vasc Surg, (2010).

[164] Treska, V, Kocova, J, Boudova, I, et al. Inflammation in the wall of abdominal aortic aneurysm and its role in the symptomatology of aneurysm, Cytokines Cell Mol Ther, (2002). , 7, 91-97.

[165] Trollope, A, Moxon, J. V, Moran, C. S, & Golledge, J. Animal models of abdominal aortic aneurysm and their role in furthering management of human disease, Cardiovasc Path, (2011). , 20, 114-123.

[166] Tsuruda, T, Kato, J, Hatakeyma, K, et al. Adrenomedullin in mast cells of abdominal aortic aneurysm, Cardiovasc Res, (2006).

[167] Tunaci, A, Berkmen, Y. M, & Gokmen, E. Thoracic involvement in Behcet's disease: pathologic, clinical, and imaging features, AJR Am J Roentgenol, (1995). , 164, 51-56.

[168] Venugopal, S. K, Devaraj, S, & Jilal, I. Macrophage conditioned medium induces the expression of C-reactive protein in human aortic endothelial cells, Am J Pathol, (2005). , 166, 1265-1271.

[169] Viscardi, F, Vergara, C, et al. Comparative finite element mode; analysis of ascending aortic flow in bicuspid and tricuspid aortic valve, Artificial Organs, (2010). , 34(12), 1114-1120.

[170] Waller, B. F, Clary, J. D, & Rohr, T. Noneoplastic diseases of aorta and pulmonary trunk- part II, Clin Cardiol, (1997). , 20, 798-804.

[171] Wang, M, Lee, E, Song, W, et al. Genetic deficiency of cyclooxygenase-2 attenuates abdominal aortic aneurysm formation in mice, Cardiovasc Res, (2007). , 73, 227-236.

[172] Youn, Y. H, Feng, J, Tessarollo, L, et al. Neural crest stem cell and cardiac endothelium defects in the TRKC null mouse, Mol Cell Neurosci, (2003). , 24, 160-170.

[173] Zanjani, L. S, & Niwa, K. Aortic dilatation and aortopathy in congenital heart diseases, J Cardiol, (2013). , 61(1), 16-21.

[174] Zhu, L, Vranckx, R, et al. Mutations in myosin heavy chain 11 cause a syndrome associating thoracic aortic aneurysm/aortic dissection and patent *ductus arteriosus*, Nat Genet, (2006). , 38(3), 343-349.

Chapter 2

Aortic Aneurysm in Children and Adolescents

Cemşit Karakurt

Additional information is available at the end of the chapter

http://dx.doi.org/10.5772/53383

1. Introduction

Aortic aneurysm involves the aorta which is one of the large arteries through which blood passes from the heart to the rest of the body. Aortic aneurysm is a relatively common finding in the elderly patients because of aging, hypertension, or atherosclerosis, but it is rarely seen in childhood. In the adult population, the incidence of aortic aneurysm has been estimated to be 5.9 cases per 100000 person-years. However, there are no real data about the incidence of aortic aneurysm in childhood [1]. Aortic aneurysm is mostly seen in the ascending aorta, but it may also be seen in the descending aorta and /or aortic branches [2, 3]. Although it is rare, aortic aneurysm can be important cause of mortality in children and adolescents. Aortic aneurysm may be related to hereditary diseases (Marfan syndrome, Loeys –Dietz syndrome, Ehler-Danlos syndrome, Arterial Tortuosity Syndrome, Cutis laxa syndrome, Alagille syndrome, and Noonan Syndrome), or non genetic diseases (bicuspid aortic valve, coarctation of aorta, tetralogy of Fallot, and aortitis syndromes). In this review, causes, clinical findings, diagnostic methods, and treatment modalities of aortic aneurysm in children and adolescents have been discussed.

2. Genetic causes of aortic aneurysm

2.1. Marfan syndrome

Marfan syndrome, characterized by otosomal dominant inheritance, I was first described in 1986. The syndrome is due to more than 500 mutations in the fibrillin 1 gene on chromosome 15q21. Expression of the disease is variable and 30% of cases represent new mutation. Although cardiovascular manifestations are variable, the incidence (35-80%) of aortic root dilatation, mitral regurgitation in Marfan patients depends on the patient's age. In Marfan syndrome, fibrillin-1 gene mutation leads to elastic fiber fragmentation and cystic medial necrosis. Fibrillin-1 is a matrix glycoprotein and a constituent of fibrils. Apart from structural abnormalities, a defective subenthelial fibrillin leads to decreased distensibility, and increased aortic stiffness was showed in patients with Marfan syndrome. Excessive transforming growth factor β(TGFβ) activity, defect in gene encoding TGF β receptor and complex interaction between the fibrillin, microfibrils, TGFβ and its receptor have been proposed hypothesis of defective arterial wall matrix. Aortic dilatation may be related to arterial muscle cell apoptosis due to angiotensin-II receptor signalling pathways. Aortic stiffness has been showed to be an independent predictor for progressive aortic dilatation and dissection [4]. Beta blocker and ACE inhibitor therapy have been showed to decrease aortic stiffness and delay aortic surgery [5].

Clinical findings of Marfan syndrome are variable. Although most of the patients are diagnosed after 10 years, physical findings may be present at birth. The height of the patient increases. An arm span exceeds the height. Marfan patients have hypermobile joints, chest deformities, long and thin fingers, kyphoscoliosis, high palates, inguinal hernias, and dental abnormalities. Figure 1 shows long and thin fingers; figure 2 shows increased arm length and height in a Marfan syndrome patient. Ocular abnormalities such as lens subluxation, and/or myopia may be present in nearly 75% of the patients. Cardiovascular manifestation including aortic aneurysm, mitral valvar prolapse less severe in children than adults. Ghent nosology has been developed for diagnosis of Marfan syndrome in 1996. The 1996 Ghent criteria were adopted worldwide, but diagnostic criteria were revised in 2010, highlighting aortic root aneurysm and lens subluxation more [6, 7].

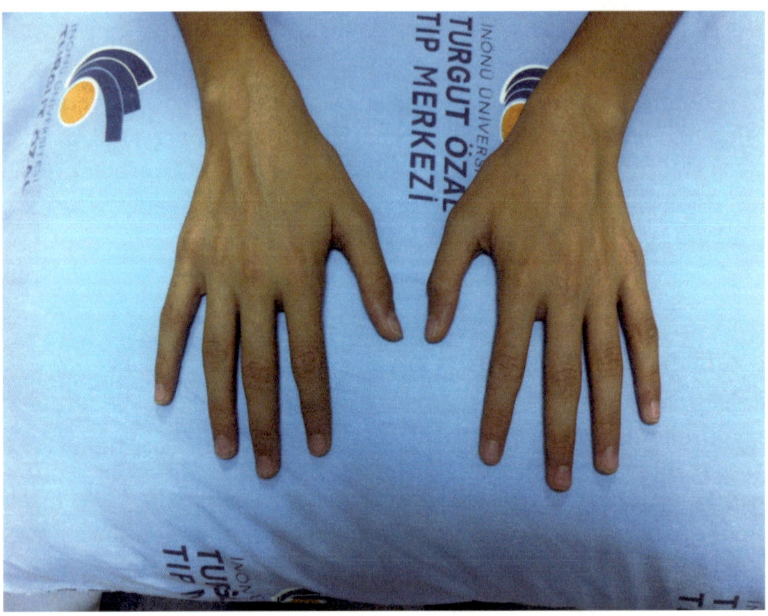

Figure 1. shows long and thin fingers in a 13-years-old patient with Marfan syndrome

http://dx.doi.org/10.5772/53383

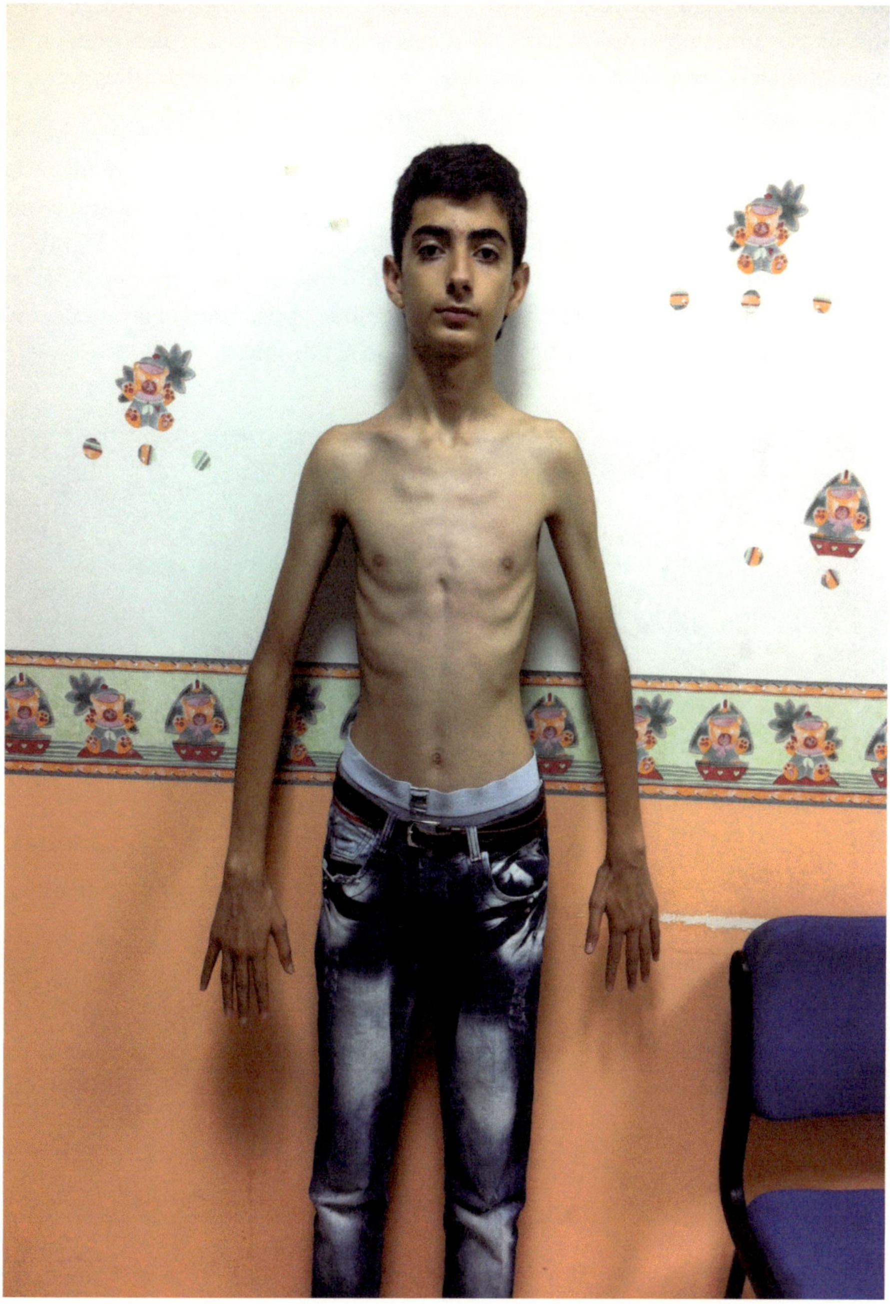

Figure 2. shows increased height and arm length in a 13-year-old patient with Marfan syndrome

According to Ghent's criteria, positive family history of Marfan syndrome (known fibrillin 1 mutation in the parent(s) or siblings), cardiac findings including aortic root dilatation, aortic dissection, and lumbosacral dural ectasia are the major criteria. Mitral valvar prolapse, calcific mitral annulus (age< 40 years), other aortic dilatations or dissections (age <50 years), spontaneous pneumothorax, apical blebs, skin abnormalities including recurrent or incisional hernias, and stria atrophicae are considered minor criteria. Recently, diagnostic criteria were revised nosology established for adult Marfan population [8, 9, 10].

Cardiovascular manifestations, especially aortic aneurysm and dissection, are the most common causes of mortality. Aortic aneurysms are usually located in the ascending aorta but it may also be located in the abdominal aorta or aortic branches [11, 12, 13]. Figure 3 and 4 show an aneurysm in the right renal artery and multiple aneurysm in the hepatic artery in a 16-year-old Marfan patient. Figure 5 shows intraoperative appearance of an aneurysm in the ascending aorta in an 18-year-old patient with Marfan syndrome.

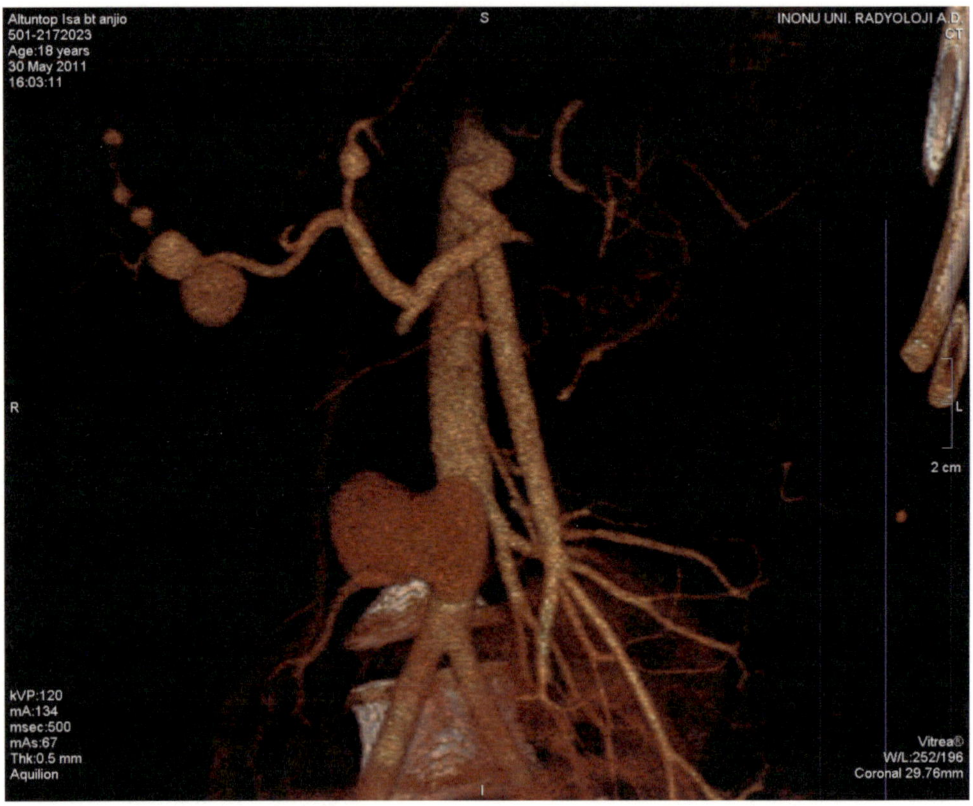

Figure 3. shows a large aneurysm in the right renal artery of a 16-year-old patient with Marfan syndrome

Elective root replacement should be seriously considered in any Marfan patient with significant root dilatation. Reoperation is required for half of Marfan syndrome patients [14]. Risk of sudden death or aortic dissection remains low in patients with Marfan syndrome and aortic diameter between 45-49 mm. Aortic diameter of 50 mm appears to be reasonable threshold for prophylactic surgery [15, 16].

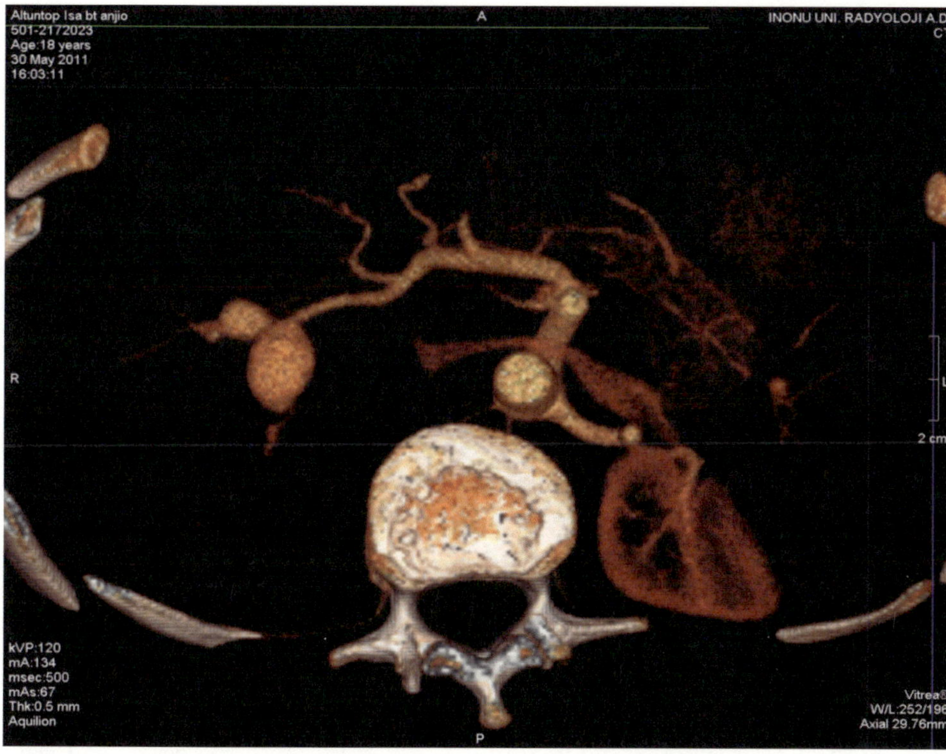

Figure 4. shows multiple aneurysms in the hepatic artery of a 16- year- old patient with Marfan syndrome

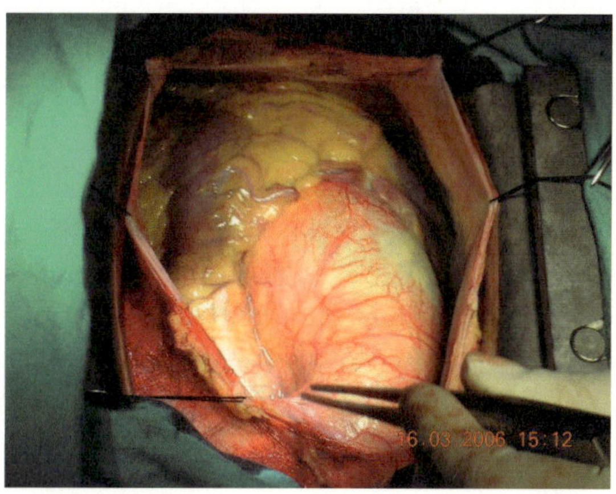

Figure 5. shows intraoperative appearance of the ascending aorta aneurysm in an 18- year-old patient with Marfan Syndrome (By courtesy of Prof Dr Nevzat Erdil)

The findings extend the mutation spectrum of Marfan syndrome, and that mutations at the F-helix in the kinase domain of TGFBR2 may be associated with the development of severe cardiovascular and skeletal lesions and minor ocular disorders [17, 18]. For patients with Marfan syndrome, failed aortic surveillance and consequent emergency dissection repair have important long-term implications with regard to the status of distal aorta; they need multiple procedures for better quality of life. These findings emphasize the importance of aortic surveillance and timely elective aortic root aneurysm repair for patients with Marfan syndrome [19, 20]. Prophylactic propranolol treatment delays progression of aortic root dilatation. Because the patogenetic role of angiotensin II receptor signaling pathway and TGFβ in Marfan syndrome is clearly understood, angiotensin converting enzyme inhibitors should be started in patients with Marfan syndrome. Timing of surgery including aortic root surgery and/or valve replacement must be determined according to the risk and benefit of the surgery. Because annual mortality rate is 5% in patients with an aortic root greater than 50 cm, elective surgery must be performed before aortic root reaches 55 mm. For patients with a family history of aortic dissection and likelihood of pregnancy, elective surgery should be performed while the aortic root is in a smaller size. Upon diagnosis of Marfan syndrome, echocardiographic evaluation should be done, and beta blocker treatment and angiotensin converting enzyme inhibitors should be started after aortic root measurement. Patients with this syndrome should be followed up with echocardiograph periodically, and if it is necessary, with magnetic resonance imaging. Patients with Marfan syndrome who remain undiagnosed until adulthood are more likely to require surgical intervention. Early diagnosis of Marfan syndrome can improve the long-term outcome [21].

Infantile form of Marfan syndrome is a rare condition in which the ocular and skeletal abnormalities are similar to those in the adult form. Myxomatous changes of mitral and tricuspid valves and chordaes with elongation of chordae tendineas are seen commonly in infantile form. Pulmonary emphysematous changes are also seen. Cardiovascular morbidity is commonly related to mitral and tricuspid valve disease rather than aortic aneurysm and dissection. Family history is rare and death commonly occurs in 2 years after diagnosis [22, 23].

2.2. Loeys-Dietz syndrome

Loeys-Dietz syndrome, which was first described in 2005, resembles Marfan syndrome, which is also inherited otosomal dominant, aortic aneurysm, and vascular pathology in Loeys-Dietz syndrome is more probable than in Marfan patients. It is caused by heterozygous mutations in the genes encoding type I and II transforming growth factor-β (TGFBR1, TGFBR2) and is characterized by hyperteleroism, bifid uvula, cleft palate, arterial tortuosity, aneurisms of the ascending aorta, and dissection. Despite phenotypical resemblance, Loeys-Dietz syndrome can be differentiated from Marfan syndrome by palatal involvement and hyperteleroism. Aneurysms may occur in young ages and lead to aortic dissection in Loeys-Dietz Syndrome. Elective surgery is recommended at an aortic root diameter of 40 mm. In Loeys-Dietz syndrome, defective microfibrils due to excessive activity of Transforming Growth Factor β activity lead to defective formation of matrix in the arterial wall and thus, aortic aneurysms [24, 25, 26].

Valve sparing operation of the aortic root is ideal in treating young patients with aortic root aneurysm with normal or minimally diseased aortic cusps to avoid the disadvantages of prosthetic valve replacements [27, 28].

Loeys-Dietz syndrome is an aggressive aortic aneurysm syndrome that can be addressed by prophylactic aortic root replacement with low operative risk. Valve-sparing procedures have encouraging early and midterm results, similar to Marfan syndrome, and are an attractive option for young patients [29, 30, 31].

2.3. Ehler-Danlos syndrome

The other genetic cause of aortic aneurysm is Ehler-Danlos syndrome. Ehler-Danlos syndrome is a genetically heterogeneous disorder of collagen and extracellular matrix and it is characterized by abnormal collagens. Although more than 10 subtypes have been described, 90% of patients with Ehler –Danlos Syndrome encompass six subtypes. Hyper extensibility of joints and skin, distinctive facial appearance, easy bruising, poor healing of wounds, smooth and rubbery palm and soles, blue sclera, epicanthal folds, lens subluxation, poor muscle tone are clinical findings of Ehler-Danlos. Premature death can occur in the most severe forms due to poor muscle tones. Cardiovascular findings are seen in subtype IV. In Ehler Danlos type IV collagen type III α-1 gene mutation leads to abnormal type III collagen in the vascular wall, skin and other organs. These patients carry aortic dissection risk and it does commonly occur after the 3rd decade. Aortic aneurysm can be seen in Ehler-Danlos type IV patients, but dissection is a rare condition in these patients [32, 33, 34, 35].

2.4. Arterial tortuosity syndrome

Arterial tortuosity syndrome is an autosomal recessive disorder characterized by tortuosity of the aorta and its major branches due to SLC2A 10 genes that encodes for the glucose transporter GLUT10. Coucke et al reported location of the arterial tortuosity syndrome locus to 20q13 to a 1.2 Mb region containing 7 genes. Aortic aneurysms can also be seen in Arterial tortuosity syndrome patients [36, 37, 38].

2.5. Turner syndrome

Turner syndrome is an aneuploidy syndrome [45, XO) characterized by short stature, webbed neck, and infertility. Bicuspid aortic valve, coarctation of the aorta, aortic dilatation, pseudocoarctation, aortic aneurysm, and dissection are common in Turner patients. Histological evidence of cystic medial necrosis has been reported in Turner syndrome. The prevalence of aortic dilation and aneurysm is lower in the young girls and women with Turner syndrome than in older Turner syndrome population [39, 40].

2.6. Noonan syndrome

Noonan syndrome is characterized by hypertelorism, a downward eyeslant, and low-set posterior rotated ears, short stature, short neck with webbing, cardiac anomalies, epicanthic folds, deafness, motor delay, and bleeding diathesis. Noonan syndrome is similar to Turner syndrome but a genetically heterogeneous disease (PTPN11, RAS-MAPK mutations) characterized by dysplastic pulmonary valve, pulmonary stenosis [41,42]. Aortic aneurysm and dissection are rarely seen in Noonan syndrome [43].

2.7. Alagille syndrome

Alagille syndrome is an autosomal dominant syndrome that has been defined as paucity of intrahepatic bile ducts, cholestasis, cardiac disease, skeletal abnormalities, ocular abnormalities and characteristic facial appearance, ocular and renal abnormalities caused by heterozygous mutation in the Jagged -1 gene on chromosome 20p12. Another form of Alagille syndrome is caused by mutation in the NOTCH2 gene. Basillary artery aneurysm, middle cerebral artery aneurysm, aortic coarctation and aortic aneurysms have been reported in Alagille patients [44, 45, 46].

2.8. Cutis laxa

Cutis laxa is rare genetically heterogeneous disorder characterized by loose, sagging disease from early age. Autosomal dominant and recessive forms of cutis laxa have been described. In patients with cutis laxa, skin is loose and appears to be larger for the body [47]. Cutis laxa phenotypically resembles Ehler –Danlos syndrome due to hypermobile joints, fragility of skin, and easy bruising. However, the skin slowly recoils after it is stretched. Inguinal hernias and rectal prolapses may be seen [48]. Pulmonary stenosis, pulmonary emphysema, cor pulmonale, mitral regurgitation, dysplastic valvar disease and aortic aneurysm have also been reported in cutis laxa syndrome.

Fibulin-4 is a member of the fibulin family, a group of extracellular matrix proteins predominantly expressed in medial layers of large veins and arteries. Fibulin-4 deficiency has been showed in autosomal recessive cutis laxa patients [49].

2.9. Aneurysms-osteoarthritis syndrome

Aneurysms-osteoarthritis syndrome (AOS) is a new autosomal dominant syndromic form of thoracic aortic aneurysms and dissections caused by mutations SMAD3 gene, characterized by the presence of arterial aneurysms and tortuosity, mild skeletal, craniofacial and cutaneous anomalies, and early onset osteoarthritis [50]. Smooth muscle alpha-actin (ACTA2] mutations have been determined to be associated with aortic aneurysm and dissection in some families [51].

3. Non-genetic causes of aortic aneurysm

Non genetic causes of aortic aneurysm are bicuspid aorta, coarctation of aorta, aortitis syndromes, systemic hypertension, and vasculitis.

3.1. Bicuspid aortic valve

Congenitally bicuspid aortic valve is the most common congenital anomaly, with a prevalence of 0.5 to 2 in 100 individuals. A bicuspid aortic valve with a fused commisure and an eccentric orifice accounts for the most common form of aortic stenosis. Bicuspid aortic valve patients have also variable degrees of aortic insufficiency and aortic aneurysm in addition to aortic stenosis (figure 6). Cystic medial necrosis has been reported in the aortic wall. Thereby, aortic aneurysm may lead to aortic dissection [52, 53]. Hope et al determined that four-dimensional flow MR imaging showed helical systolic flow in the ascending aorta of patients with bicuspid aortic, including those without aneurysm or aortic stenosis. They stated that identification and characterization of eccentric flow jets in these patients may help identify those at risk for development of ascending aortic aneurysm [54].

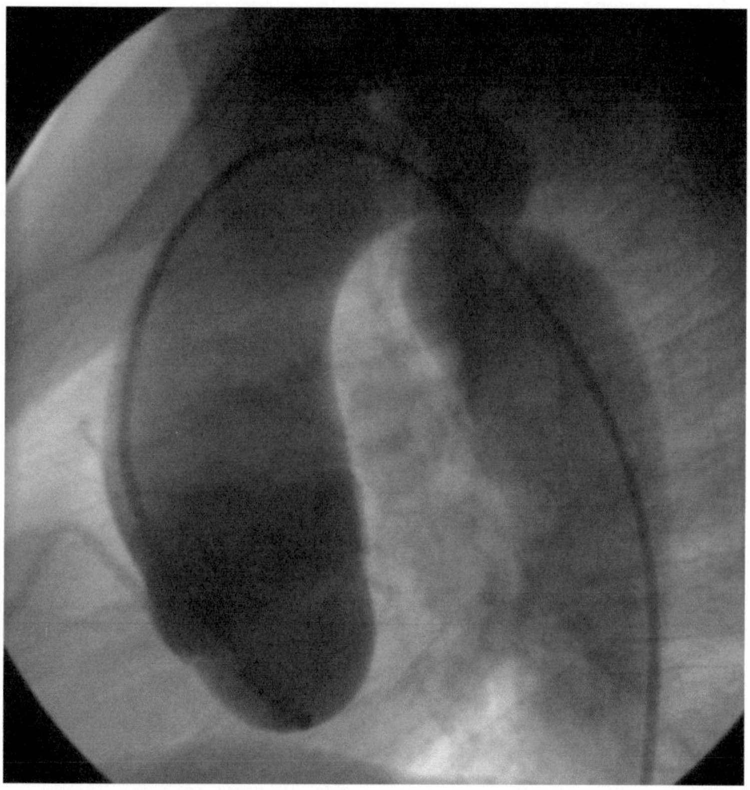

Figure 6. shows aneurysm of the ascending aorta secondary to bicuspid aortic valve and pseudocoarctation in a 13-year-old patient.

3.2. Coarctation of aorta

Coarctation of aorta occurs in 8% to 10% of all congenital heart defects. As many as 85% of patients with aortic coarctation patients have a bicuspid aortic valve. Aortic aneurysm can be seen in untreated coarctation of aorta patients, after balloon dilatation and after surgical treatment or infective endocarditis. Aneurysm formation at the site of the dilatation with balloon angioplasty markedly in different series, but in generally rare. In the earlier era of balloon angioplasty, the incidence of aneurysm was high due to over dilatation with balloon catheter but recent series showed that aneurysm incidence decreased after balloon angioplasty. The pathology in the aneurysms that were operated was tears through the intima and media of the aorta. Aneurysm of the aorta is rare but can be seen after surgical repair especially with patch aortoplasty. When discrete aneurysm was determined after surgical repair or balloon angioplasty, it should be followed closely with CT, MRI, or angiographic imaging. A discrete aneurysm can be treated by using a covered stent [55]. Aortic aneurysms are less reported but may be rarely seen after bare stent implantation [56]. Aortic aneurysm formation complicating aortic coarctation carries a risk of rupture with high mortality. Covered stents are a safe and effective treatment with low risk of complications for the treatment of coarctation associated with aortic wall aneurysm [57, 58, 59].

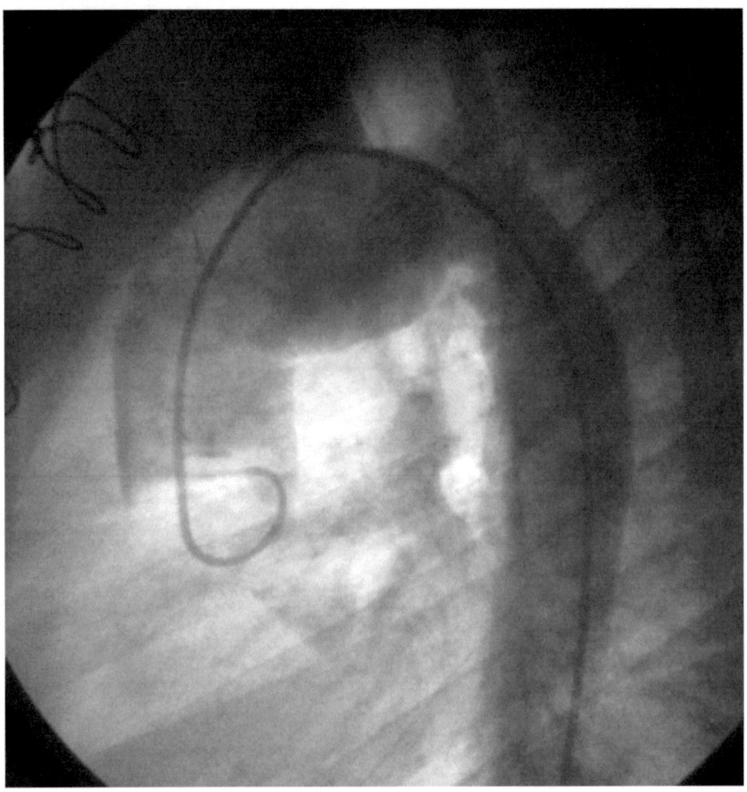

Figure 7. shows aortic aneurysm in a 14-year-old patient with operated tetralogy of Fallot.

3.3. Tetralogy of Fallot

Tetralogy of Fallot occurs in 10 % of all congenital heart defects. Although tetralogy of Fallot include ventricular septal defect, overriding of aorta, and right ventricular outflow tract obstruction, it can present with a pulmonary atresia, absent pulmonary valve. Tetralogy of Fallot patients also have variable degrees of aortic dilatation; it sometimes leads to aortic aneurysm and dissection due to volume overload, abnormalities of tunica media, elastic fibers and collagen in the aortic wall [60]. Histological abnormalities of aortic wall characterized by medial necrosis, fibrosis, and elastic fragmentation of the aortic root and ascending aorta lead to subsequent aortic root dilatation and aneurysm in patients with tetralogy of Fallot [61]. Aortic aneurysm has also been described after aortic arch repair [62].

3.4. Aortitis syndromes

Aortic aneurysm can be seen in aortitis syndromes related to syphilis, inflammatory bowel disease, and vasculitic syndromes. The primary systemic vasculitis is a group of autoimmune conditions characterized by occlusion, stenosis or aneurysmal dilations secondary to inflammation [63, 64, 65]. Aortic aneurysm may also be related to infective endocarditis (figure 8) or septicemia [66, 67, 68, 69, 70, 71].

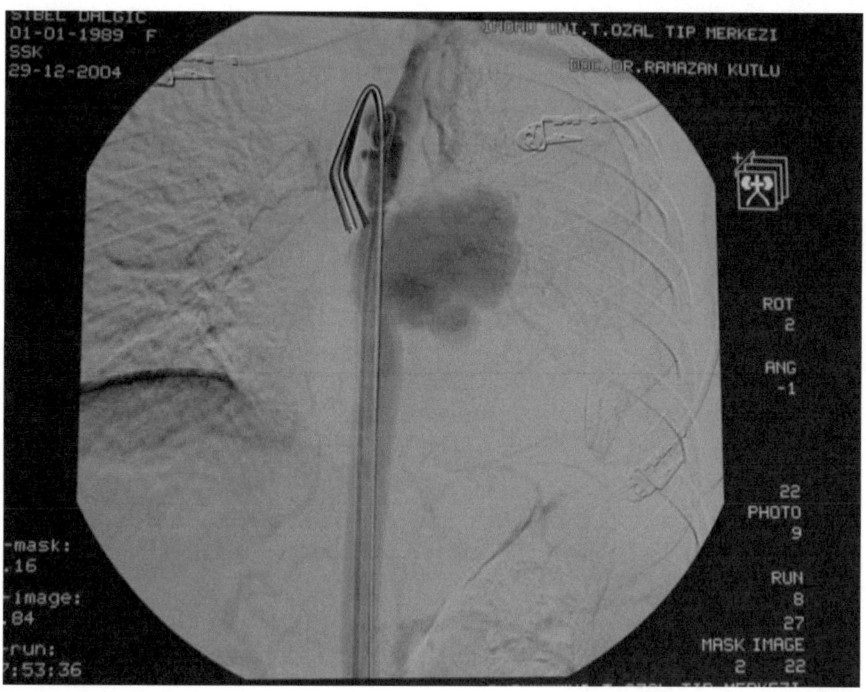

Figure 8. shows mycotic aneurysm at the postcoarctation area in a 16-year-old patient with coarctation of the aorta and infective endocarditis.

Aortic aneurysm has also been rarely described with Wiskott-Aldrich syndrome but real cause is not known [72].

3.5. Homosystinuria

Homosystinuria is an autosomal recessive metabolic disorder due to deficiency of cystathionin synthase which phenothpically resembles Marfan syndrome. Major cardiovascular complication of homosystinuria is premature atherosclerotic changes in the vascular system. Vitamin B6 and folic acid treatment helps reduce homocystein levels [73, 74].

4. Clinical presentation and diagnosis

Clinical presentation of aortic aneurysm depends on underlying disease, size, and location of aneurysm as well as presence of aortic dissection. Patients with aortic aneurysm related to genetic cause have specific phenotypical appearance such as having hypermobile joints, chest deformities, long and thin fingers, kyphoscoliosis, high palate, inguinal hernias, and/or aracnodactilia (Figure 1, 2). If patients have Marfan like appearance, family history should be sought. Decreased femoral pulsus, systolic ejection murmur in the aortic area can be detected during cardiac examination in patients with aortic aneurysm related to coarctation of the aorta or bicuspid aortic valve. Diastolic murmur can be heard secondary to aortic insufficiency or apical pansystolic murmur can be heard secondary to mitral valve insufficiency related to mitral valve prolapse. It is important to evaluate aortic dissection if presence of sharp chest and abdominal pain in patients who have aortic aneurysm.

Transthorasic and transesophageal echocardiographic evaluation is the first step evaluation for the aortic aneurysm. On transtorasic echocardiography, proximal ascending, thoracic aorta and proximal abdominal aorta can be visualized by using parasternal long axis, suprasternal views, and subcostal views. Echocardiographic evaluation can show mitral valve proplapse, aortic aneurysm, left ventricular and/or left atrial enlargement secondary to the mitral valve or aortic insufficiency, bicuspid aortic valve or coarctation of the aorta. 2D and colour-coded echocardiographic pictures from the parasternal long axis and apical four chamber view show mild aortic enlargement at the sinotubular junction, mitral valve prolapsus and mitral insufficiency in a 13-year-old patient with Marfan syndrome (figures 9, 10, 11, 12). Aortic aneurysm patients are also evaluated by transesopagheal echocardiography.

The other imaging modalities are cardiac catheterization, magnetic resonance imaging and computed tomography (figure 3, 4, 6, 7, 8). With the increasing availability of whole body imaging, the role of magnetic resonance imaging and multidetector computed tomography are increasing diagnostic modalities in patients with aortic aneurysm/dissection [75, 76, 77, 78].

http://dx.doi.org/10.5772/53383

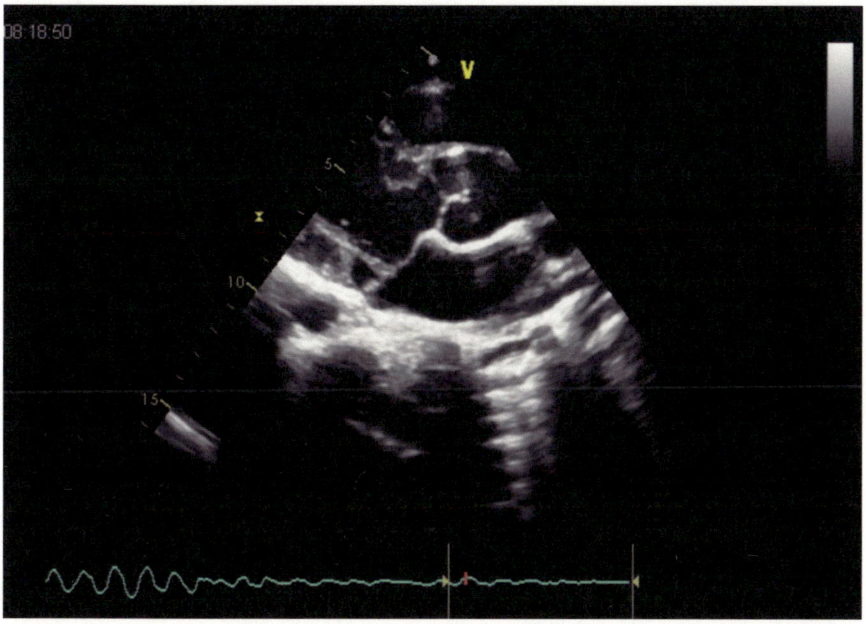

Figure 9. Long axis echo picture shows mild sinotubular junction in a 13-year-old patient with Marfan syndrome

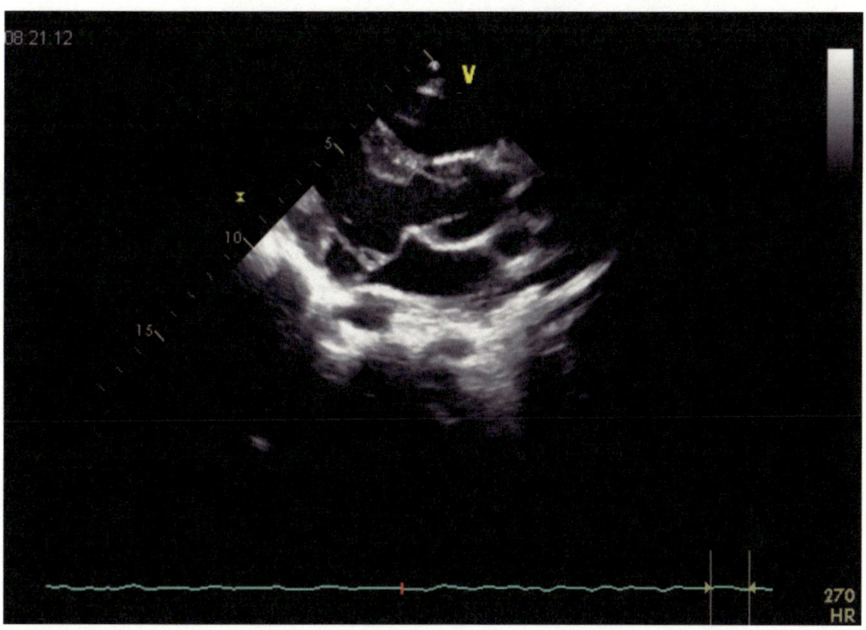

Figure 10. Long axis echo picture shows mitral valve prolapse in a 13-year-old patient with Marfan syndrome

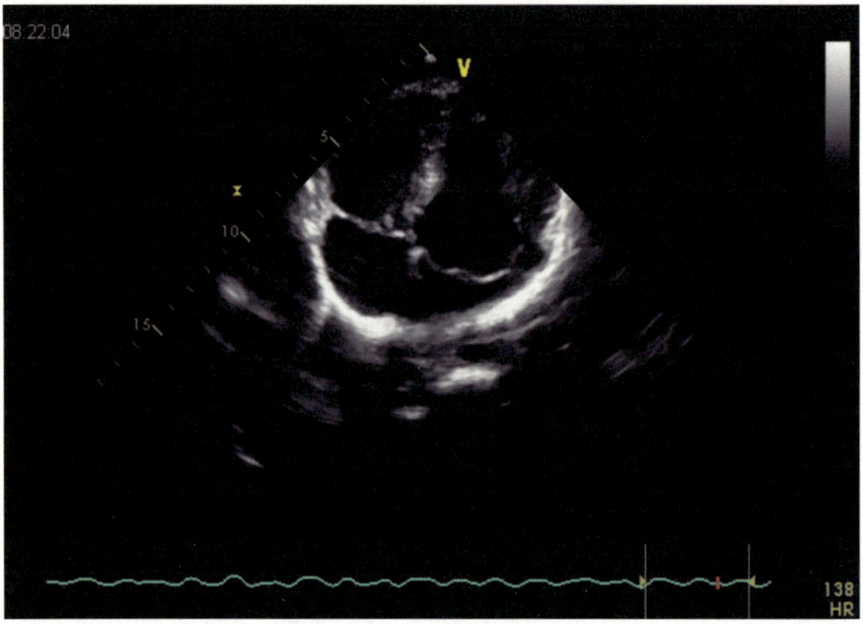

Figure 11. Apical four chamber echo picture shows mitral valve prolapse in a 13-year-old patient with Marfan syndrome

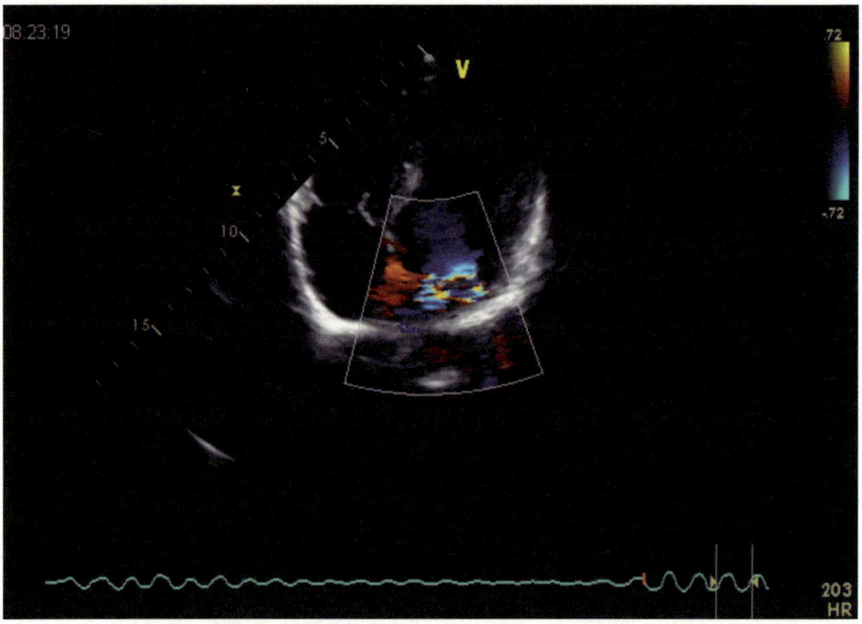

Figure 12. Apical four chamber echo picture shows mitral insufficiency secondary to mitral valve prolapse in a 13-year-old patient with Marfan syndrome

5. Treatment

Treatment of the cell cultures with dexamethasone induced remarkable up-regulation in the expression of tropoelastin, fibulin 1 and fibulin 4 encoding mRNAs, leading to normalization of elastic fiber production in fibroblasts with TGFβ-R1 mutations [78].

Among children who have aortic aneurysm, timing of surgical treatment should be weighed against life expectancy, underlying disease, the size and location of aneurysm and presence of dissection. It has been showed that beta blocker and ACE inhibitor therapy delay aortic surgery in patients with aortic aneurysm related Marfan syndrome.

The indications of surgical treatment are aortic size over 5 cm, aneurysm growth rate exceeding 1 cm per year, progressive aortic insufficiency, and familial history of early aortic dissection for most of aortic aneurysm patients. However, since the risk of dissection is higher in Loeyz-Dietz syndrome, surgery is indicated even at lower diameters of the aorta.

In conclusion, aortic aneurysm is a rare but a lifethreatening condition in childhood. It is generally related to genetic hereditary syndromes. The patients who have predisposition to aortic aneurysm should be followed-up closely.

Author details

Cemşit Karakurt

Inonu University Faculty of Medicine, Department of Pediatric Cardiology, Malatya, Turkey

References

[1] Bickerstaff. LK, Pairolero PC, Hollier LH, et al. Thoracic aortic aneurysms: a population- based study. Surgery. 1982; 92: 1103-8.

[2] Ye C, Yin H, Lin Y, Zhou L, Ye R, Li X, Han A, Wang S. Abdominal aorta aneurysms in children: a single –center experience of six patients. Ann Thorac Surg.2012; 93(1): 201-5.

[3] Mukkannavar SB, Choudhary SK, Talwar S, Makhija N, Gulati GS, Kabra SK. Aneurysmal circumflex aortic arch. J Card Surg. 2011; 26(5):515-8.

[4] Baumgartner D, Baumgartner C, Matyas G, Steinmann B, Löfller-Ragg J, Schermer E, Schweigmann U, Baldissera I, Frischhut B. Diagnostic power of aortic elastic properties in young patients with Marfan syndrome. J Thorac Cardiovasc Surg. 2005129(4): 730-9.

[5] Ramirez F, Dietz HC. Marfan syndrome: From molecular pathogenesis to clinical treatment. Curr Opin Genet Dev. 2007; 17(3)252-8.

[6] De Paepe A, Devereux RB, Dietz HC, Hennekam RC, Pyeritz RE. Am J Med Genet. 1996; 62(4):417-26.

[7] Faivre L, Collod-Beroud G, Ades L, Arbustini E et al: The new Ghent criteria for Marfan syndrome: what do they change? Clin Genet. 2012; 81(5):433-42.

[8] Radonic T, de Witte P, Groenink M et al. Critical appraisal of revised Ghent criteria for diagnosis of Marfan syndrome. Clin Genet. 2011 doi 10.1111/j. 1399-0004.2011.01646.4).

[9] Loeys BL, Dietz HC, Bravermen AC, Callewaert BL, De Backer J, Devereux RB, Hilhorst-Hofstee Y, Jondeau G, Faivre L, Milewicz DM, Pyeritz RE,Sponsoller PD, Wordsworth P, de Paepe AM: The revised Ghent nosology for the Marfan syndrome. J Med Genet. 2010; 47(7):476-85.

[10] Lachhab A, Doghmi N, Ouenzar M, Bennani R, Amri R, Cherti M. Cardiovascular manifestations of Marfan syndrome. Presse Med.2012; 41(3Pt1):328-30). Myers PO, Aggoun Y, Tissot C.

[11] Myers PO, Aggoun Y, Tissot C. Giant aortic root aneurysm in Marfan syndrome: a rare complication in early childhood. J Thorac Cardiovasc Surg.2011; 141(1):293-4.

[12] Ozdemir O, Olgunturk R, Kula S, Tunaoğlu FS. Echocardiographic findings in children with Marfan syndrome. Cardiovasc J Afr.2011; 22(5):245-8.

[13] Espinola-Zavaleta N, Iqbal FM, Nanda NC, Enrique-Rodriguez E, Amezcua-Guerra LM, Bojalil-Parra R, Reyes PA, Soto ME. Echocardiographic study of a Mestizo-Mexican population with Marfan syndrome. Echocardiography.2010;27(8):923-30.

[14] Geisbuesch S, Schray D, Bischoff MS, Lin HM, Di Luozzzo G, Griepp RB. Frequency of reoperations in patients with Marfan syndrome. Ann Thorac Surg. 2012; 93(5): 1496-501.

[15] Jondeau G, Detaind D, Tubach F et al. Aortic event rate in Marfan population: a cohort study. Circulation. 2012; 17:125(2) 226-32.

[16] Miyahara Y, Kasahara S, Takagaki M, Sano S. Successful aortic reimplantation in a three-year-old child with Marfan syndrome. Interact Cardiovasc Thorac Surg.2010; 11(2):218-20.

[17] Dietz HC.TGF-beta in the pathogenesis and prevention of disease: A matter of aneurysmic proportions.J Clin Invest.2010; 120(2):403-7.

[18] Zhang L, Gao LG, Zhang M, Zhou XL. Genotype-phenotype analysis of F-helix mutations at the kinase domain of TGFBR2, including a type 2 Marfan syndrome familial study. Mol Vis 2012; 18:55-63.

[19] Song HK, Kindem M, Bavaria JE, Dietz HC et al. Long term implications of emergency versus elective proximal aortic surgery in patients with Marfan syndrome in the genetically triggered thoracic aortic aneurysms and cardiovascular conditions consortium registry. J Thorac Cardiovasc Surg. 2012; 143(2):282-6.

[20] David TE, Maganti M, Armstrong S. Aortic root aneurysm: Principles of repair and long term follow-up. J Thorac Cardiovasc Surg.2010; 140(6):S14-9.

[21] Willis L, Roosvelet GE, Yetman AT. Comparison of clinical characteristics and frequency of adverse outcomes in patients with Marfan syndrome diagnosed in adulthood versus childhood. Pediatr Cardiol: 2009; 30(3):289-92.

[22] Pernot C, Worms AM, Marçon F, Menard O, Nassi C, Floquet J. Malignant quadrivalvular dysplasia of Marfan syndrome in a neonate. Arch Mal Coenur Vaiss.1989; 82(5):797-801.

[23] Abdel-Massih T, Goldenberg A, Vouhe P, Iserin F, Acar P, Villain E, Agnoletti G, Sidi D. Marfan syndrome in the newborn and infant less than 4 months: a series of 9 patients. Arch Mal Coeur Vaiss.2002; 95(5):462-72.

[24] Yang JH, Ki CS, Han H, Song BG, Jang SY, Chung Ty, Sung K, Lee HJ, Kim DK. Clinical features and genetic analysis of Korean patients with Loeys-Dietz syndrome. J Hum Genet. 2012; 57(1):52-6.

[25] Vida VL, Padalino MA, Motta R, Micciolo M, Cerutti A, Milanesi O, Stellin G. Traumatic aortic dissection in a boy with Loeys-Dietz syndrome. Ann Thorac Surg. 2011; 92(4):1520-2.

[26] Ha JS, Kim YH. A sporadic case of Loeys-Dietz syndrome type I with two novel mutations of theTGBR2 gene. Korean J Pediatr.2011; 54(6):272-5.

[27] Ozker E, Vuran C, Saritas B, Türköz R. Valve-sparing replacement of the ascending aorta and aortic arch in a child with Loeys-Dietz syndrome. Eur J Cardiothorac Surg. 2012; 41(5):1184-5.

[28] Valverde I, Simpson J, Beerbaum P. Magnetic resonance imaging findings in Loeys-Dietz syndrome. Cardiol Young.2010; 20(2):210-3.

[29] Patel ND, Arnaotakis GJ, George TJ, Allen JG, Alejo DE, Dietz HC, Cameron DE, Vricella LA. Valve sparing aortic root replacement in Loeys-Dietz syndrome. Ann Thorac Surg. 2011; 92(2):556-60.

[30] Rodrigues VJ, Elsayed S, Loeys BL, Dietz HC, Yousem DM. Neuroradiologic manifestations of Loeys-Dietz syndrome type 1. AJNR.2009; 30(8):1614-9.

[31] Everitt MD, Pinto N, Hawkins JA, Mitchell MB, Kouretas PC, Yetman AT. Cardiovascular surgery in children with Marfan syndrome or Loeys-Dietz syndrome. J Thorac Cardiovasc Surg.2009; 137(6):1327-32.

[32] Beighton P, De Paepe A, Steinmann B, Tsipouras P, Wenstrup RJ. Ehlers-Danlos syndromes: revised nosology, Villefranche, 1997. Am J Med Genet.1998; 77:31-37.

[33] Byers PH, Barsh GS, Holbrook KA. Molecular mechanism of connective tissue abnormalities in the Ehlers-Danlos syndrome. Collagen Res.1981; 5:475-489.

[34] Germain DP, Herrera-Guzman Y. Vascular Ehlers-Danlos syndrome. Ann Genet. 2004; 47:1-9.

[35] Kontusaari S, Tromp G, Kuivaniemi H, Romanic AM, Prockop DJ. A mutation in the gene for type III procollagen (COL3A1) in a family with aortic aneurysms. J Clin Invest.1990; 86:1465-1473.

[36] Coucke PJ, Willaert A, Wessels M et al. Mutations in the facilitative glucose transporter GLUT10 alters angiogenesis and cause arterial tortusity syndrome. Nature Genet.2006; 38:452-457.

[37] Beuren AJ, Hort W, Kalbfleisch H, Muller H, Stoermer J. Dysplasia of the systemic and pulmonary arterial system with tortusity and lengthening of the arteries: new entity, diagnosed during life, and leading to coronary death in early childhood. Circulation.1969; 39:109-115.

[38] Cine N, Basaran M, Guzelmeric F, Sunar H. Repair of ascending aortic aneurysm in a patient with arterial tortuosity syndrome. Interact Cardiovasc Thorac Surg.2011; 12(6):1051-3.

[39] Cleemann L, Mortensen KH, Holm K, Smedegaard H, Skouby SO, Wieslander SB, Leffers AM, Leth-Espensen P, Pedersen EM, Gravholt CH. Aortic dimensions in girls and young women with Turner syndrome: a magnetic resonance imaging study. Pediatr Cardiol.2010; 31(4):497-504.

[40] Prandstraller D, Mazzani L, Giardini A, Lovato L, Tamburrino F, Scarano E, Cicognani A, Fattori R, Picchio FM: Correlations of phenotype and genotype in relation to morphologic remodelling of the aortic root in patients with Turner's syndrome. Cardiol Young; 19(3)264-71.

[41] Allonson JE. Noonan syndrome. J Med Genet.1987; 24:9-13. Mendez HM, Opitz JM. Noonan syndrome: a review. Am J Med Genet.1985; 21:493-506.

[42] Mendez BR, Opitz JM. Noonan syndrome: a review. Am J Med Genet. 1985; 21:493-506.

[43] Power PD, Lewin MB, Hannibal MC, Glass IA. Aortic root dilatation is a rare complication of Noonan syndrome. Pediatr Cardiol.2006; 27(4):478-80.

[44] Alagille D, Estrada A, Hadchouel M, Gautier M, Odihvre M, Dommergues JP. Syndromic paucity of interlobular bile ducts (Alagille syndrome or arteriohepatic dysplasia): review of 80 cases. J Pediat.1987; 110:195-200.

[45] Boyer –Di Ponio J, Wright-Crosnier C, Groyer-Picard MT, Driancourt C, Beau I, Hadchouel M, Meunier-Rotival M. Biological function of mutant forms of JAGGED1 proteins in Alagille syndrome: inhibitory effetc on Notch signalling. Hum Molec Genet. 2007; 16:2683-2692.

[46] Kamath BM, Spinner NB, Emeric KM, Chudley AE, Booth C, Piccoli DA, Krantz ID. Vascular anomalies in Alagille syndrome. Am J Med Genet.2002; 112:176-180.

[47] Hutchagowder V, Sausgruber N, Kim KH, Angle B, Marmorstein LY, Urban Z. Fibulin-4: a novel gene for an autosomal recessive cutis laxa syndrome. Am J Hum Genet. 2006; 78:1075-10880.

[48] Dasouki M, Markova D, Garola R, Sasaki T, Charbonneasu NL, Sakai LY, Chu ML. Compound heterozygous mutations in fibulin-4 causing neonatal lethal pulmonary artery occlusion, aortic aneurysm, arachnodactyly and mild cutis laxa. Am J Med Genet. 2007; 143A:2635-2641.

[49] Renard M, Holm T,Veith R, Callewaert BL, Ades LC, Pickart A, Dasouki M, Hoyer J, Rauch A, Trapane P, Earing MG, Coucke PJ, Sakai LY, Dietz HC, De Paepe AM, Loeys BL. Altered TGFbeta signalling and cardiovascular manifestations in patients with autosomal recessive cutis laxa type I caused fibulin-4 deficiency.Eur J Hum Genet.2010; 18(8):895-901.

[50] Van der Laar IM, Vand der Linde D, Oei EH et al. Phenotypic spectrum of the SMAD 3 related aneurysms-osteoarthritis syndrome. J Med Genet. 2012; 49(1):47-57.

[51] Disabella E, Grasso M, Gambarin FI, Narula N, Dore R, Favalli V, Serio A, Antoniazzi E, Mosconi M, Pasotti M, Odero A, Arbustini E. Risk of dissection in thoracic aneurysm associated with mutations of smooth muscle alpha-actin 2 (ACTA2). Heart. 201; 97(4):321-6.

[52] Amazcua-Guerra L, Santiago C, Espinola-Zavaleta N, Pineda C. Bicuspid aortic valve: a synergistic factor for aortic dilation and dissection in Marfan syndrome.Rev Invest Clin.2010; 62(1):39-43.

[53] Binnetoglu K, Yildiz CE, Babaoğlu K, Altun G, Cetin G. Management of an ascending aortic aneurysm associated with a bicuspid aortic valve and a coarctation in an adolescent. J Card Surg.2011; 26(6):635-7.

[54] Hope MD, Hope TA, Meadows AK, Ordovas KG, Urbania TH, Alley MT, Higgins CB. Bicuspid aortic valve: a four dimensional MR evaluation of ascending aortic systolic flow patterns. Radiology.2010; 255(1):53-61.

[55] Yuan SM, Raanani E, Late complications of coarctation of the aorta. Cardiol J.2008; 15(6):517-24.

[56] Thanopoulos BD, Giannakoulas G, Giannaopoulos A, Galdo F, Tsaoussis GS. Initial and six–year results of stent implantation for aortic coarctation in children. Am J Cardiol.2012; 109(10):1499-503.

[57] Butera G, Heles M, MacDonald ST, Carminati M. Aortic coarctation complicated by wall aneurysm: the role of covered stents. Catheter Cardiovasc Interv.2011; 78(6): 926-32.

[58] Chakrabarti S, Kenny D, Morgan G, Curtis SL, Hamilton MC, Wilde P, Tometzki AJ, Turner MS, Martin RP. Balloon expandable stent implantation for native and recurrent coarctation of the aorta-prospective computed tomography assessment of stent integrity, aneurysm formation and stenosis relief. Heart.2010; 96(15):1212-6.

[59] Careage-Reyna G, Ramirez-Vargas AF, Hernandez-Magro RM, Arguero-Sanchez R. Thoracic aortic aneurysm associated with aortic coarctation without previous surgery: report of two cases.Cir Cir.2009;77(1):61-3.

[60] Ramayya AS, Coelho R, Sivakumar K, Radhakrishan S. Repair of tetralogy of Fallot with ascending and proximal aortic arch aneurysm: case report. J Card Surg.2011; 26(3):328-30.

[61] Niwa K. Aortic root dilatation in tetralogy of Fallot long-term after repair-histology of the aorta in tetralogy of Fallot: evidence of intrinsic aortopathy. Int J Cardiol.2005; 103(2):117-9.

[62] Ghosh A, Liu A, Mora B, Egarwala B. Giant aortic aneurysm after interrupted aortic arch repair. Pediatr Cardiol: 2010; 31(7):1104-6.

[63] Mukhtyar C, Brogan P, Lugmani R. Cardiovascular involvement in primary systemic vasculitis. Best Pract Res Clin Rheumatol.2009; 23(3):419-28.

[64] Bolin E, Moddie DS, Fraser CD Jr, Guirola R, Warren R, Eldin KW: Takayashu arteritis presenting as severe ascending aortic arch dilation and aortic regurgitation in a 10-year-old female. Congenit Heart Dis.2011; 6(6):630-3.

[65] Karakurt C, Koçak G, Selimoğlu A, Özen M. Aortic aneurysm: a rare complication of ulserative colitis. Anadolu Kardiyol Derg.2007; 7(4):461-2.

[66] Lin Q, Min Y, Song XX, Ren Y, Ding YY, Xu QQ, Li XZ. Childhood staphylococcus aureus septicemia complicated by aortic aneurysm: a cse report. Zhongguo Dang Dai Er Ke Za Zhi. 2011; 13(12):1005-6.

[67] Andersen ND, Bhattacharya SD, Williams JB, McCann RL, Hughes GC. Mycotic aneurysm of thoracoabdominal aorta in a child with end-stage renal disease. J Vasc Surg.2011; 54(4):1161-3.

[68] Zhu WH, Shen LG, Neubauer H. Clinical characteristics, interdisciplinary treatment and follow-up of 14 children with Takayasu arteritis. World J Pediatr.2010; 6(4):342-7.

[69] Schwartzs SB, Fisher D, Reinus C, Shahroor S. Infectious aortitis: a rare cause of chest pain in a child. Pediatr Emerg Care. 2011; 27(7):654-6.

[70] Erkut B, Becit N, Kantarci M, Ceviz N. Mycotic pseudo aneurysm of the ascending aorta following purulent pericardial effusion diagnosed by multi-slice computed tomography. Cardiovasc J Afr.2011; 22(3):143-4.

[71] Haas B, Wilt HG, Carlson Km, Lofland GK. Streptococcus pneumoniae causing mycotic aneurysm in a pediatric patient with coarctation of the aorta. Congenit Heart Dis. 2012; 7(1):71-5.

[72] Pellier I, Dupuis Girod S, Loisel D, Benabidahallah S, Proust A, Malhlaoui N, Picard C, Najioullah, de Saint Basile G, Blanche S, Rialland X, Casanova JL, Fischer A. Occurence of aortic aneurysms in 5 cases of Wiskott-Aldrich syndrome. Pediatrics.2011; 127(2):e498-504.

[73] Yap S, Boers GH, Wilcken B, Wilcken B, Wilcken DE, Brenton DP, Lee PJ, Walter JH, Howard PM, Naughten ER. Vascular outcome in patients with homocystinuria due to cystathionine beta-synthase deficiency treated chronically: a multicenter observational study. Arterioscler Thromb Vasc Biol; 21(12):2080-5.

[74] Almgren B, Eriksson I, Hemmingsson A, Hillerdal G, Larssson E, Aberg H.Acta Chir Scand.1978;190(1):8-10.

[75] Shon GH, Jang SY, Moon JR, Yang JH, Sung K, Ki CS, Oh JK, Choe YH, Kim DK. The usefulness of multidetector computed tomographic angiography for the diagnosis of Marfan syndrome by Ghent criteria. Int J Cardiovasc Imaging. 2011; 27(5):679-88. Suarez B, Caldera A, Castillo M. Imaging and clinical features in a child with Loeys-Dietz syndrome. A case report. Interv Neuroradiol. 2011; 17(1):9-11.

[76] Garg SK, Mohan S, Kumar S. Diagnostic value of 3D contrast-enhanced magnetic resonance angiography in Takayasu's arteritis: a comparative with digital substraction angiography. Eur Radiol.2011; 21(8):1658-66.

[77] Tsai SF, Triverdi M, Boettner B, Daniels CJ. Usefulness of screening cardiovascular magnetic resonance imaging to detect abnormalities after repair of coarctation of the aorta. Am J Cardiol.2011; 107(2):297-301.

[78] Barnett CP, Chitayat D, Bradley TJ, Wang Y, Hinek A.Dexamethasone normalizes aberrant elastic fiber production and collagen 1 secretion by Loeys-Dietz syndrome fibroblasts: a possible treatment? Eur J Hum Genet.2011; 19(6):624-33.

Chapter 3

Visceral Artery Aneurysms

Petar Popov and Đorđe Radak

Additional information is available at the end of the chapter

http://dx.doi.org/10.5772/52814

1. Introduction

In clinical practice relatively rare vascular entity, visceral artery aneurysms (VAA) can thrombose, embolise and rupture, causing high morbidity and mortality [1]. Splanchnic aneurysms pose a difficult therapeutic challenge especially in emergency cases. Almost 22% of VAA patientswith mortality as high as 8.5%,are diagnosed after rupture with variable clinical manifestations that raise the risk of misdiagnosis and unwarranted treatment [2]. Frequent use of imaging techniques and especially computed tomography scanning have significant impact on the overall increase in the number of new cases. Mostly, VAA are being discovered incidentally during assessment for abdominal pain or other disorders. Regardless of how VAA are discovered, the choice of treatment depends on clinical presentation, underlying etiology, location, general health status, and comorbidity factors. For many years surgical treatment, involving either aneurysm resection with bypass or ligation, were the only therapeutic options, especially in emergency cases [3]. At the present time, however, endovascular techniques are considered the method of choice for first-line treatment and good results have been obtained in emergency cases [4,5].

An estimated 3000 cases have been reported in the literature with an incidence of 1% in the general population and 0.1% to 10% in autopsy series [2]. VAA are described in the literature 200 years ago, and the first successful surgical resection was performed by Cooley and DeBakey in 1949. [6]. The most commonly involved arteries are the splenic artery aneurysms in 60% of cases and the hepatic artery aneurysms in about 20% of cases. Other splanchnic artery aneurysms are discovered in 20-40% of cases. Other sites include the superior mesenteric artery (SMA-5.5%), celiac trunk and gastric artery (4%), gastroepiploic artery, jejunal artery, ileal artery, and colonic artery (3%), and, inferior mesenteric artery, pancreaticoduodenal artery and pancreatic arteries (2%) [2,7,8,9] (Figure 1, Table 1).

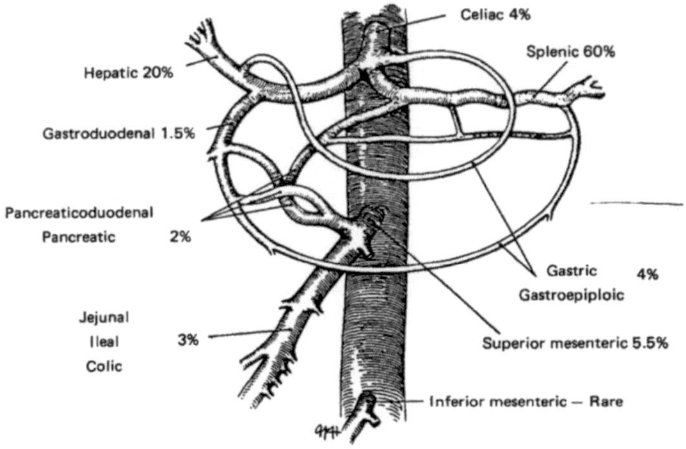

Figure 1. Visceral artery aneurysms distribution.

Aneurysm localization	Frequency	M/W	Rupture rate	Mortality
Splenic artery	60%	1:4	2%	25% nopregnent 70% mother 75% fetus
Hepatic arteries	20%	2:1	20%	35%
SMA	5.5%	1:1	rare	50%
Truncus caeliacus	4%	1:1	13%	50%
Gastric, Gastroepiploic	4%	3:1	90%	50%
Jejunal, Ileal, Colic	3%	1:1	30%	70%
Pancreaticoduodenal Gastroduodenal	2%	4:1	75% inflammatory 50% noninflammat.	50%

Table 1. Visceral artery aneurysms, frequency and distribution.

The earliest recorded work that describes visceral artery aneurysmswas announced by French physician, Beaussiera,1770, who presented the splenic artery aneurysm in 60-year-old female cadaver during an autopsy demonstration after injection contrast into the aorta and femoral veins [10].

The first record of clinical symptoms of VAA recorded Quinkue in 1871, when he described the classic "triad" of symptoms: abdominal pain, obstructive jaundice and hemobila, caused by hepatic artery aneurysm existence [11,12,13].

The first successful surgical treatment of the common hepatic artery aneurysms by artery ligation has been noted by Kehr in 1903 [14]. Thirty years later, in 1932 Lindboa was the first who preoperatively successfully diagnosed SAA, which is then surgically resolved [15].

Although visceral artery aneurysms are rare they are certainly clinically significant pathological changes, with an incidence of 0.01% to 0.2% in routine autopsies, with increasing tendency of appearance in aging population [2]. By the early nineties, diagnosis and therapeutic management of splanchnic arterial aneurysms weren't enough successful which resulted in the rupture, and the detection of these lesions only on the autopsy table. Advances in surgical and endovascular techniques have led to numerous and qualitative change in the approach to treatment of these lesions.

1.1. Aneurysm of the splenic artery

Splenic artery aneurysm is the most common splanchnic aneurysms (58-67% of all cases), the third most prevalent in the abdomen, after aneurysms of the abdominal aorta and iliac arteries. They are usually asymptomatic in nature (27% is associated with pain in the abdomen) [14]. The first splenic artery aneurysm is described Beaussier (1770) [10]. At the middle of the last century (1953), Owens and Coffey gave an extensive review of previously reported SAA in the literature and described 262 cases [16]. American history records the death (1881) President James A. Garfield as a result of rupture of splenic artery aneurysm, two months after he was wounded in the stomach during the assassination attempt [17].

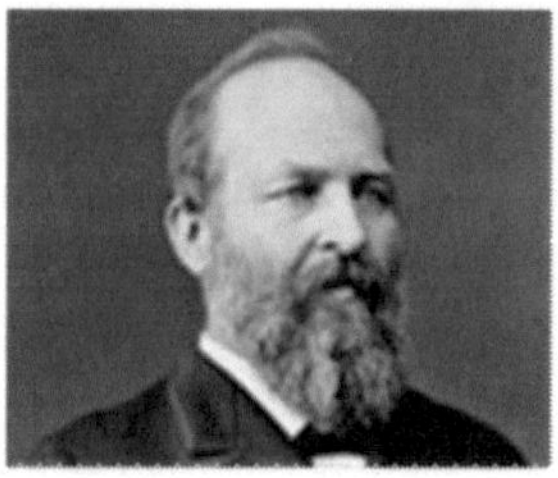

In Anglo-Saxon literature the incidence of occurrence lineal artery aneurysm ranges from 0.7% to 10.4% of the total population based on data obtained from the autopsy report.In the literature, reported splenic aneurysm diameter was found 30 cm in diameter but they are usually less than 3 cm. SAA are usually solitary, saccular in shape and localized in the distal third of artery, the bifurcation region, the splenic hilum.Splenic aneurysms are more common in women (4:1), in the sixth decade of life, as much as 80% of all cases are older than 50 years. One third of those patients have multiple aneurysm localization [19-21].

1.2. Clinical presentation

SAA are usually incidental, unexpected findings on the control, the native image of the abdomen, CT scan or angiography. When patients have symptoms, they describe vague pain in the left upper abdominal quadrant and left thigh.Since 40-50% of patients have moderate splenomegaly, and in about 10% of patients auscultation soundness of the left upper quadrant of the abdomen. Rare are those in which the pulsatile tumefaction took hold in the region under [20, 22].

1.3. The pathogenesis, formation causes

Of these aneurysms are not completely clear, but increased blood flow through the splenic artery may be a risk factor (hypertension, pregnancy). Some researchers claim that these hemodynamic instability lead to irreversible damage of tunica media and thus represent a predisposing factor for aneurysm formation. Subsequent muscular dystrophy and calcification of damaged artery wall is a secondary process [23, 24]. The recorded incidence of SAA in patients with liver cirrhosis and portal hypertension ranges from 7 to 20% and 8-13% of patients waitingfor liver transplantation and after liver transplantation because of the large portosystemic shunt, which causes the increase in splenic artery volume [25]. Other possible causes are essential hypertension, septic embolus, blunt trauma, the weakening of the arterial wall as a result of local inflammation (pancreatitis), subacute bacterial endocarditis. Less common causes are inherited diseases characterized by the development of visceral artery aneurysms multiple or associated with the appearance of polycystic kidney disease and systemic lupus erithematodus.SAA can also occur as a consequence of renal artery fibromusculardysplasia [26].

After all, arteriosclerosis is the most common histopathological findings and probably postaneurysmaticphenomenon rather than a primary cause of the aneurysm

The risk of *rupture* is difficult to estimate. Until 1980, about 10% of SAA was ruptured at the time of diagnosis, but in more recent series the incidence of rupture is at the level of 3% [2,8,19].

When rupture, SAA usually cause acute abdominal pain, irradiating in the left flank, back and subscapular region and can cause shock, abdominal distension, and finally death. Aneurysms can rupture into free space or omentum minus. The phenomenon of "double" rupture was reported in 20-30% of cases. In these patients if we do not take anything, the initial bleeding in omentum minus can provoke pain and transient hypotension and continues on a further rupture in the peritoneal cavity, which happens in the next 48 hours [19, 27, 28]. This "guard" period between the initial and subsequent bleeding gives room for the timely diagnosis and intervention. Overall mortality from ruptured SAA should be between 10 and 25%. Symptomatic, large and/or rapidly growing aneurysms, pregnancy, portal hypertension, liver transplantation and portocaval shunts are associated with increased risk of aneurysm rupture. Rupture rarely occurs when the diameter is less than 2.5 cm [28]. Pregnancy is associated with 20 to 50% of rupture rate, usually in the third trimester or early postpartum period [24]. *Barretin* his coworkers, reported rupture rate of 12% in the first two trimester, 69% in the third, 13% during labor, and 6% were recorded in puerperiumu. Mortality rate of ruptured SAA during pregnancy is about 75% of mothers and 95% for fetus. On the other hand, the mortality rates in women who are not pregnant are considerably less [29].

1.4. Treatment

Different therapeutic options are available for patients with SAA, including conventional surgery, endovascular treatment, and, more recently, laparoscopic surgery. Choice of treatment depends primarily on clinical presentation, aneurysm location, associated risk factors, and overall patient status [30, 31, 32].

Patients who arrive with signs of rupture, hemorrhagic shock or unstable hemodynamic status require urgent treatment. In such situations some authors used the endovascular approach in solving problems; otherwise, ligation of the splenic artery without further reconstruction was the most used technique [33].

Recently, we use a new, promising option: endovascular coil embolization approach (figure 2,3), stent-graft application and the laparoscopic approach to splenic artery ligation. Selective splenic artery catheterization and coil embolization of aneurysmal sac is proposed in high-risk patients or the rupture of the aneurysm [33,34].

Numbers of patients who are treated in this way are rapidly increasing. The data obtained from follow-up investigations are still insufficient to be able to make a final doctrine, especially concerning the possibility of re-creating an even greater place in the aneurysmal sac as a result of recanalization. When the embolization is technically challenging or contraindicated primarily by close contact of the aneurysm with the spleen, there are the possible options for open surgery (figure 4, 5) or laparoscopic artery ligation.

Treatment is indicated when the aneurysm is symptomatic, with diameter greater than 3 cm, and in pregnant women or women of childbearing age want to get pregnant [28].

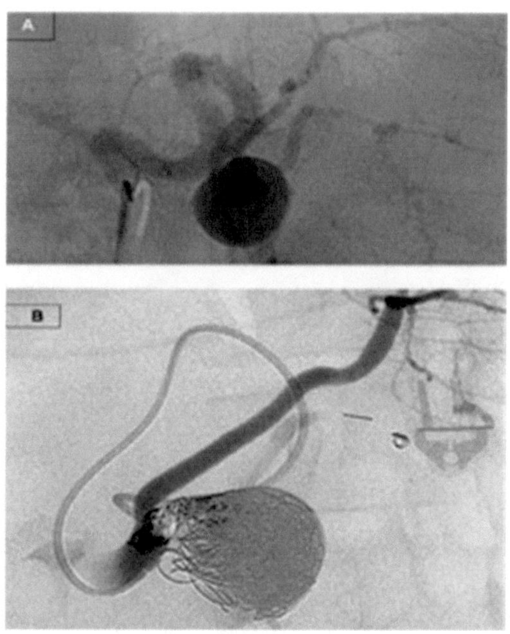

Figure 2. Splenic artery aneurysm embolization

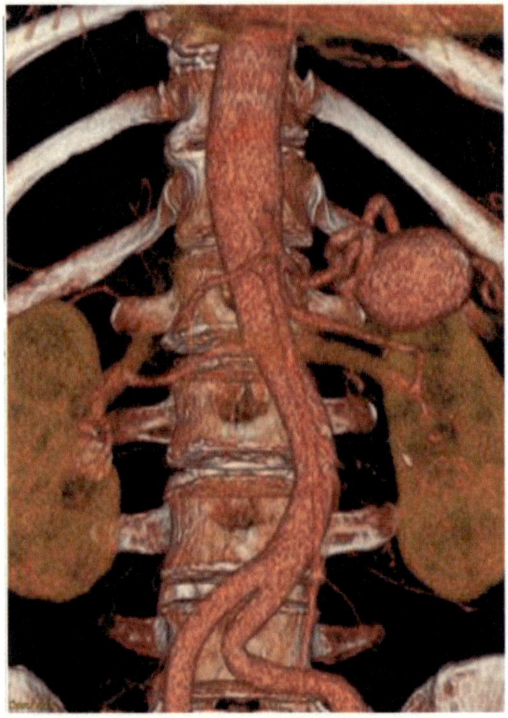

Figure 3. Splenic artery aneurysm. MSCT

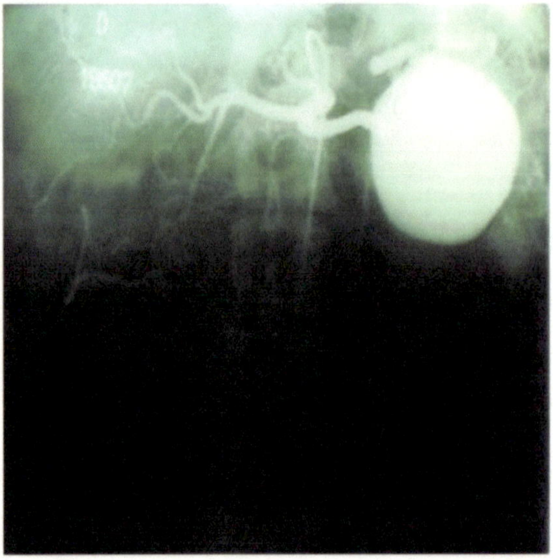

Figure 4. Splenic artery aneurysm angiography before and after surgical reconstruction

http://dx.doi.org/10.5772/52814

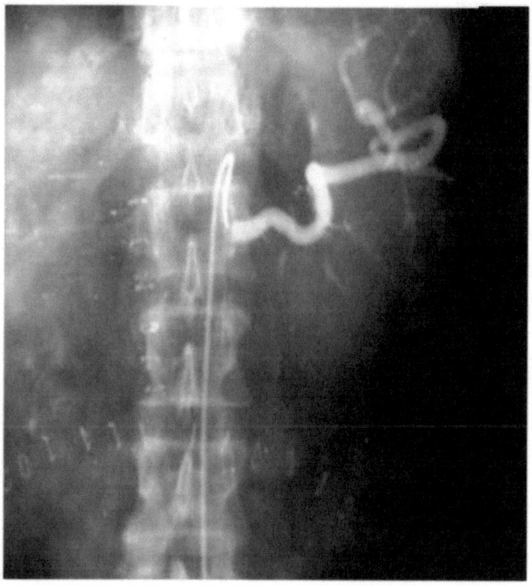

Figure 5. Splenic artery aneurysm angiography before and after surgical reconstruction

1.5. Hepatic Artery Aneurysms

Hepatic artery aneurysms (HAA) is second in height among VAA, accounting for 20% of all splanchnic artery aneurysms. In 1819, Wilson was the first who described it. Historically at the beginning, before antibiotic era, mycotic aneurysms were dominantly presentamong discovered and treated HAA, but now has been reduced to 10% of all. Most of these aneurysms was admitted to the state of rupture or accidentally discovered during autopsy [2,3,8].

Atherosclerosis is considering a basic cause in about 30-50% occurrence of HAA, while still posing as a secondary process. Less common causes of these lesions are vasculitis, such as polyarthritis nodosa, inflammatory processes caused by cholecystitis or pancreatitis, Marfan's syndrome,Ehlers-Danlos syndrome,fibromuscular dysplasia, cystic medial necrosis (24%) and trauma (22%) [35].

Posttraumatic false aneurysms accounts for about 20%, they are the most often the result or penetrating andcrush injuries or wounds, surgical procedures, liver transplantation or occurring after percutaneous needle biopsy of the liver (transhepatic cholangiography) [36].

Aneurysms are more common in man (2:1) and mostly extrahepatic located (80%). Of that, extrahepatic HAA 60% are located on common hepatic artery, 30% involve the right hepatic artery and 5% the left hepatic artery.Right incidence of HAA is unknown. Of the 2,091,965 patients reviewed at the Mayo Clinic for 18 years, hepatic aneurysms were seen in only 36 patients (12% of all VAA), the incidence was 0.002%.There is still some controversy about the incidence of hepatic aneurysm rupture and should be 20% to 80% [36].

Stanley describes in his research 162 HAA cases, 75% were located extrahepaticaly, of which 63% of aneurysms were located on common hepatic artery,28% on the right hepatic artery and 5% on the left, and finally 4% in both hepatic arteries. Atherosclerotic aneurysms are almost exclusively positioned extrahepaticalyof which 96% were placed on common hepatic artery. The remaining 25% HAA were intrahepaticaly located, predominantly pseudoaneurysm arising mainly as a result of vascular injury and trauma [1].

Hepatic aneurysms become clinically apparent when there is erosion of the biliary tree and/or portal vein with subsequent development of portal hypertension, rupture in the retroperitonel space and/or peritoneal cavity. Bleeding into the abdominal cavity is a catastrophic event, with a mortality rate of 82% [37- 39]. *Quincke's* classic triple symtoms: jaundice, biliary colic's and gastrointestinal bleeding suggests hemobilia that occurs in one third of patients [36].

HAA are often symptomatic. The most common symptom is accompanied by malaise or right-hand abdominalnmi radiating to the back, sometimesepigastric pain. Palpable masses are rare finding.

Native rontgen examinations of the abdomen or upper gastrointestinal tract by contrast medium may indicate the presence of HAA, especially if it is visible calcification in the wall of the aneurysmal sac in the right hypohondrium or the existence of a defect in the filling of the duodenum [40].

Technological advances in the field of ultrasonography and multi slice scanning (MSCT) easily and accurately allow the diagnosis of aneurysms. Magnetic resonance imaging (MRI) also gives the extraordinary results in the diagnosis of HAA.

Color duplex scan is very important and helpful diagnostic tool in showing intrahepatic lesions. It significantly contributes to the precise detection of the blood flow inside the anerysmatic sac and allows visualization of the portal system arterialization when the fistula is present. Ultrasound also has their place in monitoring of the previously embolized intrahepatic aneurysms to confirm occlusion of the sac [41].

1.6. Therapy

Basically, treatments of these lesions today consider selective endovascular embolization of the "feeding" arteries, proximal to the HAA. Different substances are in use successfully, also arterial stents and detachable silicone balloons [40].

In intact hepatic artery pseudoaneurysm (HAP), occlusion is achieved successfully by percutaneous embolization in 88% -100% cases (figure 8, 10). Good results are recorded with embolization of HAP caused by pancreatitis and ruptured HAP. Repeated embolization is necessary in 30-40% of patients. Rare reports of hepatic necrosis are noted and probably are the result of inadequatecatheter placement or embolization, particularly when the portal vena is occluded. Surgical resolution of HAP is solution when endovascular attempt fails, especially for orthostatic liver transplantation (OLT) associated with pseudocysts [39-41].

http://dx.doi.org/10.5772/52814

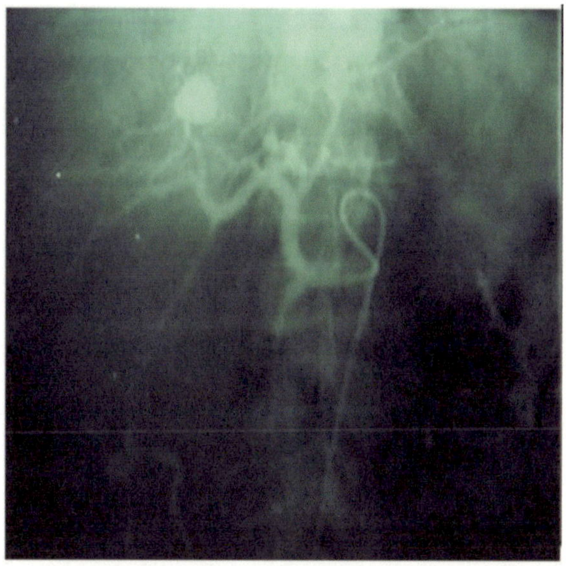

Figure 6. Hepatic artery aneurysms- angiography

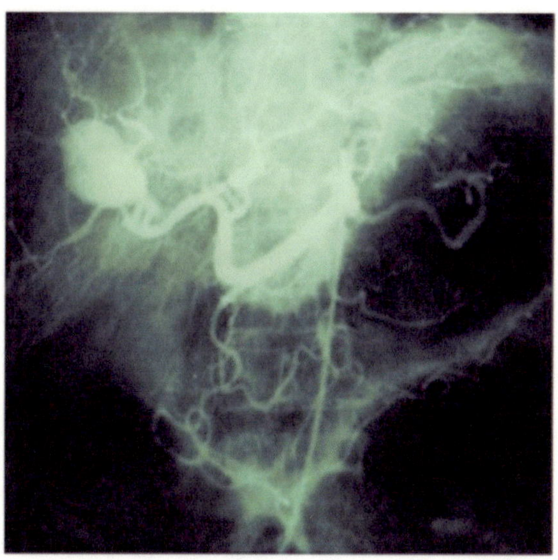

Figure 7. Hepatic artery aneurysms- angiography

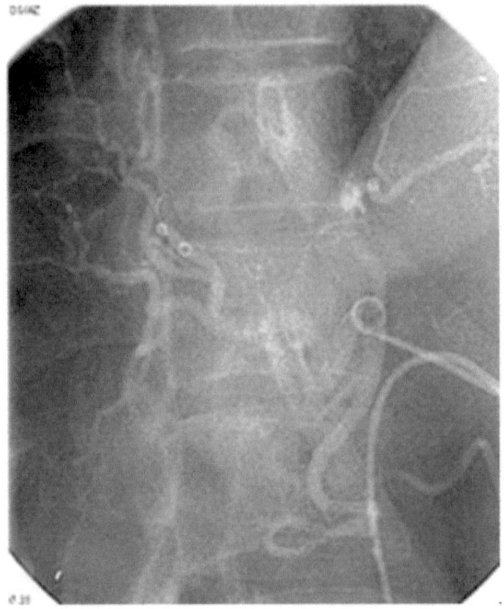

Figure 8. Hepatic artey aneurysms- percutaneous coils embolization

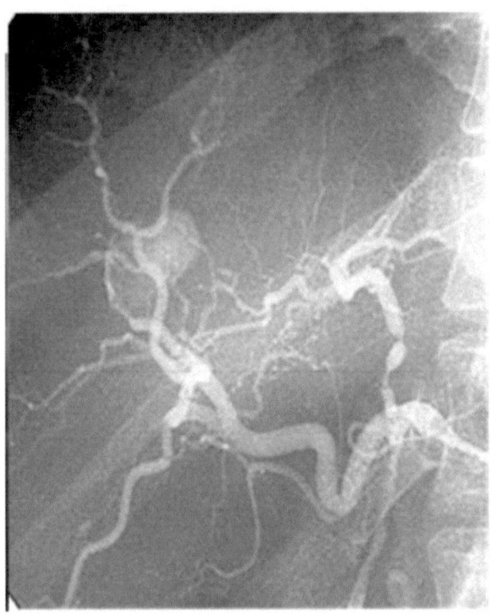

Figure 9. Hepatic artey aneurysms- percutaneous coils embolization

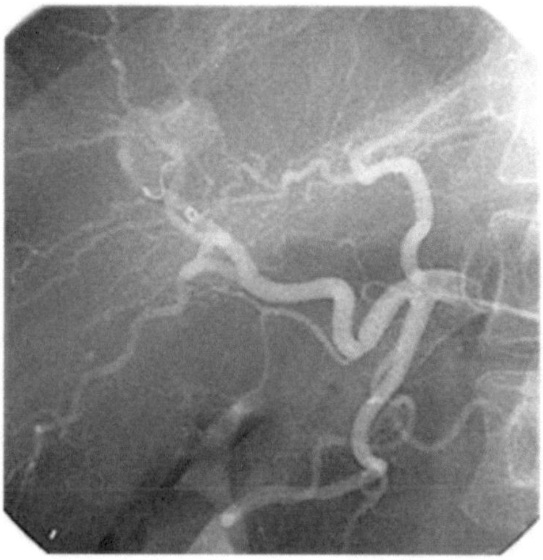

Figure 10. Hepatic artey aneurysms- percutaneous coils embolization

1.7. Celiac artery aneurysm

Aneurysms of celiac trunk represent one of the rarest forms of splanchnic artery aneurysms (3.6% to 4% of all VAA). The incidence of occurrence ranges from 0.005% to 0.01%. Since this anomaly was first described in 1745, fewer than 200 cases were registered in the World Series (Figure 11 - 13) [1 - 3,8, 42].

Although the incidence of rupture was previously 70-85% (first half of the 20th century), advances in diagnosis and early surgical and endovascular intervention significantly reduced the rupture rate on today 7%. Timely diagnosis and proper treatment are crucial for survival, because the operative mortality of ruptured cases fell down from 40% to only 5% [43, 45].

Today 85% of aneurysms were disclosed by angiography, while only 7% by autopsy.There issignificant frequency in a joint appearance between celiac trunk aneurysm and other peripheral aneurysms. In the first half of last century, the average age of diagnosed patients was 40 years. Men outnumber women nine times, and syphilis (Treponema pallidum) was a major cause in 30% of cases. Other recognized causes are arteriosclerosis and medial degeneration. Since that time, the average age of newly diagnosed patients has increased to 55 years and women now comprise almost half of all cases [43, 44, 46].

Existence of the celiac trunk aneurysm by itself is a sufficient indication for surgical reconstruction or endovascular treatment. Simple artery ligation could be final solution sometimes accompanied by the hepatic ischemia.

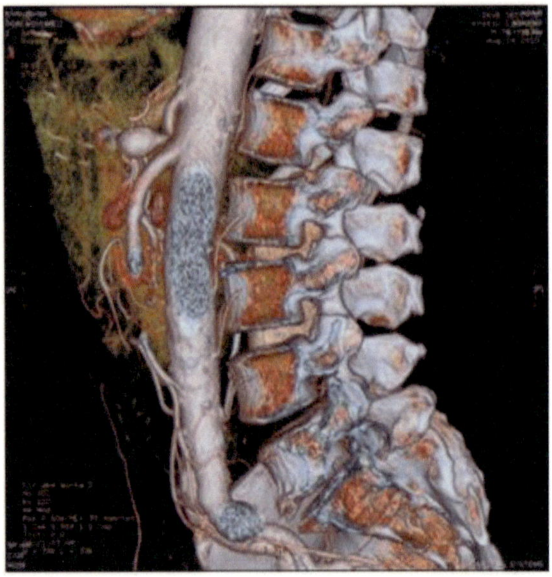

Figure 11. Coeliac artery aneurysms

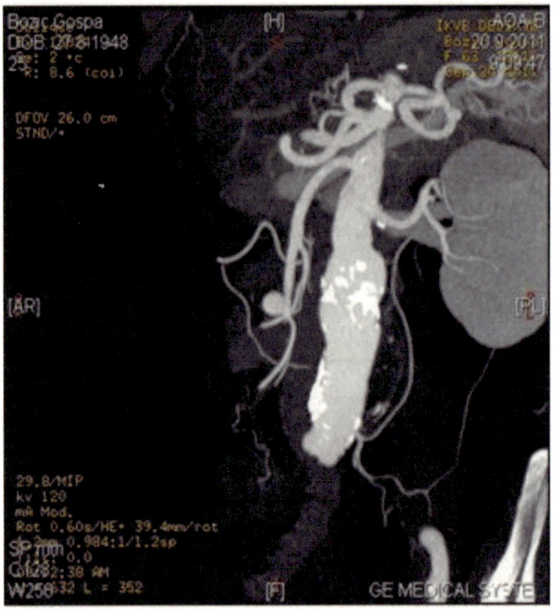

Figure 12. Coeliac artery aneurysms

http://dx.doi.org/10.5772/52814

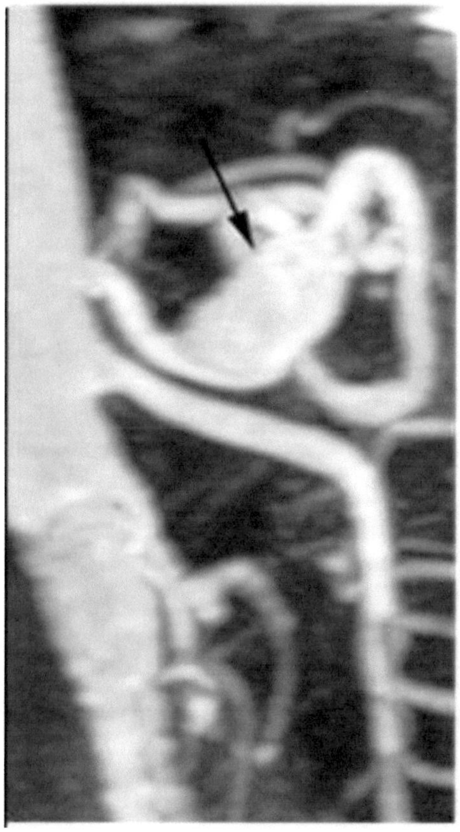

Figure 13. Coeliac artery aneurysms

First celiac trunk aneurysm resection was performed in 1958 by Shumacker. Celiac artery occlusion by coil embolization or stent graft implantation are promising way in reating these lesions [5, 45, 46].

2. Superior mesenteric artery aneurysms

SMA (figure 14-16) is located on the third most prevalent places among VAA.Until now, sixty percent's of all detected aneurysms are mycotic by etiology [1-3]. It is believed that atherosclerosis is basic cause of the SMA aneurysms occurrence. Other etiological factors are: septic embolus, polyarteritis nodosa, Bechet's syndrome, systemic lupus erithematosus, endocarditis, systemic connective tissue disorders, vasculitis, trauma, cystic medial necrosis, neurofibromatosis and history of intravenous drug abuse.*Stevenson* was made the first surgical attempt to solve the problem. The first successful, surgical treatment of SMA aneurysm was conducted by *DeBakey* and *Cooley*in 1949 [6,47].

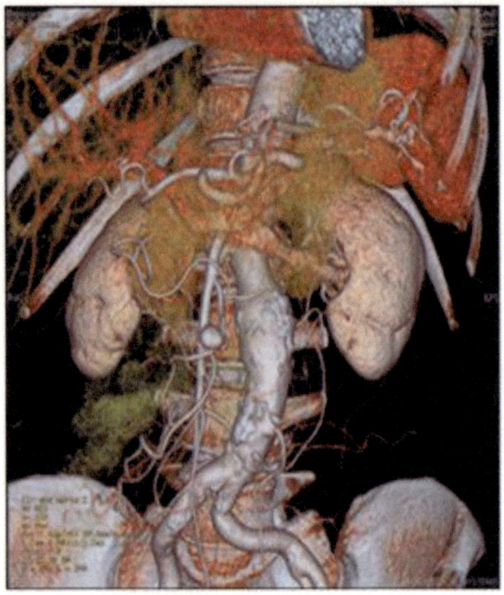

Figure 14. Superior mesenteric artery aneurysms- MSCT

Symptoms are generally vague and unclear, accompanied by pain after meals. Diagnostic procedures are the same as for other VAA. Surgical way of dealing with SMA aneurysms has previously been the main way of solving problems.SMA transcatheter embolization of aneurysm sac is particularly suitable for hemodynamically stable patients and more often is the first choice of treatment [48,49].

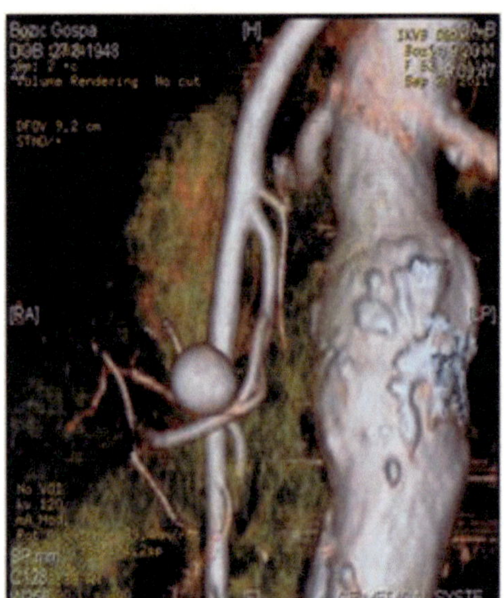

Figure 15. Superior mesenteric artery aneurysms- MSCT

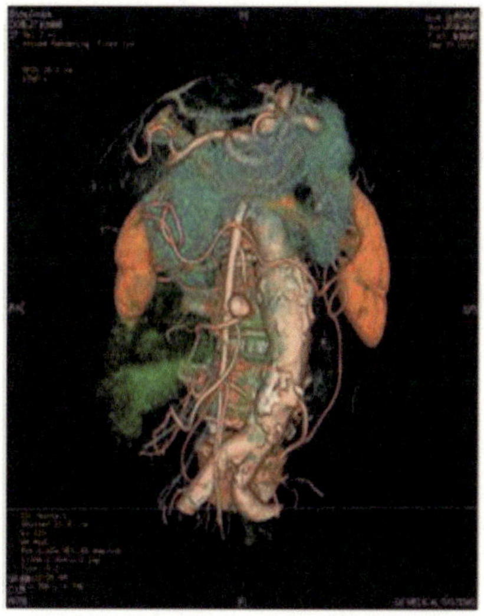

Figure 16. Superior mesenteric artery aneurysms- MSCT

Inferior mesenteric artery aneurysms

About 1% of total number recorded VAA are aneurysms of the inferior mesenteric artery (IMA)(Figure 17,18). They are usually asymptomatic in nature and the incidence of occurrence is unknown. Basically, the occurrence of atherosclerosis in aneurysms may occur as a secondary consequence of arteritis: Takayasu's arteritis, polyarteritis nodosa, segmental mediolitic arteritis, Behcetov syndromes.Common finding in patients with IMA aneurysms are celiac trunk occlusion and SMA stenosis (''jet disorder'' fenomen) [2,3].

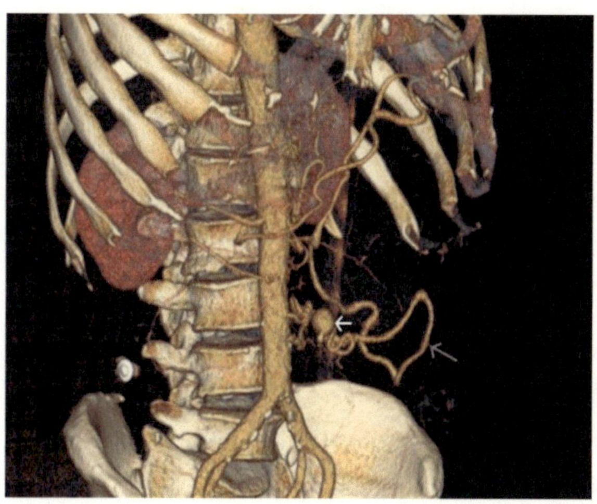

Figure 17. Inferior mesenteric artery aneurysms

The most common ways of terating these lesions are surgery and in recent years endovascular procedures such as embolization and graft stenting [50,51].

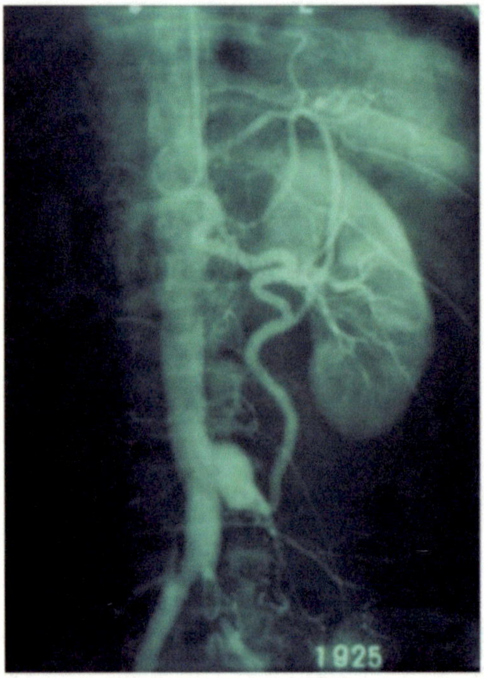

Figure 18. Inferior mesenteric artery aneurysms

Pancreticoduodenal, Gastroduodenal, and less frequent visceral artery aneurysms

Pancreatico-duodenal artery aneurysm (PDAA) are very rare (less than 2% of all VAA) and usually symptomatic splanchnic aneurysm. Symtoms are abdominal pain, nausea, vomiting, yaundice and somethimes hemorrhage in the digestive system.The different symptoms are probably the result of enlargement and/or rupture of the aneurysm, so it's sometimes difficult to properly characterize and assess the symptoms and diagnose the condition [52,53].

Gastroduodenal artery (GDA) is the least common place has been developing visceral aneurysms (1.5%) Most of GDA aneurysms are pseudoaneurysms,actually a complication of acute or chronic pancreatitis. Other key factors for development of both aneurysms are atherosclerosis, fibromuscular displasia, autoimmune disease (systemic lupus eritematosis, Wegener granulomatosis, polyarteritis nodosa), infection and the extreme rare conditions such as congenital absence of celiac trunk [52-55].

http://dx.doi.org/10.5772/52814

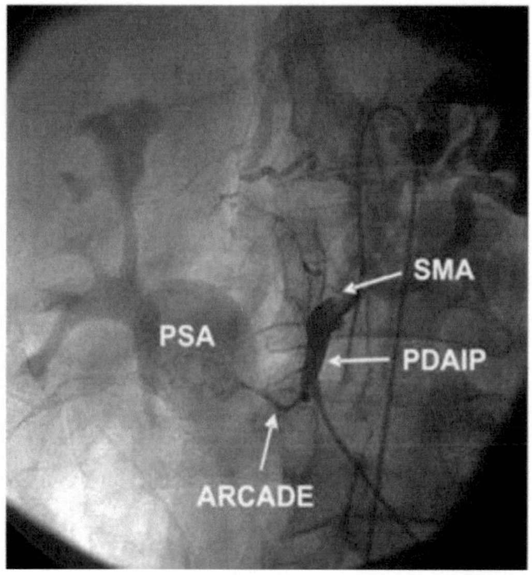

Figure 19. Pancreaticoduodenal inferior posterior artery (PDAIP) selective angiography. PSA at the level of the PDAIP and the pancreaticoduodenal superior anterior artery anasthomosis. High-grade hepatic artery stenosis relieved by balloon dilatation and placing two stents-Selfx 8.0x32 mm and Wave max Abbot 7.0x28 mm (a,b). Upper aneurysm sack entrance was closed using: Vortx-18 Diamond Shape fiber platinum coils and Vortex Diamond fiber coil 2/4 mm x 4.1 cm.

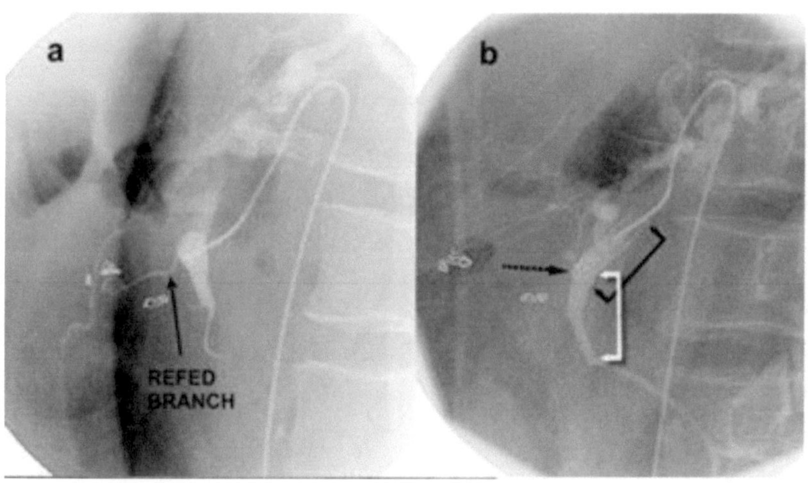

Figure 20. Pancreaticoduodenal inferior posterior artery (PDAIP) selective angiography. PSA at the level of the PDAIP and the pancreaticoduodenal superior anterior artery anasthomosis. High-grade hepatic artery stenosis relieved by balloon dilatation and placing two stents-Selfx 8.0x32 mm and Wave max Abbot 7.0x28 mm (a,b). Upper aneurysm sack entrance was closed using: Vortx-18 Diamond Shape fiber platinum coils and Vortex Diamond fiber coil 2/4 mm x 4.1 cm.

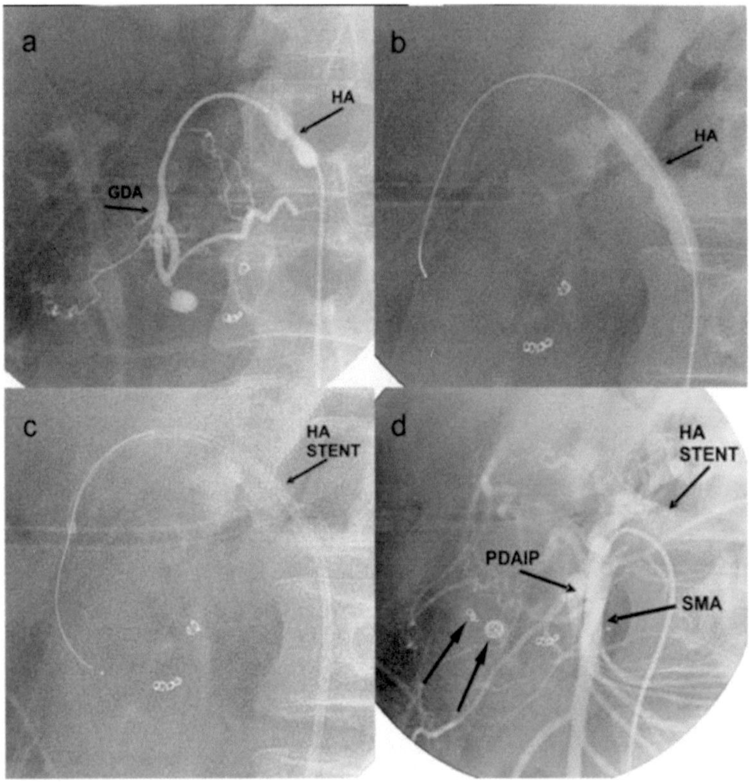

Figure 21. Pancreaticoduodenal inferior posterior artery (PDAIP) selective angiography. PSA at the level of the PDAIP and the pancreaticoduodenal superior anterior artery anasthomosis. High-grade hepatic artery stenosis relieved by balloon dilatation and placing two stents-Selfx 8.0x32 mm and Wave max Abbot 7.0x28 mm (a,b). Upper aneurysm sack entrance was closed using: Vortx-18 Diamond Shape fiber platinum coils and Vortex Diamond fiber coil 2/4 mm x 4.1 cm.

GDA, PDAA and other less frequent visceral aneurysms should be treated regardless of their size and simptomatology. Endovascular techniques have numerous advantages over surgery, such as the precise anatomic localization of the aneurysm, easy access to collateral circulation, the possibility that the procedure be done under local anesthesia, fewer postoperative complications and shorter hospital stay (figure 18-20) [56].

3. Conclusion

Splanhnic artery aneurysms are relatively rare, uncommon clinical entities, although their detection in last decades is rising due to an increased use of sofisticated imaging and sreening programs for abdominal aortic aneurysms. Potentially most devastating complication is rupture, highly associated with unwanted morbidity andmortalityrates;however, the urgent repair of these lesions is still associated with elevated mortality.Elective treatment inchosen patient, should be part of therapeutic strategy.For many years surgical repair and reconstructionwas the gold treatment method.Recently, endovascular coil embolization,*embolotherapy*,and balloon expandable stent-grafts placement has remarkable success rates and represents the first-line treatment for anatomically suitable visceral artery aneurysms and pseudoaneurysm.It is already proved that endovascular treatment associates lower morbidity and mortality rates, lower recurrence andshorter hospital stay than surgical one.

Author details

Petar Popov[1*] and Đorđe Radak[2]

*Address all correspondence to: popov1960@yahoo.com

1 Cardiovascular Institute Dedinje, Vascular department, Belgrade, Serbia

2 Cardiovascular Institute Dedinje, Vacular department Belgrad, Serbia

References

[1] Stanley, J. C., Wakefield, T. W., Graham, L. M., Whitehouse Jr, W. M., Zelenock, G. B., & Lindenaure, S. M. (1986). Clinical importance and management of splanchnic artery aneurysms. *J VascSurg*, 3, 836-840.

[2] Carr, S. C., Pearce, W. H., Vogelzang, R. L., Mc Carthy, W. J., Nemcek, A. A., & Jr Yao, J. S. (1996). Current management of visceral artery aneurysms. *Surgery*, 120, 627-33.

[3] Schanley, C. J., Shah, N. L., & Messina, L. M. (1996). Common splanchnic artery aneurysms: splenic, hepatic, and celiac-review. *Ann Vasc Surg*, 10, 315-22.

[4] Reidy, J. F., Rowe, P. H., & Ellis, F. G. (1990). Splenic artery aneurysm embolization-the preferred technique to surgery. *Clin Radiol*, 41, 281-2.

[5] Gabelmann, A., Gorich, J., & Merkle, E. M. (2002). Endovascular treatment of visceral artery aneurysms. *J. Endovasc. Ther*, 9, 38-47.

[6] De Bakey, M. E., & Cooley, D. A. (1953). Successful resection of mycotic aneurysm of superior mesenteric artery: Case report and review of literature. *Am Surg*, 19, 202-212.

[7] Sabiston Text Book Of Surgery. 16th Edition; Vascular and visceral artery aneurysm. Section 12,, 2209.

[8] Carmeci, C., Wisconsin, M., & Mc Clenathan, J. (2000). Visceral artery aneurysms as seen in a community hospital. *Am J Surg*, 179, 486-489.

[9] Smith, J. A., Macleish, D. G., & Collier, N. A. (1989). Aneurysms of the visceral arteries. *Aust. N. Z. J. Surg*, 59, 329-334.

[10] Beaussier, M. (1770). Sur un anevrisme de l'artere splinque dont les parnis se sont ossifiees. *Journal Medical Toulose*, 32, 157.

[11] Abbas, M. A., Fowl, R. J., Stone, W. M., Panneton, J. M., Oldenburg, W. A., Bower, T. C., Cherry, K. J., & Gloviczki, P. (2003). Hepatic artery aneurysm: factors that predict complications. *J VascSurg*, 38, 41-45.

[12] Lumsden, A., Samer, G., Mattar, Allen. R. C., & Bacha, E. A. (1996). Hepatic Artery Aneurysms: The Management of 22 Patients. *Jour Surg Res*, 60, 345-350.

[13] Hulsberg, P., Garza-Jordan, L., Jordan, R., Matusz, P., Tubbs, R. S., & Loukas, M. (2011). Hepatic aneurysm: a review. *Am Surg*, 77(5), 586-91.

[14] Harlaftis, N. N., & Akin, J. T. (1977). Hemobilia from ruptured hepaticarteryaneurysm: Report of a case and review of the literature. *Am Jour Surg*, 33(2), 229-232.

[15] Trastek, V. F., Pairolero, P. C., Joyce, J. W., et al. (1982). Splenic artery aneurysms. *Surgery*, 91, 694-699.

[16] Steinberg, I., & Lord, J. W. (1960). Splenic artery aneurysm. Diagnosis by intravenous abdominal aortography. *JAMA*, 174(1), 74-77.

[17] New York Times. (1881). How Dr. Bliss Got His Name; Rutkow (2006), James A. Garfield, p.85;Baxter (1891), History of the city of Grand Rapids, Michigan, p. 699; Lamb (1909). *History of the Medical Society of the District of Columbia*, 227, 1817-1909.

[18] de Vries, J. E., Schattenkerk, M. E., & Malt, R. A. (1982). Complications of the splenic artery aneurysm other than intraperitoneal rupture. *Surgery*, 91, 200-3.

[19] Sandeep, P., Dave, B., Ernane, R. , Azhar, M. D., Hossain, Peter., Taub, J., Kerstein, M., & Hollier, L. (2000). Splenic Artery Aneurysm in the 1990s. *Ann VascSurg*, 14, 223-229.

[20] Nishida, O., Moriyasu, F., Nakamura, T., et al. (1986). Hemodynamics of splenic artery aneurysm. *Gastroenterology*, 90, 1042-6.

[21] Mattar, S. G., & Lumsden, A. B. (1995). The management of splenic artery aneurysms: experience with 23 cases. *Am J Surg*, 169, 580-584.

[22] Spittel, J. A., Fairbairn, J. F., Kincaid, O. W., & Remine, W. H. (1961). Aneurysm of the splenic artery. *JAMA*, 175, 452-456.

[23] Stanley, J. C., & Fry, W. J. (1974). Pathogenesis and clinical significance of splenic artery aneurysms. *Surgery*, 76, 898-909.

[24] Lowry, S. M., O'Dea, T. P., Gallagher, D. I., et al. (1986). Splenic artery aneurysm rupture: the seventh instance of maternal and fetal survival. *ObstetGynecol*, 62, 665-666.

[25] Ayalon, A., Wiesner, R. H., Perkins, J. D., Tominaga, S., Hayes, D. H., & Krom, R. A. (1988). Splenic artery aneurysms in liver transplant patients. *Transplantation*, 45, 386-9.

[26] Tazawa, K., Shimoda, M., Nagata, T., et al. (1999). Splenic artery aneurysm associated with systemic lupus erythematosus: report of a case. *Surg Today*, 29, 76-79.

[27] Agrawa, G. A., Johnson, P. T., & Fishman, E. K. (2007). Splenic artery aneurysms and pseudoaneurysms: Clinical distinctions and CT appearances. *Am J Roentgenol*, 188, 992-9.

[28] Abbas, M. A., Stone, W. M., Fowl, R. J., et al. (2002). Splenic artery aneurysms: two decades experience at Mayo clinic. *Ann VascSurg*, 16, 442-449.

[29] Selo-Ojeme, D. O., & Welch, C. C. (2003). Review: spontaneous rupture of splenic artery aneurysm in pregnancy. EurJ ObstetGynecolReprodBiol , 109, 124-127.

[30] Arepally, A., Dagli, M., Hofmann, L. V., Kim, H. S., Cooper, M., & Klein, A. (2002). Treatment of splenic artery aneurysm with use of a stent-graft. *J VascIntervRadiol*, 13, 631-633.

[31] Guillon, R., Garcier, J. M., Abergel, A., et al. (2003). Management of splenic artery aneurysms and false aneurysms with endovascular treatment in 12 patients. *CardiovascInterventRadiol*, 26, 256-260.

[32] Kreuger, K., Zaehringer, M., & Lackner, K. (2005). Percutaneous treatment of a splenic artery pseudoaneurysm by thrombin injection. *J VascIntervRadiol*, 16, 1023-1025.

[33] Laganàa, D., Carrafielloa, G., Manginia, M., Dionigib, G., Caronnoc, R., Castellic, P., & Fugazzolaa, C. (2006). Multimodal approach to endovascular treatment of visceral arteryaneurysms and pseudoaneurysms. *Eur Jour Rad*, 59.

[34] Larson, R. A., Solomon, J., & Carpenter, J. P. (2002). Stent graft repair of visceral artery aneurysms. *J VascSurg*, 36, 1260-1263.

[35] Salcuni, P. F., Spaggiari, L., Tecchio, T., Benincase, A., & Azzarone, M. (1995). Hepatic artery aneurysm: an ever present danger. *J CardiovascSurg*, 36, 595-9.

[36] Abbas, M., Fowl, R. J., Stone, W. M., Panneton, J. M., Oldenburg, W. A., Bower, T. C., Cherry, K. J., & Gloviczki, P. (2003). Hepatic artery aneurysm: Factors that predict complications. *J VascSurg*, 38, 41-5.

[37] Dougherty, M. J., Gloviczki, P., Cherry, K. J., Bower, T. C., Hallett, J. W., & Pairolero, P. C. (1993). Hepatic artery aneurysms: evaluation and current management. *IntAngiol*, 12, 178-84.

[38] Stouffer, J. T., Weinman, M. D., & Bynum, T. E. (1989). Hemobilia in a patient with multiple artery aneurysms: a case report and review of the literature. Am. J. Gastroenter. , 84, 59.

[39] Venturini, M., Angeli, E., Salvioni, M., De Cobelli, F., Trentin, C., Carlucci, M., et al. (2002). Hemorrhage from a right hepatic artery pseudoaneurysm: endovascular treatment with a coronary stentgraft. *J EndovascTher*, 9, 221-4.

[40] Schick, C., Ritter, R. G., Jörn, O. B., Thalhammer, A., & Vogl, T. J. (2004). Hepatic artery aneurysm: treatment options. *EurRad*, 14.

[41] Riesenman, P. J., Bower, T. C., Oderich, G. S., & Bjarnason, H. (2006). Multiple hepatic artery aneurysms: Use of transcatheter embolization for rupture. *Ann VascSurg*, 20(3), 399-404.

[42] Cavallo, A., Cavallo, L., Orlandi, R., & De Albertis, P. (1991). An aneurysm of the common trunk of the celiac tripod diagnosed with echo-Doppler [in Italian]. *Radiol Med (Torino)*, 82, 694-7.

[43] Graham, L. M., Stanley, J. C., Whitehouse, W. M., Jr Zelenock, G. B., Wakefield, T. W., Cronenwett, J. L., & Lindenauer, S. M. (1985). Celiac artery aneurysms: historic (1745-1949) versus contemporary (1950-1984) differences in etiology and clinical importance. *J VascSurg*, 2, 757-64.

[44] Risher, W. H., Hollier, L. H., Bolton, J. S., & Ochsner, J. L. (1991). Celiac artery aneurysm. *Ann VascSurg*, 5, 392-5.

[45] Rengo, M., Terrinoni, V., Lamazza, A., Cosimati, A., & Bianchi, G. (1997). Treatment of an aneurysm of the coeliac axis, by transluminal steel wire occlusion. *Eur J VascEndovascSurg*, 13, 88-90.

[46] Sessa, C., Tinelli, G., Porcu, P., Aubert, A., Thony, F., & Magne, J. (2004). Treatment of visceral artery aneurysms: Description of a retrospective series of 42 Aneurysms in 34 patients. *Ann VascSurg*, 18(6), 695-703.

[47] Stevenson, W. F. (1895). Case of abdominal aneurysm treated by laparotomy and introduction of wire into sac with death. *Lancet*, 1, 22-3.

[48] Komori, K., Mori, E., & Yamaoka, T. (2000). Successful resection of superior mesenteric artery aneurysm. A case report and review of the literature. *J CardiovascSurg (Torino)*, 41, 475-478.

[49] Perhnan, M., & Golinger, D. (1967). Mycotic aneurysm of the superior mesenteric artery treated by ligation with survival. *Br J Surg*, 54, 735-8.

[50] Pérez-Vallecillos, P., Muíño, R. C. I., Seura-Jiménez, Fernández. N. M., Ferrón, J. A., García-Róspide, V., & Palma, P. (2010). Acute retroperitoneal bleeding due to inferior mesenteric artery aneurysm: Case report. *BMC Gastroenterology*, 10, 59.

[51] Davidovic, L. B., Vasic, D. M., & Colic, M. I. (2003). Inferior mesenteric artery aneurysm: case report and review of the literature. *Asian J Surg*, 26, 176-9.

[52] Neschis, D. G., Safford, S. D., & Golden, M. A. (1998). Management of pancreaticoduodenal artery aneurysms presenting as catastrophic intra-abdominal bleeding. *Surgery*, 123, 8-12.

[53] Chiesa, R., Astore, D., Guzzo, G., Frigerio, S., Tshomba, Y., Castellano, R., de Moura, M. R., & Melissano, G. (2005). Visceral artery aneurysms. *Ann Vasc Surg*, 19(1), 42-48.

[54] Spanos, P. K., Kloppedal, E. A., & Murray, C. A. (1974). Aneurysms of the gastroduodenal and pancreaticoduodenal arteries. *Am Jour Surg*, 127(3), 345-348.

[55] Popov, P., Sagic, D., Radovanovic, D., Antonic, Z., Nenezic, D., & Radak, Dj. (2008). Pancreaticoduodenal artery pseudoaneurysm embolization. *Vascular*, 16.

[56] Popov, P., Boskovic, S., Sagic, D., Radevic, B., Ilijevski, N., Nenezic, D., Tasic, N., Davidovic, L., & Radak, D. (2007). Treatment of visceral artery aneurysms : Retrospective study of 35 cases. *VASA*, 36.

Chapter 4

Preoperative Evaluation Prior to High-Risk Vascular Surgery

Santiago Garcia and Edward O. McFalls

Additional information is available at the end of the chapter

http://dx.doi.org/10.5772/52233

1. Introduction

The number of patients undergoing noncardiac surgery worldwide is growing, and annually 500,000 to 900,000 of these patients experience perioperative cardiac death, nonfatal perioperative myocardial infarction (PMI) or cardiac arrest [1]. Over 300,000 surgical revascularization procedures are performed in the US annually as part of the treatment of expanding abdominal aortic aneurysms, critical limb ischemia, and severe carotid disease [2].

The preoperative assessment of a patient in need of elective non-cardiac surgery is often a difficult task. Current guidelines consider vascular surgery a high-risk operation with an anticipated risk of major postoperative cardiac complications in excess of 5% [3]. Although the reasons relate, in part, to the hemodynamic stresses associated with aortic procedures, the prevalence of atherosclerotic coronary artery disease (CAD) in patients undergoing vascular surgery exceeds 50% and therefore, may require special attention in the preoperative period [4].

2. Pathophysiology of postoperative myocardial infarction

Unlike spontaneous myocardial infarction the majority of postoperative, or type 2, myocardial infarctions (PMI) are thought to result from an imbalance between oxygen supply and demand in the setting of severe, yet stable, coronary artery disease [5]. Several studies using continuous electrocardiographic monitoring in high-risk vascular patients undergoing surgery have shown that tachycardia-related ST-segment depression is common in the postoperative period and is associated with in-hospital as well as long-term mortality [6-7]. Peak troponin elevation correlates well with duration of ST-segment depression [8].

Angiographic and Autopsy Data: In a landmark angiographic study Hertzer et al. showed that only 8% of patients with peripheral arterial disease in need of major vascular surgery have normal coronary arteries [4]. In the CARP trial, among 1048 patients undergoing coronary angiography within 6-months of a high-risk vascular operation, the extent and severity of CAD were predictors of long-term mortality (Figure 1) [9].

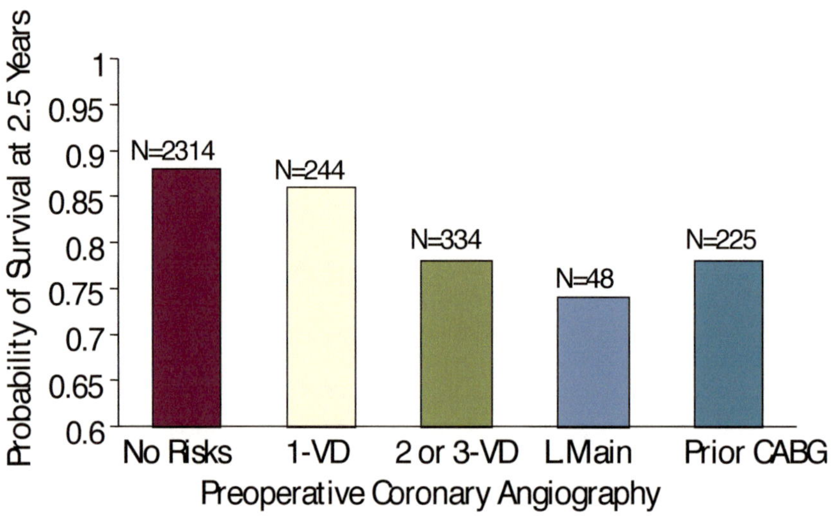

Reproduced from The American Journal of Cardiology 2008, 102: 809-13. VD= Vessel disease, CABG= coronary artery bypass grafting, L main= Left main

Figure 1. Extent of Coronary Artery Disease and Survival

The prevalence of angiographic chronic total occlusions in patients with PMI or cardiac death is 81% as opposed to only 29% of matched control patients without PMI or cardiac death [10]. On average patients with postoperative cardiac complications have 2 ±1.4 critical (>70%) coronary stenosis in contrast to patients without postoperative complications who have less disease burden (0.7 ±1.2). Two small autopsy studies reported conflicting data on the incidence of coronary plaque rupture in patients with fatal PMI [11-12]. Dawood et al. found plaque rupture in only 7% of 42 autopsied patients [11]. In contrast, Cohen et al. reported in a smaller study a higher incidence of plaque rupture (46%) [12]. Differences between studies could be explained on the basis of timing of the autopsy relative to occurrence of PMI.

Stepwise approach to preoperative risk assessment:

The approach to assessing the potential cardiac risk associated with any patient scheduled for elective non-cardiac operation includes the nature of the operation, the risk of associated coronary artery disease and the functional capacity of the patient. The initial evaluation requires an assessment of a prior history of cardiac problems and/or risk fac-

http://dx.doi.org/10.5772/52233

tors along with either classical angina or unusual symptoms such as shortness of breath or atypical chest pains. Attention should be given to clinical risk variables such as age >70 years, angina, history of congestive heart failure, prior myocardial infarction, prior cerebrovascular accident (CVA) or transient ischemic attack (TIA), history of ventricular arrhythmias, diabetes mellitus (particularly insulin dependent), and abnormal renal function (Creatinine >2.0 mg/dl) [13] (Table 1). The physical examination also provides key insight into high risk variable and include a chronic debilitated state, increased jugular venous distention, edema, S_3 gallop, significant aortic stenosis while the 12-lead electrocardiogram provides prognostic information related to the presence of abnormal Q-waves or heart rhythms other than normal sinus. Assessing the functional capacity of patients undergoing elective operations is an important ingredient to determining whether a patient can withstand the rigors of a prolonged operation. In those patients who are unable to achieve a 4-MET demand, a level compatible with routine daily activities, there is increased risk of postoperative events and additional testing may be warranted (i.e. stress test). The presence of multiple ischemic segments indicative of either multivessel coronary artery disease or left main disease is considered high risk and is associated with an increased risk of perioperative cardiac complications and reduced long-term survival [14]. Ultimately, a combined approach of utilizing clinical variables associated with stress-imaging tests is most cost-effective.

RCRI	**Derivation set (2893)**		**Validation set (n=1422)**	
	Events	Rate, 95% CI	Events	Rate, 95% CI
0	5/1071	0.5 (0.2-1.1)	2/488	0.4 (0.5-1.5)
1	14/1106	1.3 (0.7-2.1)	5/567	0.9 (0.3-2.1)
2	18/506	3.6 (2.1-5.6)	17/258	6.6 (3.9-10.3)
≥3	19/210	9.1 (5.5-13.8)	12/109	11 (5.8-18.4)

Table 1. The Revised Cardiac Risk Index (RCRI) can be used to risk-stratify patients prior to non-cardiac surgery with regard to the risk of serious cardiac complications. Adapted from Lee et al. Circulation 1999; 100:1043-1049.

3. Preventive therapies

Therapies that have been proven to reduce PMI among patients undergoing non-cardiac surgery include beta-blockers and statins.

Beta-blockers:

Mangano et al. reported a 6% absolute risk reduction in cardiac events at 6 months with atenolol among 200 male veterans undergoing noncardiac surgery [15]. Poldermans et al. reported a more dramatic 30% absolute risk reduction with bisoprolol among 173 patients undergoing vascular surgery with evidence of myocardial ischemia on stress test [16]. However, subsequent larger studies with metoprolol yielded negative results [17-19]

(Table 2). The landmark POISE trial, with over 8300 patients enrolled showed that although extended-release metoprolol 200 mg reduces PMI by 26%, it is associated with a higher risk of death and stroke. For every 1000 patients treated with extended-release metoprolol 15 non-fatal myocardial infarctions would be prevented but 5 strokes and 8 deaths would be caused by it [20]. Therefore, the POISE trial raised serious concerns about the safety of injudicious administration of high-dose beta-blockers in the perioperative period.

Study	Patients	Intervention	Findings
Mangano et al. [15]	200 Male veterans undergoing non-cardiac surgery	Atenolol begun in hospital	Cardiac events at 6 months 0% (drug) vs. 8% (placebo)
Poldermans et al. [16]	173 patients with ischemia undergoing vascular surgery	Bisoprolol 30 days before surgery	Cardiac events 3.4 % (drug) vs. 34% (placebo)
Yang et al. [17]	496 vascular surgery patients	Metoprolol begun before surgery	Cardiac events 10.2% (metoprolol) vs. 12% (placebo) (p=NS)
Juul et al. [18]	921 patients with diabetes undergoing major non-cardiac surgery	Metoprolol XL 100 mg	21 % vs. 20% (p=NS)
Brady et al. [19]	103 patients without previous MI undergoing infrarenal vascular surgery	Oral metoprolol 50 mg bid	34 % vs. 30% (p=NS)
Devereaux et al. [20]	8351 undergoing non-cardiac surgery	Oral CR- metoprolol 200 mg/d for 30 days	5.8% (drug) vs. 6.9% (placebo). Reduction in MI but increased risk of stroke and mortality with metoprolol

Table 2. Summary of clinical trials assessing the role of beta-blockers prior to non-cardiac surgery.

Statins:

In the Dutch Echocardiographic Cardiac Risk Evaluation Applying Stress Echocardiography (DECREASE-III) study high-dose fluvastatin reduced the composite of cardiovascular death and non-fatal myocardial infarction by 53% among 457 patients undergoing vascular surgery [21]. In a smaller trial involving 100 vascular patients randomly assigned to 20 mg of atorvastatin or placebo, statins reduced cardiac events from 26% to 8% at 6 months [22]. In a single center registry of patients undergoing vascular operations at our institution the use of perioperative statins was an independent predictor of long-term survival [23]. Statins may play a pivotal role in plaque stabilization by reducing circulating levels of inflammatory cytokines, increase expression of nitric oxide synthase, and reduced production of endothelin-1 and reactive oxygen species.

Role of coronary revascularization:

The Coronary Artery Prophylactic Revascularization trial (CARP) showed that a strategy of prophylactic revascularization was not superior to optimal medical therapy in preventing PMIs or improving long-term mortality among 510 Veterans undergoing elective major vascular surgery [24] (Figure 2). Despite high utilization rates of statins and beta-blockers in the CARP trial, 16% of patients suffered a PMI [24]. Moreover, among patients with multiple risk factors and/or evidence of myocardial ischemia on nuclear imaging test the incidence of PMI was 25% [25], which was unaffected by revascularization status (Figure 3). Similarly to CARP, the DECREASE-V pilot study failed to show any benefit with prophylactic revascularization among 101 patients with multivessel CAD and abnormal stress test prior to vascular surgery (death or MI at 1 year 49% vs. 44%) [26]. These high events rates despite optimal medical therapy highlight the need for additional interventions for risk reduction among high-risk patients.

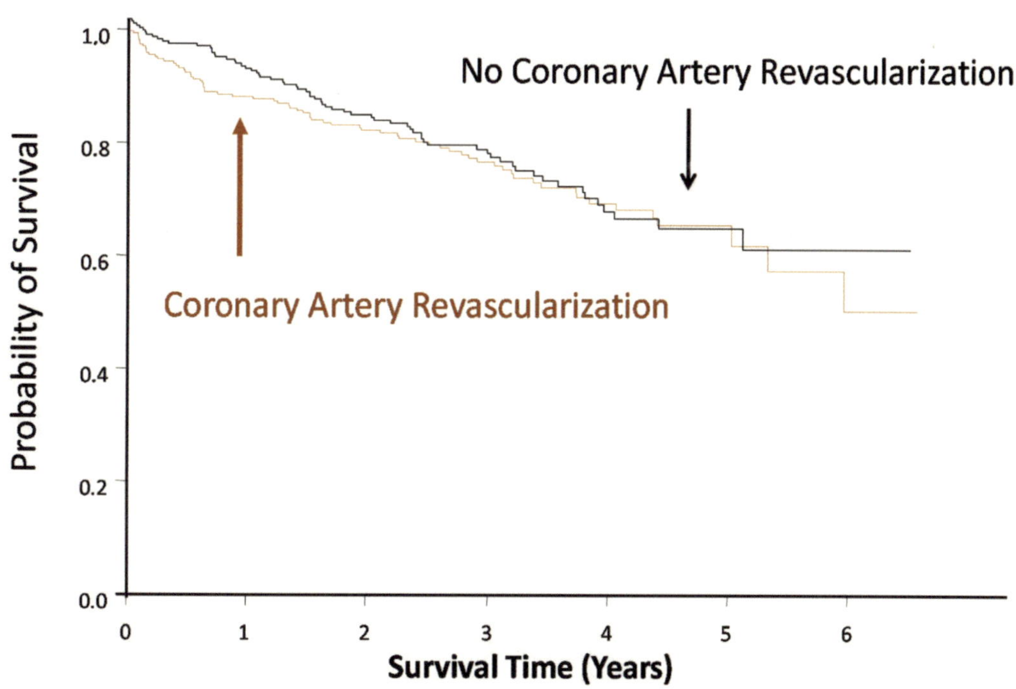

Reproduced from The New England Journal of Medicine 2004; 351:1795-804

Figure 2. Primary Outcome of the Coronary Artery Revascularization Prophylaxis (CARP) Trial

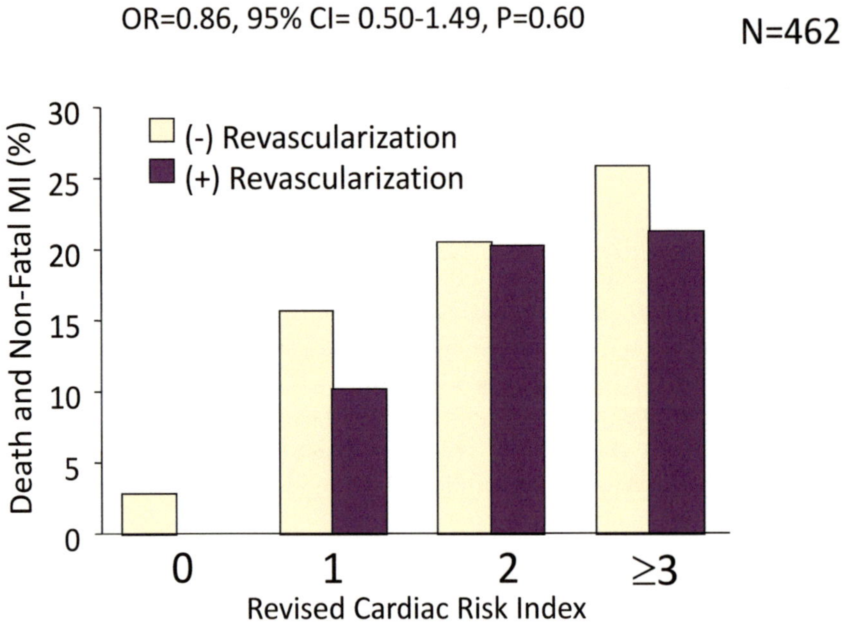

Reproduced from Circulation: Quality and Outcomes. 2009; 2: 73-77. OR= Odds Ratio, CI=Confidence Interval

Figure 3. Impact of Revascularization According to Number of Risks Enumerated in the Revised Cardiac Risk Index

4. Diagnosis

A joint ESC/ACCF/AHA/WHF Task Force has redefined myocardial infarction as an event characterized by ischemic symptoms (i.e. chest pain or dyspnea), a typical rise and fall of cardiac biomarkers (preferably troponin) with at least one value above the 99th percentile of the upper reference limit, and electrocardiographic (ECG) changes consistent with myocardial ischemia or imaging evidence of new loss of viable myocardium (i.e. new perfusion defect) or wall motion abnormality [27].

Although this definition is useful for distinguishing spontaneous coronary events (Type I MI) from events that arise at the time of coronary revascularization (Type 4 and 5 MIs), it does not take into account unique features of perioperative myocardial infarctions after noncardiac operations. First, the majority of coronary events that occur in the post-operative period are clinically silent as a result of sedation and analgesia. In a post-hoc analysis of the POISE trial 65.3% of all patients with an MI did not have any ischemic symptoms [28]. Second, the ECG is insensitive, relative to cardiac troponins, to detect myocardial ischemia in the post-operative period [29]. Finally, after vascular surgery the presence of ischemic ECG changes does not provide additional prognostic information regarding long-term mortality over and above that provided by a single peak troponin I measured within 48 hours after vascular surgery [30].

Our group, and others [31], has shown that cardiac troponins measured after surgery are independent predictors of 30-day and long-term mortality [32] (Figure 4).

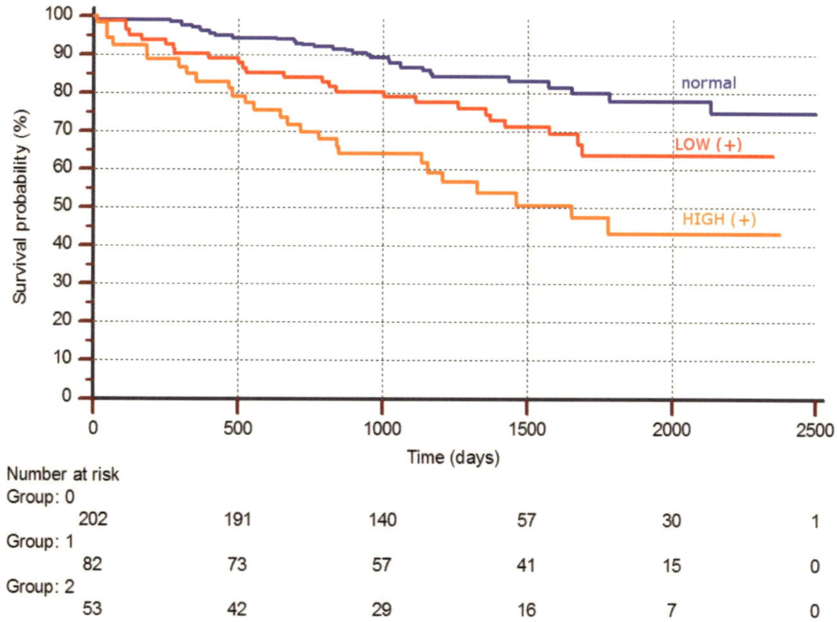

Group 0 (blue) normal, Group 1 (red) cTnI > 99th percentile but < 3 URL, Group 2 (orange) cTnI ≥ 3 URL. Adapted from Journal of Vascular Surgery. In Press.

Figure 4. Kaplan-Meier estimates of mortality after vascular surgery relative to peak cardiac troponin I levels within 72 hours post-surgery

Taken together, these observations emphasize the importance of widespread utilization of cardiac troponin in the perioperative period for the surveillance of myocardial infarction and risk-stratification.

5. Treatment

Although robust data from randomized clinical trials is lacking small studies have shown that interventions aimed at improving oxygen delivery and minimizing myocardial oxygen consumption are beneficial in this setting. The main goals of therapy are to prevent, or minimize, wide fluctuations in blood pressure and heart rate through beta-blockade, analgesia, and fluid administration with the intention to preserve optimal coronary perfusion pressure during diastole.

Martinez et al. randomized 80 patients with prolonged (≥ 20 minutes) ischemia after vascular surgery to beta-blockers, aspirin, nitrates and optimization of oxygen supply-demand balance or control. At 6 months, patients treated for ischemia had lower mortality relative to control patients (8% vs. 20%). In the post-operative period treated patients had lower median troponin values when compared to controls (3.3 ng/ml vs. 8.5 ng/ml) [33].

Anemia is an independent predictor of mortality after non-cardiac surgery in the elderly [34]. Blood transfusion improved survival in critically ill patients with CAD and hemoglobin < 10% [35]. This benefit was not seen among patients without CAD or among patients with a hematocrit > 25% with some studies reporting increased mortality and nosocomial infections associated with blood transfusions in [36].

Cardiac evaluation:

Although there is no consensus in the community with regard to the type (invasive angiography vs. imaging) and timing (in-hospital vs. 4-6 weeks after discharge) of cardiac evaluation after a PMI registry data suggest that only a minority of patients with elevated biomarkers receive cardiac work-up after the event [37].

Given the high-risk of bleeding immediately after non-cardiac surgery the use of emergency coronary angiography and stenting is usually reserved for patients with hemodynamic instability, ST-elevation or inability to control ischemic symptoms with medications. Among patients with coronary stents it is important to consider stent thrombosis in the differential diagnosis if ischemic symptoms develop after non-cardiac surgery, particularly if antiplatelet agents have been prematurely discontinued prior to the operation [38,39]. These patients have a high mortality rate and emergency coronary angiography with revascularization is appropriate.

6. Conclusions

Improving outcomes in this high-risk group of patients undergoing vascular surgery will require a paradigm shift from widespread use of cardiac imaging and procedures in the preoperative phase to rapid detection and management of cardiac complications in the post-operative setting with routine surveillance of cardiac troponins and targeted interventions.

Acknowledgements

Dr. Garcia is supported by the VA Office of Research and Development through a career development award (1IK2CX000699-01).

Author details

Santiago Garcia* and Edward O. McFalls

Minneapolis VA Healthcare System and University of Minnesota, Minneapolis, USA

References

[1] Devereaux, P. J, Goldman, L, Cook, D. J, et al. Perioperative cardiac events in patients undergoing noncardiac surgery: a review of the magnitude of the problem, the pathophysiology of the events and methods to estimate and communicate risk. *CMAJ.* Sep 13 (2005). , 173(6), 627-634.

[2] Nowygrod, R, Egorova, N, Greco, G, et al. Trends, complications and mortality in peripheral vascular surgery. J Vasc Surg (2006). , 43, 205-16.

[3] Fleisher, L, Beckman, J, Brown, K, Calkins, H, Chaikof, E, Fleischmann, K, Freeman, W, Froehlich, J, Kasper, E, Kersten, J, Riegel, B, Robb, J, Smith, S, Jacobs, A, Adams, C, Anderson, J, Antman, E, Buller, C, Creager, M, Ettinger, S, Faxon, D, Fuster, V, Halperin, J, Hiratzka, L, Hunt, S, Lytle, B, Nishimura, R, Ornato, J, Page, R, Tarkington, L, & Yancy, C. ACC/AHA 2007 guidelines on perioperative cardiovascular evaluation and care for noncardiac surgery: a report of the American College of Cardiology/American Heart Association Task Force on Practice Guidelines. Circulation (2007). , 116, 1971-1996.

[4] Hertzer, N, Beven, E, Young, J, et al. Coronary artery disease in peripheral vascular patients: A classification of 1000 coronary angiograms and results of surgical management. Ann Surg (1984). , 199, 223-233.

[5] Landesberg, G, Beattie, S, Mosseri, M, Jaffe, A. S, & Alpert, J. S. Perioperative myocardial infarction. Circulation (2009).

[6] Bottiger, B. W, Motsch, J, Teschendorf, P, et al. Postoperative 12-lead ECG predicts peri-operative myocardial ischaemia associated with myocardial cell damage. Anaesthesia (2004). , 59, 1083-90.

[7] Badner, N. H, Knil, R. L, Brown, J. E, Novick, T. V, & Gelb, A. W. Myocardial infarction after noncardiac surgery: Anesthesiology. (1998). , 88, 572-578.

[8] Landesberg, G, Maseri, M, Zahger, D, et al. Myocardial infarction following vascular surgery: the role of prolonged, stress-induced, ST-depression-type ischemia. J Am Coll Cardiol. (2001). , 37, 1839-1845.

[9] Garcia, S, Moritz, T. E, Ward, H. B, et al. Usefulness of revascularization of patients with multivessel coronary artery disease before elective vascular surgery for abdominal aortic and peripheral occlusive disease. Am J Cardiol (2008). , 102, 809-813.

[10] Ellis, S. G, Hertzer, N. R, Young, J. R, & Brener, S. Angiographic correlates of cardiac death and myocardial infarction complicating major nonthoracic vascular surgery. Am J Cardiol. May 15 (1996). , 77(12), 1126-1128.

[11] Dawood, M. M, Gutpa, D. K, Southern, J, Walia, A, Atkinson, J. B, & Eagle, K. A. Pathology of fatal perioperative myocardial infarction: implications regarding pathophysiology and prevention. Int J Cardiol. Nov 15 (1996). , 57(1), 37-44.

[12] Cohen, M. C, & Aretz, T. H. Histological analysis of coronary artery lesions in fatal postoperative myocardial infarction. *Cardiovasc Pathol.* May-Jun (1999). , 8(3), 133-139.

[13] Lee, T, Marcantonio, E, Mangione, C, et al. Derivation and prospective validation of a simple index for prediction of cardiac risk of major noncardiac surgery. Circulation (1999). , 100, 1043-9.

[14] Shaw, L, Eagle, K, Gersh, B, & Miller, D. Meta-analysis of intravenous dipyridamole-thallium-201 imaging (1985 to 1994) and dobutamine echocardiography (1991 to 1994) for risk stratification before vascular surgery. J Am Coll Cardiol (1996). , 27, 787-98.

[15] Mangano, D. T, Layug, E. L, Wallace, A, & Tateo, I. Effect of atenolol on mortality and cardiovascular morbidity after noncardiac surgery. Multicenter Study of Perioperative Ischemia Research Group. *N Engl J Med.*(1996). , 335(23), 1713-1720.

[16] Poldermans, D, Boersma, E, Bax, J. J, et al. The effect of bisoprolol on perioperative mortality and myocardial infarction in high-risk patients undergoing vascular surgery. Dutch Echocardiographic Cardiac Risk Evaluation Applying Stress Echocardiography Study Group. *N Engl J Med.* Dec 9 (1999). , 341(24), 1789-1794.

[17] Yang, H, Raymer, K, Butler, R, Parlow, J, & Roberts, R. The effects of perioperative beta-blockade: results of the Metoprolol after Vascular Surgery (MaVS) study, a randomized controlled trial. *Am Heart J* (2006). , 152, 983-90.

[18] Juul, A. B, Wetterslev, J, Gluud, C, et al. Effect of perioperative βblockade in patients with diabetes undergoing major non-cardiac surgery: randomised placebo controlled, blinded multicentre trial. BMJ (2006).

[19] Brady, A. R, Gibbs, J. S, Greenhalgh, R. M, Powell, J. T, & Sydes, M. R. Perioperative beta-blockade (POBBLE) for patients undergoing infrarenal vascular surgery: results of a randomized double-blind controlled trial. J Vasc Surg (2005). , 41, 602-609.

[20] Devereaux, P. J, Yang, H, Yusuf, S, et al. Effects of extended-release metoprolol succinate in patients undergoing non-cardiac surgery (POISE trial): a randomized controlled trial. *Lancet.* May 31 (2008). , 371(9627), 1839-1847.

[21] Schouten, O, Boersma, E, Hoeks, S. E, et al. for the Dutch Echocardiographic Cardiac Risk Evaluation Applying Stress Echocardiograpy Study Group (DECREASE). Fluvastatin and Perioperative Events in Patients Undergoing Vascular Surgery. NEJM (2009). , 361, 980-9.

[22] Durazzo, A. E, Machado, F. S, Ikeoka, D. T, et al. Reduction in cardiovascular events after vascular surgery with atorvastatin: a randomized trial. *J Vasc Surg.* May (2004). discussion 975-966, 39(5), 967-975.

[23] Marston, N, Brenes, J, Garcia, S, et al. Peak postoperative troponin levels outperform preoperative cardiac risk indices as predictors of long-term mortality after vascular surgery troponins and postoperative outcomes. *J Crit Care.* (2012). , 27, 66-72.

[24] Mcfalls, E, Ward, H, Moritz, T, Goldman, S, Krupski, W, Littooy, F, Pierpont, G, Santilli, S, Rapp, J, Hattler, B, Shunk, K, Jaenicke, C, Thottapurathu, L, Ellis, N, Reda, D, & Henderson, W. Coronary-artery revascularization before elective major vascular surgery. N Engl J Med (2004). , 351, 2795-2804.

[25] Garcia, S, Moritz, T, Goldman, S, et al. Perioperative complications after vascular surgery are predicted by the revised cardiac risk index but are not reduced in high-risk subsets with preoperative revascularization. Circulation: Cardiovasc Qual Outcomes (2009). , 73-77.

[26] Poldermans, D, Schouten, O, Vidakovic, R, et al. A clinical randomized trial to evaluate the safety of a noninvasive approach in high-risk patients undergoing major vascular surgery: the DECREASE-V Pilot Study. *J Am Coll Cardiol.* (2007). , 49(17), 1763-1769.

[27] Thygesen, K, Alpert, J, & White, H. Universal Definition of Myocardial Infarction. Circulation (2007). , 116, 2634-2653.

[28] Devereaux, P. J, Xavier, D, Pogue, J, et al. Characteristics and short-term prognosis of perioperative myocardial infarction in patients undergoing noncardiac surgery: A cohort study. *Ann Intern Med.* (2011). , 154, 523-528.

[29] Rinfret, S, Goldman, L, Polanczyk, C. A, Cook, E. F, & Lee, T. H. Value of immediate postoperative electrocardiogram to update risk stratification after noncardiac surgery. Am J Cardiol (2004). , 94, 1017-22.

[30] Garcia, S, Marston, N, Brenes, J, et al. Troponin Elevation, Ischemic Electrocardiographic Changes and Prognosis after a Postoperative Myocardial Infarction. Circulation. 124:A9218.

[31] The Vascular Events in Noncardiac Surgery Patients Cohort Evaluation (VISION) Study InvestigatorsJAMA. (2012). , 307(21), 2295-2304.

[32] Garcia, S, Marston, N, Sandoval, Y, et al. Prognostic value of lead electrocardiogram and peak troponin I level following vascular surgery. J Vasc Surg. 2012 Sep 10. [Epub ahead of print]. PMID: 22862805, 12.

[33] Martinez, E, Kim, L, Rosenfeld, B, et al. Early detection and real-time intervention of postoperative myocardial ischemia: the STOPMI (Study for the Treatment of Perioperative Myocardial Ischemia) Study. Abstract presented at: Association of University Anesthesiologists; May (2008). Durham, NC., 16-18.

[34] Wu, W. C, Schifftner, T. L, Henderson, W. G, et al. Preoperative hematocrit levels and postoperative outcomes in older patients undergoing noncardiac surgery. *JAMA.* (2007). , 297(22), 2481-2488.

[35] Deans, K. J, Minneci, P. C, Suffredini, A. F, et al. Randomization in clinical trials of titrated therapies: unintended consequences of using fixed treatment protocols. *Crit Care Med.* (2007). , 35(6), 1509-1516.

[36] Rao, S. V, Jollis, J. G, Harrington, R. A, et al. Relationship of blood transfusion and clinical outcomes in patients with acute coronary syndromes. *JAMA.* Oct 6 (2004). , 292(13), 1555-1562.

[37] Mcfalls, E. O, Larsen, G, Johnson, G. R, et al. Outcomes of hospitalized patients with non-acute coronary syndrome and elevated cardiac troponin level. *Am J Med.* Jul (2011). , 124(7), 630-635.

[38] Brilakis, E. S, Banerjee, S, & Berger, P. B. Perioperative management of patients with coronary stents. *J Am Coll Cardiol.* Jun 5 (2007). , 49(22), 2145-2150.

[39] Holmes, D. R. Jr., Kereiakes DJ, Garg S, et al. Stent thrombosis. *J Am Coll Cardiol.* Oct 19 (2010). , 56(17), 1357-1365.

Chapter 5

Navigation in Endovascular Aortic Repair

Geir Arne Tangen, Frode Manstad-Hulaas,
Reidar Brekken and Toril A. N. Hernes

Additional information is available at the end of the chapter

http://dx.doi.org/10.5772/55097

1. Introduction

The formation and growth of an aortic aneurysm may lead to rupture resulting in life threatening haemorrhage. Aortic replacement, either by open surgery or endovascular aortic repair (EVAR), is recommended when the maximum diameter of the aneurysm increases rapidly or exceeds 55mm for the thoracic aorta or 50-55mm for the abdominal aorta (Brewster et al., 2003; Hiratzka et al., 2010; Lederle et al., 2002; Moll et al., 2011).

In EVAR, instruments and the aortic prosthesis (stent graft) are normally inserted from the femoral arteries and into the aneurysmatic aorta under the guidance of fluoroscopy and digital subtraction angiography (DSA). Although mandatory in all endovascular procedures, radiation and contrast medium constitute some of the most important disadvantages in endovascular aortic repair in regards to skin erythema and contrast media-induced nephropathy (Geijer et al., 2005; Morcos et al., 2005). The radiation exposure to staff during endovascular procedures is low (Ho et al., 2007), but not negligible. It is possible to treat complex aortic aneurysms (e.g. juxtarenal and thoracoabdominal aneurysms) with endovascular technique, but the stent grafts usually have to be patient specific and may contain scallops, fenestrations or directional cuffs. Since the fluoroscopic and DSA images are 2-dimensional, the impression of depth is insufficient, making challenging procedures more time consuming. Poor opacification in some regions of the aorta and increased use of radiation and contrast medium constitute limitations in the endovascular approach to complex aneurysms (Greenberg et al., 2006).

In surgical *navigation*, pre-operative three-dimensional (3D) medical images are combined with a positioning system that is able to track the position of different instruments during intervention. The instruments can then be visualized within the 3D images, giving the physician a better spatial visualization and understanding of the patient's vascular anatomy, including the position and orientation of instruments. At the same time the use of radiation and contrast medium is reduced.

In this chapter we give a brief introduction to the development of the guidance techniques currently used during EVAR, before the present state-of-the-art and future navigation technology for EVAR are emphasized. Finally, we will discuss future clinical potential technological possibilities and challenges related to navigation in EVAR.

2. Current image guidance in EVAR

The visual information required during EVAR is common for all image-guided procedures; the operator needs to see the instrument(s) and the surrounding anatomy. In EVAR, this means that the catheters, guide wires, stent grafts and the vascular anatomy has to be sufficiently presented to the operator. This can be achieved by using X-rays, both without and in combination with a contrast medium.

In 1948 Coltman (Coltman et al. 1948) invented the first image intensifier, a device that made it possible to view X-ray images directly in daylight. If radiation was applied continuously, the movement of an object could be followed. Since the image intensifier was based on a fluorescent screen (Phosphor), the visualization technique became known as "fluoroscopy". Today the flat panel detector with increased sensitivity to X-rays and better temporal resolution has replaced the image intensifier.

When a contrast medium is injected into the vascular system, in interventional radiology usually through a catheter directly into the vessel(s) of interest, an angiogram is acquired. However, in the original angiogram all other anatomical structures are overlaying the contrast-filled vessels. During the 1970s the digital video subtraction was developed, a technique that made it possible to subtract a pre-contrast X-ray image from a post-contrast X-ray image. Then only the contrast-loaded structures were presented. The digital video subtraction was originally developed for intravenously injected contrast medium, but Crummy et al. (Crummy et al. 1982) presented in 1981 a work where the technique was applied on intra-arterial catheter-based injections. This technique, today known as digital subtraction angiography (DSA), reduced the need for contrast medium and made it possible to obtain a vascular "roadmap".

Fluoroscopy, angiography, DSA and roadmaps are used during EVAR to guide the instruments and facilitate an optimal positioning and alignment of the stent graft. Special attention is given to branching vessels to avoid vessel occlusion or compromised circulation. Despite that fluoroscopy and DSA are 2 dimensional images, they have until the present remained cornerstones in all image guided vascular interventions, including EVAR. Perhaps we are facing a paradigm shift?

3. Navigation technology in EVAR

Minimal invasive procedures require new technology for navigation. In procedures without direct visual access to the operating field, the operator depends on updated images of the related anatomy. Using 2D images with limited contrast information can be a challenge to the operator. Extensive experience is required to be able to interpret the image information and relate it to the 3D anatomy and at the same time guide the instruments with high precision. The procedures can be time-consuming and result in considerable contrast and radiation dose to the patient and contribute to the accumulated radiation dose to the medical staff. These issues are addressed in modern navigation technology solutions.

The introduction of the stereotactic frame by Horsley and Clarke (Clarke & Horsley, 1906) made it possible for the surgeons to precisely target anatomical structures deep inside the brain during neurosurgery. After the invention of medical imaging technology, such as the computed tomography (CT) scanner in early 1970s and some years later the magnetic resonance imaging (MRI) scanner, the concept of image guided surgery/therapy has evolved immensely. Especially the introduction of the personal computer (PC) around 1980, when computing power became more available to researchers and the general public, contributed to the development of navigation technology. From its humble start in neurosurgery, image guided technology has gradually made its way into other areas of medicine like oncology, orthopedics etc., and can today be found as an integrated part in multiple medical disciplines.

3.1. Imaging and visualization technology

The technologic development in computer science, image processing and robot technology results in continuous advances in medical imaging equipment. The high-resolution 3D imaging only available in a CT lab a few years ago, now finds its way into the operating rooms (OR). Modern hybrid angiography suites are fully equipped ORs, reducing the complexity of patient logistics. An emergency patient today can in many cases be transferred directly to the angiography suite (or OR with intraoperative imaging equipment) without stopping at the separate CT lab, and thus save valuable time. In the angiography suite, a Cone-Beam CT acquires an advanced 3D image of the patient. The 3D image provides diagnostic information and can be used for navigation during the EVAR procedure. A 3D CT can also be acquired intra-operatively, presenting an updated 3D map of the relevant anatomy to the operator during the operation (Eide et al. 2011).

The advances in registration technology have made it possible to display a combination of image modalities to the EVAR operator. One example is the Syngo iPilot (Siemens, Medical Solutions, Erlangen, Germany), which combines 2D fluoroscopy/roadmap images with preoperative 3D CT models in real time, helping the operator navigate complex 3D vessel anatomy.

Modern computer graphics hardware and algorithms enables visualisation of high quality 3D renderings of image data in real-time. Surfaces can be extracted from the image data and visualized as polygon data objects. Image data can be visualized directly through 2D slices or as 3D voxel data with volume rendering techniques as shown in figure 1.

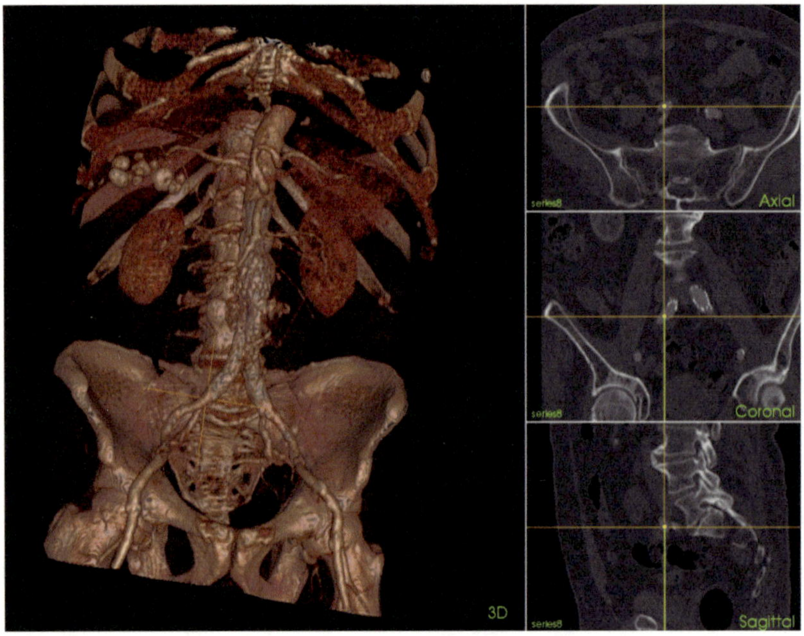

Figure 1. Visualization of vascular anatomy for an AAA patient. Left showing volume rendering and right showing orthogonal 2D slices

3.2. Position tracking systems

Mechanical systems for navigation, like the stereotactic frame, are feasible when fixed anatomical references like the skull is available. Optical position tracking systems and frameless stereotactic surgery has since taken over as preferred tracking technology. These systems supports sensors that can be integrated with most surgical equipment and provide position data with sub-millimeter precision. For endovascular applications the problem has been the line-of-sight limitation of optical systems, making tracking of flexible instruments inside the body difficult. The introduction of electromagnetic tracking systems have made navigation systems an option also for endovascular applications and other clinical areas where position tracking of needles, endoscopes, catheters or other flexible instruments inside the body is required. Aurora (Northern Digital Inc, Waterloo, ON, Canada), shown in figure 2, and 3D Guidance medSAFE (Ascension Technology Corp., Burlington, Vermont, USA) are commercial products that can be integrated into navigation systems.

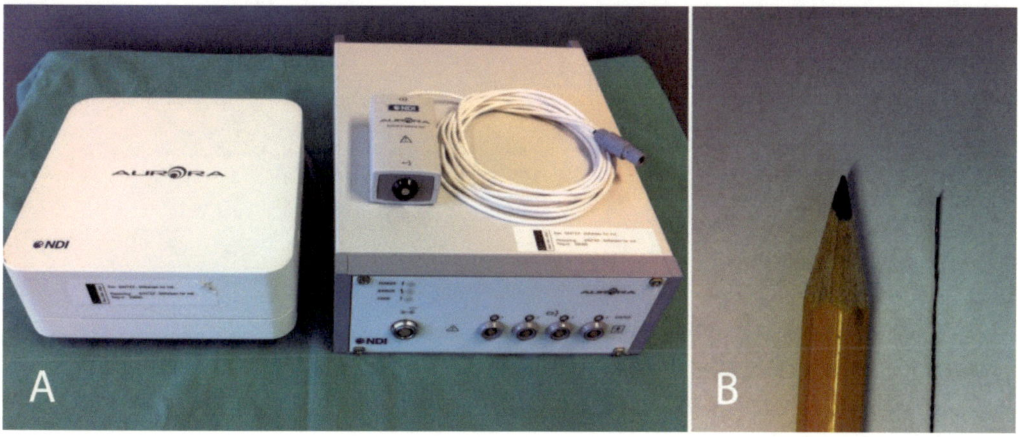

Figure 2. A) Electromagnetic tracking system - NDI Aurora. (B) Tracking sensor – 0.5 mm diameter

However, electromagnetic tracking systems are sensitive to disturbances created by metallic objects and electromagnetic noise. For Endovascular applications this is specially challenging since the X-ray/fluoroscopy imaging equipment represents a substantial dynamic disturbance (Bø et al., 2012). To make navigation feasible in these cases either the disturbing equipment (i.e. X-ray equipment) must be moved to a safe distance during navigation or a correction scheme must be applied. Several methods for compensating the disturbances have been reported in literature. The most common approach is to sample reference points throughout the tracking volume. The same points are sampled with and without disturbances present and this is used to map the deformation field caused by the disturbance (Kindratenko, 2000).

3.3. Registration

In order to use 3D images for accurate navigation inside a patient the position coordinates output from the tracking system must be matched to the exact same location in the medical images. That is, the 3D coordinate system of the tracking system needs to be transformed to the coordinate system of the 3D medical image dataset. This has traditionally been done by performing a rigid registration, meaning that the two coordinate systems are matched by translation and rotation of one of them, no deformation is involved. This can be implemented as a point-pair registration using fiducial markers or using visible anatomical landmarks etc. Figure 3 shows an example from our research (Manstad-Hulaas et al, 2010 & 2012) were a tracked reference plate containing radio opaque fiducial markers is attached to the patient. The tracked fiducial marker coordinates are visualized as green spheres and the same markers show up as intensity spots in the CT image. By matching these two pointsets to eachother, by the use of the navigation system, we perform a registration between the tracking system and the CT images.

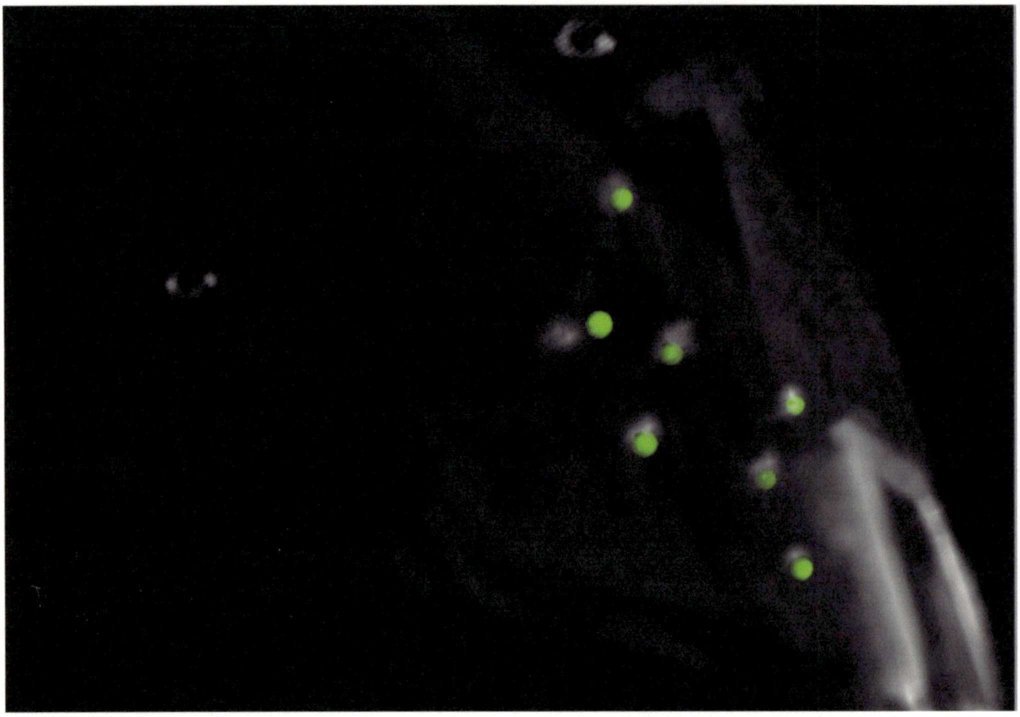

Figure 3. Registration by the use of fiducial markers. Green indicators show the positions in the position tracking systems coordinate system. Intensity spots show the corresponding marker positions in the images.

Registration can also involve matching images from different modalities to each other or matching images from the same modality acquired at different points in time. For endovascular applications augmenting the small intraoperative Cone Beam CT volume with information from a larger high-quality preoperative CT volume can give us a better navigation map for the guiding procedures. In our research we have compared two algorithms for image registration of Cone Beam CT to CT, and achieved a registration match of 5.05 ± 4.74 mm and 4.02 ± 1.52 mm. This can be sufficient for navigation if we use the intraoperative Cone Beam CT volume as the basis for high accuracy navigation and the preoperative CT information to provide overview etc. (Manstad-Hulaas et al, 2010).

3.4. Navigation systems

Visualization, position tracking, registration and control software are essential parts of a navigation system. In a wide range of medical specialties the use of navigation systems based on 3D images and tracked instruments and tools have been tested and to some degree taken into clinical practice. Examples include transbronchial biopsies, laparoscopic ultrasound and radiofrequency ablation, neuronavigation, orthopedic surgery and cardiac ablation (Eberhardt et al., 2010; Harms et al., 2001; Hayhurst et al., 2009; Hildebrand et al., 2008; Hernes et al., 2006; Knecht et al., 2008; Tigani et al., 2009; von Jako et al., 2009; Wood et al., 2007). Abi-Jaoudeh et al. (2010) showed in an animal trial the feasibility of inserting a thoracic stent graft using a navigation system based on 3D images and electromagnetic tracking, but in general the use of navigation systems during endovascular procedures have been sparse.

4. Future possibilities and challenges

4.1. Research within navigation in AAA

In our research we have used a prototype navigation system for 3D navigation, CustusX (SINTEF, Dept Medical Technology, Trondheim, Norway), which has been developed for minimally invasive procedures. CustusX evolved through the cooperating partners SINTEF, St Olav's Hospital and Norwegian University of Science and Technology (NTNU). The activity in usage of navigation for guidance of surgical procedures, started in 1995 to support research studies in the operating room, mainly within neurosurgery, vascular surgery and laparoscopic surgery. It has since then evolved into new clinical areas such as spine surgery and lung biopsy applications.

The research within usage of navigation for guidance of endovascular treatment of AAA was in our research group, based on pre-operative CT-images in combination with an electromagnetic tracking system. The feasibility and accuracy of the navigation system was studied in a series of paper (Manstad-Hulaas et al. 2007, 2010 & 2011). The authors concluded that the navigation system had sufficient accuracy and was easy to use. Manstad-Hulaas et al. (2012) reported use of the navigation system in a study comprising patients scheduled for EVAR. Successfully catheterizations of the contralateral cuff with an electromagnetically tracked catheter were achieved in 6 of 7 patients (86%). In the control group, successful placement of a catheter within the main stent graft was achieved in 8 of 10 patients (80%). Maximum 8 attempts were needed to insert the guide wire correctly in the intervention group vs. 33 in the control group. A navigation system visualizing instruments in a 3D image of the vascular system was shown to be a reliable and useful tool during minimally invasive treatment of the aorta. Other examples on groups doing research using navigation in endovascular applications are as mentioned in previous chapter, Abi-Jaoudeh et al. A very interesting work is done by (Sidhu et al, 2012) reporting a new method for arterial cannulation using a tracked guidewire and the StealthStation navigation system (Medtronic Inc., USA).

4.2. Integration with medical imaging equipment

Solutions that integrate imaging and navigation have recently become commercially available. Some manufacturers have integrated 3D visualization into the angiography equipment, such as the syngo iPilot from Siemens. This might be a technique to enhance spatial information and reduce the use of contrast medium.

St. Jude Medical is performing clinical testing of a system called MediGuide (Gaspar et al, 2012) that supports electromagnetic tracking of catheter position, integrating this with existing angiography equipment. This enables the position of the catheter/instrument to be superimposed as a marker on the live fluoroscopy images. 3D models of arteries etc. can also be augmented on the live images, simplifying the navigation in complex vascular structures. Other research groups are also working on how to integrate electromagnetic tracking with catheter position extracted from fluoroscopy images for accurate navigation (Azizian M. et al, 2011).

3D ultrasound scanners with integrated electromagnetic tracking systems exists today. Examples are PercuNav (Phillips, Eindhoven, Netherlands) and SonixGPS (Ultrasonix, Toronto, ON, Canada), enabling fusion of pre-operative images with tracking and real-time 3D ultrasound for image guidance of needle tracking procedures (nerve blocks, biopsies, vascular access etc.).

4.3. Steerable tools and robot-assisted procedures

There have been increasing activity during the last years towards steerable tools and robot-assisted procedures, especially within the cardiac field to treat arrhythmias and atrial fibrillation. The motivation for this is to improve catheter stability and control and to achieve correct placement of the catheters during complex cardiac arrhythmia procedures. Normally the operators have had to use several catheters with different properties (preshaped tip and stiffness etc.). Multiple sequences with "catheter-over-wire" technique are performed to switch between the different guidewires and catheters. This increases the danger of trauma to the vessel wall, with risk of embolization etc. that can lead to stroke when working in the aortic arch or the coronary arteries (Nordon et al, 2010). The friction caused by the instrument resting against the vessel wall can also make it impossible to maneuver by twisting and pushing the guidewire/catheter. Also, the anatomy can be challenging when the operator must maneuver through tortuous iliac arteries etc. This can result in prolonged procedure time, extended use of radiation and require highly skilled and experienced operators.

Hansen Medical (Mountain View, CA, USA) has commercialized a robotic system for electrophysiology called Sensei. (Riga et al., 2010). The operator can control a steerable catheter consisting of an inner guide (11F outer diameter, 8.5F inner diameter) within an outer guide sheat (14F outer diameter, 11F inner diameter) from a remote control station with a joystick. Ablation therapy is performed through the catheter. The catheter also has force sensors integrated and force quantification is displayed to the operator to minimize the risk of trauma to the vessel. (Riga et al, 2010) has shown the feasibility of this robotic solution for advanced EVAR with fenestrated stent graft procedure with promising results. The last year Hansen has also released a product called Magellan with smaller dimension catheter (6F – 2 mm) targeting peripheral vascular interventions.

Hansen Medicals solution is based on mechanical steering of the catheter. Another alternative is magnetic steering (Remote Magnetic Navigation). The company Stereotaxis (St. Louis, MO, USA) has developed a robotic solution named Niobe where two large magnets placed beside the patient controls the movement of the tip of a catheter. The system is operated from a remote control station. Since the system directly controls the tip of the instrument they claim that the risk for complications like perforation is minimized. The technology has been licensed to Siemens and Phillips which both have integrated the navigation system in their electrophysiology product line.

http://dx.doi.org/10.5772/55097

5. Conclusions

Navigation provides the operators with more anatomic information and makes EVAR safer and more accurate. Steerable catheters and accurate navigation technology can speed-up operating time and increase the possibilities for use of EVAR in more complex aneurysms.

Conflict of interest

The authors have no conflict of interest regarding commercial products mentioned in this text.

Acknowledgements

This work was funded by the Ministry of Health and Social Affairs of Norway, through the National Centre for 3D Ultrasound in Surgery (St. Olavs University Hospital, the Norwegian University of Science and Technology, SINTEF Trondheim, Norway), project 196726=V50 eMIT (Enhanced minimally invasive therapy, FRIMED program),

Author details

Geir Arne Tangen[1,2], Frode Manstad-Hulaas[1,3], Reidar Brekken[1,2] and Toril A. N. Hernes[1,2]

1 Norwegian University of Science and Technology, Dept. Circulation and Medical Imaging, Trondheim, Norway

2 SINTEF, Dept. Medical Technology, Trondheim, Norway

3 St. Olav's University Hospital, Trondheim, Norway

References

[1] Abi-jaoudeh, N, Glossop, N, Dake, M, Pritchard, W. F, Chiesa, A, Dreher, M. R, et al. Electromagnetic navigation for thoracic aortic stent-graft deployment: a pilot study in swine. Journal of Vascular and Interventional Radiology. (2010). Jun;, 21(6), 888-95.

[2] Azizian, M, & Patel, R. Data Fusion for Catheter Tracking using Kalman Filtering: Applications in Robot-Assisted Catheter Insertion. Presented at the Medical Imaging (2011). Visualization, Image-Guided Procedures, and Modeling, SPIE.

[3] Brewster, D. C, Cronenwett, J. L, & Hallett, J. W. Jr., Johnston KW, Krupski WC, Matsumura JS. Guidelines for the treatment of abdominal aortic aneurysms. Report of a subcommittee of the Joint Council of the American Association for Vascular Surgery and Society for Vascular Surgery. J Vasc Surg. (2003). May;, 37(5), 1106-17.

[4] Bø, L. E, Leira, H. O, Tangen, G. A, Hofstad, E. F, Amundsen, T, & Langø, T. (2012). Accuracy of electromagnetic tracking with a prototype field generator in an interventional OR setting. *Medical physics*, *39*(1), 399.

[5] Clarke, R. H, & Horsley, V. On a method of investigating the deep ganglia and tracts of the central nervous system cerebellum, Br Med J (1906).

[6] Coltman, J. W. Fluoroscopic image brightening by electronic means. Radiology. (1948). Sep;, 51(3), 359-6.

[7] Crummy, A. B, Stieghorst, M. F, Turski, P. A, Strother, C. M, Lieberman, R. P, Sackett, J. F, et al. Digital subtraction angiography: current status and use of intra-arterial injection. Radiology. (1982). November 1, 1982;, 145(2), 303-7.

[8] Eberhardt, R, Morgan, R. K, Ernst, A, Beyer, T, & Herth, F. J. Comparison of suction catheter versus forceps biopsy for sampling of solitary pulmonary nodules guided by electromagnetic navigational bronchoscopy. Respiration. (2010). , 79(1), 54-60.

[9] Eide, K. R, Ødegård, A, Myhre, H. O, Hatlinghus, S, & Haraldseth, O. DynaCT in pre-treatment evaluation of aortic aneurysm before EVAR. *European journal of vascular and endovascular surgery : the official journal of the European Society for Vascular Surgery*, ((2011).

[10] Gaspar, T, Kircher, S, Arya, A, Sommer, P, Rolf, S, Hindricks, G, & Piorkowski, C. Enhancement of intracardiac navigation by new GPS-guided location system (MediGuide Technologies). *Europace : European pacing, arrhythmias, and cardiac electrophysiology : journal of the working groups on cardiac pacing, arrhythmias, and cardiac cellular electrophysiology of the European Society of Cardiology*, (2012). *Suppl 2*, iiii25., 24.

[11] Geijer, H, Larzon, T, Popek, R, & Beckman, K. W. Radiation exposure in stent-grafting of abdominal aortic aneurysms. British Journal of Radiology. (2005). Oct;, 78(934), 906-12.

[12] Greenberg, R. K, West, K, Pfaff, K, Foster, J, Skender, D, Haulon, S, et al. Beyond the aortic bifurcation: branched endovascular grafts for thoracoabdominal and aortoiliac aneurysms. J Vasc Surg. (2006). May;discussion 86-7., 43(5), 879-86.

[13] Harms, J, Feussner, H, Baumgartner, M, Schneider, A, Donhauser, M, & Wessels, G. Three-dimensional navigated laparoscopic ultrasonography: first experiences with a new minimally invasive diagnostic device. Surg Endosc. (2001). Dec;, 15(12), 1459-62.

[14] Hayhurst, C, Byrne, P, Eldridge, P. R, & Mallucci, C. L. Application of electromagnetic technology to neuronavigation: a revolution in image-guided neurosurgery. J Neurosurg. (2009). Dec;, 111(6), 1179-84.

[15] Hildebrand, P, Schlichting, S, Martens, V, Besirevic, A, Kleemann, M, Roblick, U, et al. Prototype of an intraoperative navigation and documentation system for laparoscopic radiofrequency ablation: first experiences. European Journal of Surgical Oncology. (2008). Apr;, 34(4), 418-21.

[16] Hiratzka, L. F, Bakris, G. L, Beckman, J. A, Bersin, R. M, Carr, V. F, Casey, D. E, et al. ACCF/AHA/AATS/ACR/ASA/SCA/SCAI/SIR/STS/SVM guidelines for the diagnosis and management of patients with Thoracic Aortic Disease: a report of the American College of Cardiology Foundation/American Heart Association Task Force on Practice Guidelines, American Association for Thoracic Surgery, American College of Radiology, American Stroke Association, Society of Cardiovascular Anesthesiologists, Society for Cardiovascular Angiography and Interventions, Society of Interventional Radiology, Society of Thoracic Surgeons, and Society for Vascular Medicine. Circulation. (2010). Apr 6;121(13):e, 266-369.

[17] Ho, P, Cheng, S. W, Wu, P. M, Ting, A. C, Poon, J. T, Cheng, C. K, et al. Ionizing radiation absorption of vascular surgeons during endovascular procedures. Journal of Vascular Surgery. (2007). Sep;, 46(3), 455-9.

[18] Von Jako, R. A, Carrino, J. A, Yonemura, K. S, Noda, G. A, Zhue, W, Blaskiewicz, D, et al. Electromagnetic navigation for percutaneous guide-wire insertion: accuracy and efficiency compared to conventional fluoroscopic guidance. Neuroimage. (2009). Aug;47 Suppl 2(2):T, 127-32.

[19] Kindratenko, V. A survey of electromagnetic position tracker calibration techniques. Virtual Reality, ((2000).

[20] Knecht, S, Skali, H, Neill, O, Wright, M. D, Matsuo, M, & Chaudhry, S. GM, et al. Computed tomography-fluoroscopy overlay evaluation during catheter ablation of left atrial arrhythmia. Europace. (2008). Aug;, 10(8), 931-8.

[21] Lederle, F. A, Wilson, S. E, Johnson, G. R, Reinke, D. B, Littooy, F. N, Acher, C. W, et al. Immediate repair compared with surveillance of small abdominal aortic aneurysms. N Engl J Med. (2002). May 9;, 346(19), 1437-44.

[22] Manstad-hulaas, F, Ommedal, S, Tangen, G. A, Aadahl, P, & Hernes, T. N. Side-branched AAA stent graft insertion using navigation technology- a phantom study. Eur Surg Res. (2007). , 39(6), 364-71.

[23] Manstad-hulaas, F, Tangen, G. A, Dahl, T, Hernes, T. A, & Aadahl, P. Three-Dimensional Electromagnetic Navigation vs. Fluoroscopy for Endovascular Aneurysm Repair: A Prospective Feasibility Study In Patients. J Endovasc Ther. (2012). Feb;, 19(1), 70-8.

[24] Manstad-hulaas, F, Tangen, G. A, Demirci, S, Pfister, M, Lydersen, S, & Hernes, T. N. Endovascular Image-Guided Navigation- Validation of Two Volume-Volume Registration Algorithms. Minim Invasive Ther Allied Technol. (2010). Nov 24.

[25] Manstad-hulaas, F, Tangen, G. A, Gruionu, L. G, Aadahl, P, & Hernes, T. A. Three-Dimensional Endovascular Navigation with Electromagnetic Tracking- Ex Vivo and In Vivo Accuracy. J Endovasc Ther. (2011). Apr;, 18(2), 230-40.

[26] Moll, F. L, Powell, J. T, Fraedrich, G, Verzini, F, Haulon, S, Waltham, M, et al. Management of abdominal aortic aneurysms clinical practice guidelines of the European society for vascular surgery. European Journal of Vascular and Endovascular Surgery. (2011). Jan;41 Suppl 1(1):SS58., 1.

[27] Morcos, S. K. Prevention of contrast media-induced nephrotoxicity after angiographic procedures. Journal of Vascular and Interventional Radiology. (2005). Jan;, 16(1), 13-23.

[28] Nagelhus Hernes TALindseth F, Selbekk T, Wollf A, Solberg OV, Harg E, et al. Computer-assisted 3D ultrasound-guided neurosurgery: technological contributions, including multimodal registration and advanced display, demonstrating future perspectives. Int J Med Robot. (2006). Mar;, 2(1), 45-59.

[29] Nordon, I. M, Hinchliffe, R. J, Holt, P. J, Loftus, I. M, & Thompson, M. M. The requirement for smart catheters for advanced endovascular applications. *Proceedings of the Institution of Mechanical Engineers Part H, Journal of engineering in medicine,* ((2010).

[30] Riga, C. V, Cheshire, N. J. W, Hamady, M. S, & Bicknell, C. D. The role of robotic endovascular catheters in fenestrated stent grafting. *Journal of vascular surgery : official publication, the Society for Vascular Surgery [and] International Society for Cardiovascular Surgery, North American Chapter,* ((2010).

[31] Sidhu, R. Weir-McCall, J., Cochennec, F., Riga, C., DiMarco, A., & Bicknell, C. D. Evaluation of an electromagnetic 3D navigation system to facilitate endovascular tasks: a feasibility study. *European journal of vascular and endovascular surgery : the official journal of the European Society for Vascular Surgery,* ((2012).

[32] Tigani, D, Busacca, M, Moio, A, & Rimondi, E. Del Piccolo N, Sabbioni G. Preliminary experience with electromagnetic navigation system in TKA. Knee. (2009). Jan;, 16(1), 33-8.

[33] Wood, B. J, Locklin, J. K, Viswanathan, A, Kruecker, J, Haemmerich, D, Cebral, J, et al. Technologies for guidance of radiofrequency ablation in the multimodality interventional suite of the future. Journal of Vascular and Interventional Radiology. (2007). Jan;18(1 Pt 1):9-24.

Chapter 6

Endovascular Treatment of Descending Thoracic Aortic Aneurysms

Gioachino Coppi, Stefano Gennai,
Roberto Silingardi, Francesca Benassi and
Valentina Cataldi

Additional information is available at the end of the chapter

http://dx.doi.org/10.5772/54692

1. Introduction

The first series of patients treated with the endovascular technique for descending thoracic aortic aneurysm (DTAA) was published by Dake et al in 1994 [1]. Since then, the use of endografts has been affirmed as a valid alternative to traditional surgery, above all in elderly and high surgical risk patients. The progress of experience has evidenced advantageous immediate and mid term results, above all when compared with traditional surgery. However, this advantage has not been found in results at a distance.

The mobilization of the often extremely tortuous thoracic aorta, which is not supported by nearby internal organs and which extends into three spacial plains, are factors which determine through time an extreme strain on materials. This wear and tear can be responsible for stent rupture, and the evolution of complications such as stent migration and endoleak. Further, the anatomic contiguity of the bronchi and the esophagus, and the fragility of the diseased thoracic aortic wall, pose serious doubts on the development of catastrophic complications such as aorta-bronchial and aorta-esophageal fistula through time.

Aneurysms are distinguished as either true, where the aortic wall is constituted by all 3 layers (tunica intima, media and adventitia), or false, where only the adventitia and/or a perivascular connective tissue is present. They are classified according to either the pathogenesis: atherosclerotic (degenerative), post-traumatic, micotic, or inflammatory, or based on the morphology: sacciform or fusiform. The most frequent form of aneurysm is atherosclerotic, with an incidence of 10 cases per 10,000 adults, of which 30-40% are limited to the descending tract of the thoracic aorta. [2] The pathogenesis of the descending thoracic aorta is similar to the frequent infra-renal aneurysm, and is due to the progressive degeneration of the media. Some authors indicate treatment for aneurysms of a diameter greater than 5.5 cm, but the universal indications specify a diameter of greater than or equal to 6 cm. The indications are based on the annual exponential risk of rupture [3], dissection or death associated with aneurysms greater than 6 cm reaching 16%. [4] True rupture or radiographic signals of imminent rupture with associated symptoms, also constitute an absolute indication for treatment.

2. Materials and methods

From May 1995 to July 2012, 170 consecutive patients presented at this centre with thoracic aortic pathologies which were subsequently treated with endovascular solutions. A total of 109 (64.1%) patients were treated in election, and 61 (35.9%) in emergency. The types of treated thoracic diseases in election included atherosclerotic aneurysms, chronic dissection and chronic post-traumatic. In emergency, pathologies included ruptured atherosclerotic aneurysm, acute dissection, aorto-esophageal fistula (AEF), aorto-bronchial fistula (ABF), acute pseudoaneurysm, acute post-traumatic and penetrating ulcer.

2.1. Patient selection

Patient selection for elective treatment at this centre includes rapid aneurysm expansion (> 10 mm in 1 year) or absolute size. For fusiform aneurysms, the minimum diameter was 5.5 cm, and for saccular aneurysms a protrusion of at least 2 cm from the disease free aortic wall or a total aortic size of 5 cm was considered an indication for treatment.

2.2. Emergency patient management

All patients treated in emergency are assisted by a vascular surgeon and an anaesthesiologist from their presentation through to the operating room. Permissive hypotension is practised with prudent fluid resuscitation to keep systolic blood pressure around 80 mm Hg, in order to avoid a recommencement of, or increase in bleeding. Patients are assessed by computed tomographic angiography (Angio-CT), 5 mm slices. Rupture is defined as visible spilling of blood outside the aneurysm as evident by Angio-CT images, and in some cases of extreme urgency, by intra-operative angiography and IVUS. During the Angio-CT scanning process, the operating room is prepared, in order to further reduce delay.

2.3. Pre-operative evaluation

The patients' anatomic suitability for emergency TEVAR is determined by Angio-CT. The maximum time taken to execute an Angio-CT in emergency is between 5 - 7 minutes at this centre (total time delay of 15 – 20 minutes). The diameter and length of the aneurysms are evaluated directly by the vascular surgeon from the screen. Transferred patients from other hospitals, with previously performed CT scans, are evaluated during patient transport, with images delivered via a diacom intranet system.

http://dx.doi.org/10.5772/54692

Elective patients are evaluated for TEVAR suitability according to the most appropriate modality:

- Computed tomographic angiography (Angio-CT)

The volumetric angio-CT (Angio-CTV) is currently considered the best diagnostic tool for the evaluation of the aorta and its branches. [5-6] The Angio-CTV is non invasive, has a high spatial resolution and densitometry, which allows the study of the vessels on any spatial plain (the submillimeter isotropic voxels of the recent Angio-CTV consents the elaboration of the oblique images to a quality equal to that obtained at axial images).

In endovascular treatment of the DTAA, the Angio-CTV correlated with adequate multi-plain reconstruction, allows an accurate evaluation of aortic caliber and length, essential information for the choice of endograft, and the presence of tortuosity, thrombosis and atherosclerotic lesions. The evaluation of the condition of the accesses is also of fundamental importance.

The limits of the Angio-CTV are common to all imaging methods which utilize ionizing radiation and iodized contrast mediums:

- exposure to elevated doses of radiation, especially for patients with a long life expectancy who will require programmed check-ups. Compared to the annual level of natural radiation a person is exposed to (2 mSv), a single thoracic Angio-CT delivers a dosage equivalent to that absorbed in 3.6 years (8mSv), which increases to an equivalent of 4.5 years (10 mSv) if the exam is extended to include the abdomen and the pelvis.

- the risk of allergic reactions to iodized compounds (which is less frequent since the introduction of non-ionic contrasts)

- nephrotoxicity from iodized contrast, partly resolvable by reducing the toxic chemical compounds (non ionic iso-osmolar) and the quantity of contrast injected.

- Magnetic resonance angiography (Angio-MR)

Compared with the Angio-CT, the Angio-MR has the advantage of not requiring ionizing radiation and iodized contrast medium. It therefore represents an alternative for patients with allergies to contrast mediums and those affected by renal insufficiency. However, the Angio-MR has an inferior spatial resolution and a reduced capacity to highlight the presence of calcification compared with Angio-CT. The evaluation of aortic neck and aneurysmal sac diameters are often less precise, caused by the difficult visualization of the extreme limit of the aortic wall.

Further, this diagnostic examination cannot be performed in patients with iron magnetic devices (pace-maker, metallic acoustic devices, vascular ocular clips. etc...), and is contra-indicated for patients with grave renal insufficiency (GFR <30 ml/min/1.73m^2) due to the risk of systemic nephrogenic fibrosis onset associated with the administration of gadolinium. Compared to the Angio-CT, this examination methodology is less common, more costly and more time consuming, and therefore is less accessible to patients.

2.4. The TEVAR procedure

All TEVAR procedures are performed in a dedicated vascular operating room equipped with mobile C-Arm (OEC 9800, GE Medical System, Salt Lake City, UT, USA), IVUS (Volcano s5, Rancho Cordova, CA, USA) and eco-duplex scanner (Esaote AU 5, Genova, Italy). Our TEVAR team includes 3 vascular surgeons (at least 2 endovascular experts), an anaesthesiologist, an endovascular trained operating room nurse and a radiological technician.

CSF drainage is applied selectively in patients with previous or contemporary AAA treatment, programmed long coverage of the aortic tract (≥20cm), and coverage of the distal tract beyond T10-T12. In the case of a short or absent proximal neck which would require the coverage of the left subclavian artery, reimplantation (the preferred technique) or a bypass is performed pre-operatively. A preventive retrograde re-vascularization of the visceral vessels (i.e. tripode or mesenteric or renal arteries) is performed in cases of short distal neck to ensure adequate distal sealing.

In most cases, arterial access is obtained through the surgical exposure of both femoral or omeral arteries. Intra-operative angiography is performed manually through an introducer sheath inserted from the contro-lateral artery to the side chosen for the deployment of the endograft. The angiography outlines exactly the position of the supra-aortic vessels, which are then marked directly by the vascular surgeon on the C-Arm screen.

Following the insertion of a super-stiff guide wire, the endograft is deployed. Completion angiography confirms adequate proximal and distal fixation and identifies any endoleak. When required, a post-dilation is executed with a compliant balloon.

2.5. Endograft selection

The increasing frequency of DTAA has generated an intensification in endograft manufacturers interest, determining a technological breakthrough in the presentation of increasingly refined and better performing devices, each with an individual peculiarity. Nevertheless, the ideal endograft still does not exist and a single endograft has not demonstrated a clear superiority over another.

In selecting an endograft, some fundamental principles apply which should always be respected.

- An oversizing of more than 10 - 15% should not be performed. This is most important in order to reduce the risk of aorto-esophageal and aorto-bronchial fistulas. However, to date there are no studies which have demonstrated that the adoption of oversizing greater than 15% to be correlated with the above mentioned complications.
- In the case of a measurement discrepancy of greater than 10% between the proximal and distal necks, the selection of a tapered endograft is advised.
- For necks with diameters inferior to 20 mm, the use of an endograft with an uncovered proximal or distal end with the positioning of the device either at the emergence of the epiaortic or the celiac-mesenteric vessels, according to the case.

- Where possible, the use of a single segment is preferred to the "telescopic technique" in order to avoid type III endoleak from segment disconnection. In the case of multiple segments being utilized, the overlapping should be at least 5 cm.

The first generation of endografts were Stentor (Min Tec, La Ciotat, France), Vanguard (Boston Scientific Corp., Natick, MA), Aneurx (Medtronic Vascular, Santa Rosa, CA, USA). The endografts recently used in the study were commercially available, supplied by Talent (Medtronic Vascular, Santa Rosa, CA, USA), Excluder and TAG device (W.L. Gore and Associates, Inc., Flagstaff, AZ, USA), Zenith TX2 (Cook, Inc., Bloomington, IN, USA), Endofit (Endomed, Phoenix, AZ, USA) and Relay (Bolton Medical Inc., Sunrise, FL, USA).

2.6. Data collection

Patients' clinical information is collected prospectively in a dedicated database, and were retrospectively evaluated for this study.

2.7. Follow-up protocol

The post-discharge TEVAR follow-up scheme at this centre consists of routine Angio-CT at 3, 6 and 12 months, and annually thereafter in the absence of symptoms. Plain radiographs are performed at 6 months, and annually thereafter.

3. Results

From May 1995 to July 2012, 170 consecutive patients with various thoracic aortic pathologies were treated with endovascular solutions at this centre. A total of 109 (64.1%) patients were treated in election for DTA diseases, and 61 (35.9%) in emergency (Table 1). Patient mean age was 73.78 yrs old.

CSF drainage was used in 16 (9.4%) patients. A reimplantation or bypass of the left subclavian artery was performed pre-operatively for a total of 31 (18.2%) patients. In 5 (2.9%) cases, a preventive retrograde re-vascularization of the visceral vessels was performed.

Complications following treatment are outlined in Table 2. The most common intra-operative complications were access associated (15.9%). Neurological complications were observed in 7%. 30 day mortality was reported at 14.1%, with the majority of the deaths occurring among the patients treated in emergency (29.5%).

Late complications included a rate of endoleak of 20% (24 patients of the 34 cases had recurrent endoleak), rupture in 3.5%, 2 aorto-esophageal fistulas (AEF) and single cases of aorto-bronchial fistula and infection.

Reinterventions were required in 21.1%. Most were treated with endovascular solutions (91.7%). Table 3 outlines the complications for which a reintervention was required and the modality of intervention.

4. Discussion

Various studies which compare thoracic endovascular aortic aneurysm repair (TEVAR) to traditional surgery for DTAA in literature report superior results for endovascular treatment, most importantly in terms of post-operative complication rates and length of hospital stay.

A meta-analysis published in 2010 [7] including 38 comparative studies and 4 registries (5,888 patients) revealed a significant reduction in mortality for TEVAR (5.8% vs 13.8%, $p<0.00001$, OR=0.44), neurological, renal, respiratory and cardiological complications (41.4% vs 69.3%, $p<0.001$, OR=0.19) and length of hospital stay (7 days less for TEVAR).

A meta-analysis comparing the two techniques by Walsh et al. [8] including 17 published series, with a total of 1,109 patients, also concluded a significant reduction in mortality ($p=0.005$, OR=0.25) and neurological complications ($p=0.0013$, OR=0.28) for TEVAR.

A study published in 2010 [9] compared data extracted from the NIS (National Inpatient Sample) database with data of 11,669 patients. This study found that the mortality rates were identical for both TEVAR and traditional surgery (2.3%), even though the mean age of TEVAR patients was significantly higher (69.5 vs 60.2 yrs, $p<0.001$). Significant reductions were also found for TEVAR in terms of post-operative complications (60%, $p<0.001$, OR=0.39) and length of hospital stay ($p<0.001$).

4.1. Complications associated with endovascular treatment

4.1.1. Access complications

Carpenter et al. [10] reported that inadequate accesses are responsible for roughly 50% of the cases of ineligibility for TEVAR treatment.

Damage of access vessels continues to the greatest cause of grave comorbidities and even death, correlated to endovascular treatment of thoracic aorta pathologies. [11-12] It has been estimated that access related problems occur in around 28% of cases. [13-14] This is principally due to three reasons. The first reasons is that thoracic endografts generally require introducers with large calibers (20-25 Fr.), with external diameters between 22 and 27 Fr. Secondly, unlike the aneurysmatic pathology in the abdominal aorta, over 30% of the population with DTAA is female who generally present with vessels of smaller diameters. [15] The third reason is that the often advanced aged patients present with atherosclerotic steno-obstructive lesions and accentuated tortuosity, above all at the iliac axes.

In cases of small caliber vessels, the phase of the removal of the introducer is particularly crucial, which can provoke rupture and in some cases the complete detachment of the iliac artery. [16]

The preoperative examination is therefore of fundamental importance in order to plan the best access site and to be ready during the intervention for alternative operative strategies if necessary. The femoral access is suitable in 70-85% of cases, [11, 17] although in doubtful cases, the selection of a more proximal access site (iliac or aortic in extreme cases), also with the assitance of another graft, is recommended to avoid potential grave complications.

Another useful strategy includes the use of a Coons dilator (Cook Medical, Bloomington, IN) with progressively increasing diameters, incrementing 2 Fr at a time. The dilator enables both the testing of a possible passage and the progressive dilation of the artery to a diameter which adequately allows the passage of the endograft. It must also be underlined that, in cases of difficult accesses, an angiographic evaluation of the iliac arteries is absolutely necessary.

4.1.2. Neurological complications

Paraplegia and stroke represent the most devastating complications associated with the treatment of thoracic aorta pathologies.

Compared to traditional surgery, endovascular treatment appears to have significantly reduced the global incidence of paraplegia. This advantage is of particular relevance in the treatment of acute Stanford type B dissections, where the incidence associated with traditional surgery is between 14 - 19% [18-19]. Conversely, for the treatment of isolated descending thoracic aneurysms, the two treatment techniques have a comparable incidence of paraplegia, reported to be between 0-4% [20] and 2.5% [21] respectively.

The mechanisms which provoke paraplegia following TEVAR have not been fully identified. Simultaneous and previous traditional surgery of the abdominal aorta has been associated with increased risk of paraplegia. [21-23] The medullary vascularization from the lumbar and hypogastric arteries are important contributors in the risk of paraplegia. [24] Given this information, it is therefore advised by various authors [22,25] to perform eventual treatment of the abdominal and thoracic aorta in different interventions, so that a gradual establishment of a collateral medullary vascular circuit can be established. At this centre, in cases where a long segment of the thoracic aorta is planned to be covered and the hypogastric circulation is compromised, a preventive treatment is routinely performed. Embolization into major intercostal arteries due to the manipulation of the device in the aortic lumen has also been nominated as another potential risk factor. Extended coverage of the thoracic aorta has also been proven [22,26-28] to augment the risk of medullary ischemia. This risk rises further when coverage includes the region distal to T10. [22, 25, 29]

The EUROSTAR [21] study reported a significantly increased incidence of paraplegia when three or more endograft segments were used (OR, 3.5; P =.043).

A debated argument is that of the necessity to perform left subclavian revascularization when the placement of the endograft requires the coverage of the left subclavian artery. The EUROSTAR [21] study demonstrated the contribution of the subclavian/left vertebral arteries to the anterior spinal artery, and that the coverage of which determines an almost 4 times increased risk of paraplegia (OR, 3.9; P =.027). At this centre, with the exception of emergency cases, a preventative transposition of the subclavian artery is performed in all cases where treatment would require it to be covered.

Chiesa et al. [25] highlighted the importance of arterial pressure in the post-operative period: medium pressure values of 70 mmHg are associated with an increased risk of medullary ischemia. Other correlated factors include the female gender and renal insufficiency.

The causes of late onset paraplegia are more difficult to identify. A possible cause could be the onset of a secondary medullary edema due to damage such as reperfusion ischemia, which could in some cases reduce the medullary perfusion. Another possible cause could also be linked to long periods of post-operative hypotension.

The principal prevention method of medullary ischemia is cerebral spinal fluid (CSF) drainage. The use of this method however, should be weighted against the risk of complications associated with this procedure, which above all include subdural hematoma and infection. For this reason, and as suggested by other authors, the procedure is reserved for selected cases only in which a long tract of thoracic aorta is programmed to be covered (>20 cm) or in cases in which previous traditional surgery or endovascular treatment of the abdominal aorta is evidenced. Other methods utilized in the surgical environment includes medullary cooling [30] in order to reduce metabolic activity and increase the tolerance of the medulla to ischemia and the use of corticosteroids [31] with the aim of reducing edema from revascularization. This method has not found a use in TEVAR.

The incidence of stroke was reported in a literature review published in 2006 by Sullivan et al. [32] to be a mean of 2.2%. The EUROSTAR [21] study reported a 3.1% incidence of stroke in 606 patients treated with endografts for all pathologies of the thoracic aorta. It is commonly accepted that the cause of stroke during TEVAR is related to embolization caused by the manipulation of catheters and guide wires in the "dirty" aortic arch, rather than a base of hypoperfusion. [33-34]

The EUROSTAR [21] identified two significant risk factors for stroke: the duration of the procedure > 2.6 hours and female gender. Whilst the duration of the procedure is obviously connected to a greater manipulation of the guide wire and catheters in the aortic arch, the reasons explaining as to why females are more likely to develop a stroke is more difficult to understand. An hypothesized explanation is that in female patients the atherosclerotic pathology is often more advanced.

It can be deduced that the most effective mode of stroke prevention is an accurate pre-operative evaluation of the aortic arch, a careful manipulation of the catheters and guide wires attempting to limit maneuvers to those of absolute necessity, and an extensive operative strategy plan devised to reduce to a minimum the operative time.

4.1.3. Endoleak

Endoleak is the most frequent motive for reintervention following TEVAR. [35]

The rates of endoleak reported in literature vary and depend upon the type of pathology treated, and the length of the follow-up. Parmer et al. [36] reported an endoleak incidence of 29% at an average follow-up of 17 months, Ellozy et al. [37] published an incidence of 18% at roughly 15 months, and the Gore-TAG trial [38] reported only 10.6% at 5 years.

The EUROSTAR study [35] declared a 6.5% rate of need for secondary intervention due to endoleak at 2 years. Beyond single experiences, the reasoning behind this frequent complication can be explained by two fundamental factors: the prominent mobility and the frequent tortuosity of the thoracic aorta. Both of these factors force the endograft, and can provoke migration through time, disconnection and even rupture.

Parmer et al. [36] also evidenced some factors which are combined with the development of endoleak: male gender, larger diameter aneurysms, coverage of a long portion of the thoracic aorta and the usage of multiple endograft segments.

Among the various types of endoleak, the most frequent is type I proximal, reported as having an incidence in literature ranging between 0 and 44%. [39-41] The extreme variation in range can be explained by the different anatomical complexities in the aneurysms treated and therefore in the selection criteria. It is noted that the treatment of an isolated relatively small aneurysm situated in the rectilinear descending thoracic aorta, is relatively simple to treat and the development of a complication is relatively rare. Conversely, the treatment of an aneurysm which includes a part of the aortic arch is more complex and the results are less convincing. We believe that in the circumstances of complex anatomies including the aortic arch, it is necessary to construct a straight neck of at least 2 cm, which may include a by-pass or a transposition of the epi-aortic branches, in the hope of achieving aneurysm exclusion which will endure through time.

Type II endoleak are less common in the thoracic aorta compared to the incidence observed in the abdominal aortic region. In some cases, post-deployment angiography can evidence the patency of bronchial and intercostal arteries, but these arteries generally develop spontaneous thrombosis and do not require treatment.

Type III endoleak are the second most common form of endoleak. The extreme mobility of the thoracic aorta and its frequent tortuosity, especially found in large caliber aneurysms, can invoke through time the disconnection of the endograft segments and in some cases wear and tear which can lead to graft rupture. Experience has enabled the reduction in the incidence of type III endoleak, through increasing the length of device overlap in the case of multiple segments, which at this centre we believe should not be less than 5 cm, and using longer endografts rather than multiple shorter segments.

4.1.4. Aneurysm rupture

Avoiding aneurysm rupture is the ultimate objective of endovascular treatment. The percentage of rupture following endovascular treatment of abdominal aortic aneurysms (AAA) has been estimated to be around 1%.

The Stanford University group [42] reported their experience of TEVAR with a "custom-made" endograft claiming a rate of rupture at a distance of 10.7%, and a mortality rate of 91% at an average follow-up of 54 months. The EUROSTAR study [35] reported 2 cases of rupture at a distance of 12 months in 443 patients (0.5%). Other smaller experiences in literature with follow-ups ranging from 15 - 40 months presented a percentage of rupture at a distance between 1.6% and 6%. [37,43,44]

4.1.5. Aorto-Esophageal Fistula (AEF) and Aorto-Bronchial Fistula (ABF)

The AEF and the ABF are grave complications, which are almost always fatal and whose incidence is yet to be clearly defined. The Stanford University study [42], published in 2004, revealed a rate of AEF/ABF of 3%. Eggebrecht [45] also reported in 2004 an incidence equal to 5%, which were fatal in 100% of cases. Other cases of AEF/ABF following TEVAR have also been reported in more recent experiences. [38,43,46-47]

The anatomical proximity of the bronchi and the esophagus to the aorta is a factor which influences the incidence of this disastrous complication through time, due to the associated mechanical stress exercised by the endograft on the diseased aortic wall.

The use of restricted oversizing (about 10%) to reduce the mechanical stress on the aortic wall may theoretically reduce the incidence of these complications. However, this theory has not yet been proven.

4.2. Emergency treatment for ruptured thoracic aortic aneurysms

The annual incidence of rupture of the thoracic aortic aneurysm has been estimated to be at 5 cases per 100,000 inhabitants. [48-49] Around 30% of all the ruptured thoracic aortic aneurysms are localized in the descending aorta (rDTAA), with the remaining 70 % involving the arch and the ascending thoracic aorta. RDTAA represents a catastrophic event with a global mortality rate estimated to be up to 97%. [48]

In the few patients who arrive to the emergency department alive, traditional surgery has an ulterior mortality rate of 45% and a rate of systemic complications of around 50%. [50]

Endovascular treatment for rDTAA requires an endovascular emergency service with dedicated technical and nursing personnel combined with a surgical, anesthesiological and radiological team with knowledge and experience of endovascular materials. This preparation also demands the availability of advanced radiological equipment (eg. Angio CT) and an endovascular team 24hr/24hr for adequate diagnosis and treatment. The endovascular team must also be competent in traditional surgical techniques, so as to be able to treat different cases with the most appropriate surgical method. The operation room must also be equipped for an endovascular procedure, with high quality radiological and ultrasonographic machines (such as a portable C-Arm angiography and intravascular ultrasound (IVUS) and must have a large warehouse of basic endovascular materials available.

A meta-analysis [51] comparing traditional surgery and TEVAR for rDTAA included 859 patients and revealed significantly reduced mortality and paraplegia rates in favour of TEVAR. Mortality rates (11.4% vs 26.5%, p=0.13) favoring endovascular treatment were also reported by Patel et al. [52] in a comparative study.

http://dx.doi.org/10.5772/54692

5. Conclusion

Various studies have demonstrated a reduction in intra-operative mortality and neurological complications associated with endovascular treatment for DTAA pathologies compared to traditional surgery.

Technical improvements in catheters, specifically in terms of flexibility, have enabled the reduction in access related complications and the extension of the patient population to include those with more complex anatomies in terms of tortuosity. Mid and long term complications are still frequent, but are often able to be treated with ulterior endovascular procedures. A substantial rate of complications, such as rupture and AEF/ABF, are frequently fatal and often underestimated, especially in the case of fistulas.

At this centre however, endovascular treatment is considered the first choice treatment in emergency for rDTAA and in elderly patients and/or patients at high surgical risk. For patients with a long life expectancy, traditional surgery is currently our preferred treatment.

Acknowledgements

The authors would like to thank Johanna Chester for her translation and editing assistance.

Author details

Gioachino Coppi*, Stefano Gennai, Roberto Silingardi, Francesca Benassi and Valentina Cataldi

*Address all correspondence to: chirvascmo@gmail.com

Department of Vascular Surgery, University of Modena and Reggio Emilia, New Civic Hospital St. Agostino-Estense, Modena, Italy

References

[1] Dake MD, Miller DC, et al. Transluminal placement of endovascular stent-grafts for the treatment of descending thoracic aortic aneurysms. N Engl J Med. 1994;331:1729-34.

[2] Chiesa R, Civilini E, Tshomba Y, Marone EM, Bertoglio L, Coppi G, et al. Open and endovascular treatment of descending thoracic aneurysms. Best practice in vascular procedures, Ed Michale Jacobs. Edizioni Minerva Medica, Turin 2010;11:109-127.

[3] Coady MA, Rizzo JA, Hammond GL, et al. What is the appropriate size criterion for resection of thoracic aortic aneurysms? J Thorac Cardiovasc Surg 1997;113:476-491.

[4] Davies RR, Goldstein LJ, Coady MA, et al. Yearly rupture or dissection rates for thoracic aortic aneurysms: simple prediction based on size. Ann Thorac Surg 2002;73:17–28.

[5] Moore AG, Eagle KA, Bruckman D, et al. Choice of computed tomography, transesophageal echocardiography, magnetic resonance imaging, and aortography in acute aortic dissection: International Registry of Acute Aortic Dissection (IRAD). Am J Cardiol. 2002;89(10):1235-8.

[6] Sommer T, Fehske W, Holzknecht N, et al. Aortic dissection: a comparative study of diagnosis with spiral CT, multiplanar transesophageal echocardiography, and MR imaging. Radiology 1996;199(2):347-352.

[7] Cheng D, Martin J, Shennib H, et al: Endovascular aortic repair versus open surgical repair for descending thoracic aortic disease a systematic review and meta-analysis of comparative studies. J Am Coll Cardiol 55:986-1001, 2010.

[8] Walsh SR, Tang TY, Sadat U, et al: Endovascular stenting versus open surgery for thoracic aortic disease: systematic review and meta-analysis of perioperative results. J Vasc Surg 2008;47:1094-1098.

[9] Gopaldas RR, Huh J, Dao TK, LeMaire SA, Chu D, Bakaeen FG, et al. Superior nationwide outcomes of endovascular versus open repair for isolated descending thoracic aortic aneurysm in 11,669 patients. J Thorac Cardiovasc Surg 2010;140:1001-10.

[10] Carpenter JP, Baum RA, et al. Impact of exclusion criteria on patient selection for endovascular abdominal aortic aneurysm repair. J Vasc Surg 2001;34:1050-4.

[11] Criado FJ. TEVAR acess, delivery, and fixation: Key considerations and new developments to achieve optimal endograft placement. Endovascular Today, Nov 2007:45-52.

[12] Criado FJ, Clark NS, et al. Stent graft repair in the aortic arch and descending thoracic aorta; a 4 year experience. J Am Coll Cardiol 2010;55:986-1001.

[13] Melissano G, Civilini E, et al. Single centre experience with a new commercially available thoracic endovascular graft. Eur J Vasc Endovasc Surg 2005;29:579-85.

[14] Fairman RM, Velazquez O, et al. Endovascular repair of aortic aneurysms. critical events and adjunctive procedures. J Vasc Surg 2001;33:1226-32

[15] Velazquez O, Larson RA, et al. Gender-related differences in infrarenal aortic aneurysm morphologic features: issues relevant to Ancure and Talent endografts. J Vasc Surg. 2001;33(2 Suppl):S77-84.

[16] Shane S. Parmer, MD, et al. Techniques for large sheath insertion during endovascular thoracic aortic aneurysm repair. J Vasc Surg 2006;43 Suppl A:62A-68A.

[17] Matsumura J. Worldwide survey of thoracic endografts: practical clinical applications. J Vasc Surg 2005;43:20A-21A.

[18] Coselli JS, LeMaire SA, et al. Paraplegia after thoracoabdominal aortic aneurysm repair: is dissection a risk factor? Ann Thorac Surg. 1997;63:28-35.

[19] Matsumura J. Worldwide survey of thoracic endografts: practical clinical applications. J Vasc Surg 2005;43:20A-21A.

[20] Coselli JS, LeMaire SA, et al. Left heart bypass during descending thoracic aortic aneurysm repair does not reduce the incidence of paraplegia. Ann Thor Surg 2004;77:1298-303.

[21] Buth J, Harris PL, et al. Neurological complications associated with endovascular repair of thoracic aortic pathology: Incidence and risk factors. A study from the European Collaborators on Stent/Graft tehniques for Aortic Aneurysm Repair (Eurostar) Registry. J Vasc Surg 2007;46:1103-11.

[22] Gravereaux EC, Faries PL, et al. Risk of spinal cord ischemia after endograft repair of thoracic aortic aneurysms. J Vasc Surg 2001;34:997-1003.

[23] Makaroun MS, Dillavou ED, et al. Endovascular treatment of thoracic aortic aneurysms: results of the phase II multicentre trial of the GORE TAG thoracic endoprosthesis. J Vasc Surg 2005;41:1-9.

[24] Khoynezhad A, Donayre CE, et al. Risk factors of neurologic deficit after thoracic aortic endografting. Ann Thorac Surg 2007;83:S882-9.

[25] Chiesa R, Melissano G, et al. Spinal cord ischemia after elective stent-graft repair of the thoracic aorta. J Vasc Surg 2005;42:11-7.

[26] Greenberg R, Resch T, et al. Endovascular repair of descending thoracic aortic aneurysms: an early experience with intermediate-term follow-up. J Vasc Surg 2000;31:147-156.

[27] Marcheix B, Dambrin C, et al. Midterm results of endovascular treatment of atherosclerotic aneurysms of the descending thoracic aorta. J Thorac Cardiovasc Surg. 2006;132:1030-6.

[28] Bavaria JE, Appoo JJ; GORE TAG Investigators, et al. Endovascularstent grafting versus open surgical repiar of descending thoracic aortic aneurysms in low-risk patients: a multi- centre comparative trial. J Thorac Cardiovasc Surg 2007;133:369-77.

[29] Stone DH, Brewster DC, et al. Stent-graft versus open-surgical repair of the thoracic aorta: mid-term results. J Vasc Surg 2006;44:1188-97.

[30] Cambria RP, Davison JK, et al. Epidural cooling for spinal cord protection during thoracoabdominal aneurysm repair: A five-year experience. J Vasc Surg. 2000;31:1093- 102.

[31] Fowl RJ, Patterson RB, et al. Protection against postischemic spinal cord injury using a new 21-aminosteroid. J Surg Res. 1990;48:597-600.

[32] Sullivan TM, Sundt TM 3rd. Complications of thoracic aortic endografts: spinal cord ischemia and stroke. J Vasc Surg. 2006;43 Suppl A:85A-88A.

[33] Okita Y, Takamoto S, et al. Predictive factors for postoperative cerebral complications in patients with thoracic aortic aneurysm. Eur J Cardiothorac Surg. 1996;10:826-32.

[34] Blauth CI, Cosgrove DM, et al. Atheroembolism from the ascending aorta. An emerging problem in cardiac surgery. J Thorac Cardiovasc Surg. 1992;103:1104-11.

[35] Leurs LJ, Bell R; EUROSTAR; UK Thoracic Endograft Registry collaborators. Endovascular treatment of thoracic aortic diseases: combined experience from the EUROSTAR and United Kingdom Thoracic Endograft registries. J Vasc Surg. 2004 Oct;40(4):670-9; discussion 679-80.

[36] Parmer SS, Carpenter JP, et al. Endoleaks after endovascular repair of the thoracic aortic aneurysms. J Vasc Surg 2006;44:47-52.

[37] Ellozy SH, Carroccio A, et al. Challenges of endovascular tube graft repair of thoracic aortic aneurysm: midterm follow-up and lessons learned. J Vasc Surg. 2003;38:676-83.

[38] Makaroun MS, Dillavoi ED; Gore TAG Investigators. Five year results of endovascular treatment with the Gore TAG device compared with open repair of thoracic aortic aneurysms. J Vasc Surg 2008;47:912-8.

[39] Eggebrecht H, Nienaber CA, et al. Endovascular stent-graft placement in aortic dissection: a meta-analysis. European Heart Journal 2006;27:489-98.

[40] Nienaber CA, Fattori R, et al. Nonsurgical reconstruction of thoracic aortic dissection by stent-graft placement. N Engl J Med 1999;340:1539-45.

[41] Czermak BV, Waldenberger P, et al. Placement of endovascular stent-grafts for emergency treatment of acute disease of the descending thoracic aorta. AJR Am J Roentgenol. 2002;179:337-45.

[42] Demers P, Miller DC, et al. Midterm results of endovascular repair of descending thoracic aortic aneurysms with first-generation stent grafts. J Thorac Cardiovasc Surg. 2004;127:664-73.

[43] Fattori R, Nienaber CA, et al. Talent Thoracic Retrospective Registry. Results of endovascular repair of the thoracic aorta with the Talent Thoracic stent graft: the Talent Thoracic Retrospective Registry. J Thorac Cardiovasc Surg. 2006;132:332-9.

[44] Criado FJ, Abul-Khoudoud OR, et al. Endovascular repair of the thoracic aorta: lessons learned. Ann Thorac Surg. 2005;80:857-63.

[45] Eggebrecht H, Baumgart D, et al. Aortoesophageal fistula secondary to stent-graft repair of the thoracic aorta. J Endovasc Ther. 2004;11:161-7.

[46] Riesenman PJ, Farber MA, et al. Aortoesophageal fistula after thoracic endovascular aortic repair and transthoracic embolization. J Vasc Surg. 2007;46:789-91.

[47] Santo KC, Guest P, et al. Aortoesophageal fistula secondary to stent-graft repair of the thoracic aorta after previous surgical coarctation repair. J Thorac Cardiovasc Surg. 2007;134:1585-6.

[48] Hyhlik-Dürr A, Geisbüsch P, von Tengg-Kobligk H, Klemm K, Böckler D. Intentional overstenting of the celiac trunk during thoracic endovascular aortic repair: preoperative role of multislice CT angiography. J Endovasc Ther 2009;16:48-54.

[49] Attia C, Farhat F, Boussel L, Villard J, Revel D, Douek P. Endovascular repair of lesions involving the descending thoracic aorta. Mid-term morphological changes. Interact Cardiovasc Thorac Surg 2008; 7:595-9.

[50] Schermerhorn ML, Giles KA, Hamdan AD, Dalhberg SE, Hagberg R, Pomposelli F. Population-based outcomes of open descending thoracic aortic aneurysm repair. J Vasc Surg 2008;48:821-7.

[51] Xenos ES, Minion DJ, Davenport DL, Hamdallah O, Abedi NN, Sorial EE, Endean ED. Endovascular versus open repair for descending thoracic aortic rupture: institutional experience and meta-analysis. Eur J Cardio-Thor Surg 2009; 35(2);282-6.

[52] Patel HJ, Williams DM, Upchurch GR, Dasika NL, Deeb GM. A comparative analysis of open and endovascular repair for the ruptured descending thoracic aorta. J Vasc Surg 2009; 50(6);1265-70.

Chapter 7

Delayed Aneurysm Rupture After EVAR

Guido Regina, Domenico Angiletta,
Martinella Fullone, Davide Marinazzo,
Francesco Talarico and Raffaele Pulli

Additional information is available at the end of the chapter

http://dx.doi.org/10.5772/53415

1. Introduction

Endovascular repair is becoming the milestone of treatment for aneurysmal disease of the abdominal aorta, evolving over time as an attractive alternative to open repair, especially for elderly and high risk patients.

Since the introduction of endovascular aneurysm repair (EVAR) 20 years ago [1] many successful early results have been achieved with this treatment, but mid-term and long-term durability of the endograft devices that have been used remains questionable [2-5].

Endovascular techniques and technical material have improved from the initial devices and have permitted the extension of the treatment to more and more complex anatomies.

However, sustained survival benefits have not been proven because nowadays only mid-term results after EVAR have been reported, and additional procedures were required in many patients.

Late failure of endovascular repair secondary to endoleaks, endotension and sac enlargement, stentgraft migration, tear and fracture or infection continues to be a persistent problem that can result in delayed aneurysm rupture [5-8].

Large cohorts of studies have reported rates of abdominal aortic aneurysm (AAA) rupture after EVAR ranging from 0.5 to 1.2% per patient per year [9-14]. Lifetime risks are even higher because most patients live for several years after the procedure [15].

Therefore, although several randomized trials have shown lower perioperative morbidity and mortality after EVAR compared with open repair [16-19], mid and long-term complication, most of which represented by endoleaks, are quite frequent after EVAR and the risk of late rupture persists.

Availability of new generation devices, strict patient selection and respect of correct morphological criteria are crucial to obtain good outomes of EVAR, reducing the risk of postoperative complications, including delayed rupture.

2. Materials and methods

In our own series, involving one University Hospital and four Regional Hospitals, between January 2004 and December 2011, a total of 1500 patients underwent endovascular repair of AAA with a variety of commercially available stent grafts.

Emergent aortomonoiliac EVAR and crossover bypass was performed in 90 (5%) patients with ruptured AAA, while the remaining patients received elective EVAR with bifurcated (n=1020, 72.3%) or aortomonoiliac endograft with crossover bypass (n=390, 27.7%).

The mean postoperative follow-up was 30 months (range 6-72). The imaging protocol included angiogrphic computer tomography (angioTC) performed at intervals of 1, 3, 6, 12 months after the procedure and annually thereafter.

Aneurysm rupture was defined as an extravasation of blood outside the aortic wall, documented at angioCT.

3. Results

During the follow-up 22 patients (1.46%) presented with late aneurysm rupture after EVAR. These results are in consonance with the data avaiable in literature [20-24].

There were no statistical differences between patients undergoing emergent or elective EVAR and among patients undergoing bifurcated or aortomonoiliac endografting.

Causes of rupture include endoleaks in 51.3% of cases (35% type I, 15.3% type II, 0% type III and IV), while in 49.7% of cases the cause remained undetermined.

Most of the described AAA ruptures occurred within 1-3 years after endovascular repair. The mean time to rupture from the primary EVAR was 20 months. The mean initial aneurysm diameter was relatively large (62 mm).

All patients arrived alive to treatment. Eight patients had a redo EVAR, while 14 underwent open repair. Three out of 8 patients (37.5%) died after redo EVAR and 6 out of 14 patients (42.8%) treated by open repair died during the operation or in the perioperative period.

The incidence of overall mortality after rupture in this experience was 40.9 %.

http://dx.doi.org/10.5772/53415

4. Discussion

Several studies have demonstrated better peri-operative survival for endovascular over open repair of AAA, with fewer complications and a shorter recovery period [16-19].

However there are concerns about durability of endovascular repair at long-term when compared with conventional open treatment. Actually EVAR does not completely eliminate the risk of late aneurysm rupture and requires more frequent reinterventions to maintain the exclusion of the aneurysm, including conversion to open repair.

Success of the endovascular treatment depends on the strict selection of the patients, evaluating specific anatomic characteristics like diameter, lenght and angulation of the aortic neck as well as iliac morphology.

In a 2010 retrospective study involving 1768 patients undergoing EVAR, Metha et al [25] reported an incidence of additional secondary procedures of 19.2% during a mean follow-up period of 34 months (Tab. 1).

Number of patients	1,768
Mean follow-up [SD]	34 Months [30]
Secondary intervention	19.2%
Type II Endoleak	40.1%
Type I/III Endoleak	16.5%
Migration	13.6%
Limb occlusion	7.4%
Other (rupture, device defect, etc.)	8.6%

Table 1. Incidence of secondary procedures after EVAR.

In 2010 the results of the DREAM trial showed a reintervention rate of almost 30% within 6 years [26]. The most frequently reported complications include endograft migration, endoleaks, limb occlusion and rupture.

Endoleak is the Achille's heel of the EVAR, revealing associations with both early and late failure of the procedure and is the most common reason for aortic rupture and reinterventions in the follow up of EVAR.

The incidence of all endoleaks is reported in the major trials of recent years as ranging from 15.6% to 19.8% [17-19].

The endoleaks are classified into five types according to the etiology (Tab. 2) [27].

Type	Origin of the leak
I	Inadeguate seal at proximal (Ia) or distal (Ib) end of the graft
II	Retrograde flow from the inferior mesenteric artery, lumbar arteries, others collateral vessels of the aneurysm sac
III	Component disconnection (IIIa) or fabric disruption (IIIb)
IV	Graft material porosity
V	Endotension: increase of the pressare without any visibile evidente of blood in the aneurysm sac

Table 2. Endoleak classification. From: Moll FL, Powell JT, Fraedrich G, et al. Management of abdominal aortic aneurysms clinical practice guidelines of the European society for vascular surgery. Eur J Vasc Endovasc Surg 2011;41(Suppl 1):S1-S58.

One of the most frequent causes of type I endoleak is represented by the aneurysmatic evolution of the proximal aortic neck. Aortic aneurysmal degeneration can progress over time to involve the segments chosen at the time of surgery as appropriate landing zones for effective sealing. Therefore, late degeneration of the landing zones can lead to endograft migration and type I endoleak with sac enlargement.

Some authors have reported a dilatation of the landing zone after EVAR [28]. Possibile explanations could be the continuous outward radial force of the uncovered portion of the endograft, in particular in case of high oversizing, or the forces applied in this region during the implantation of the device.

Type I endoleaks can also occur as a result of stentgraft migration that may originate from unstable proximal sealing, as a consequence of wrong planning involving oversizing understimation and lack of graft radial force, especially in case of poor quality of proximal aortic neck (i.e. short lenght, severe angulation, high calcification and thrombus load).

Severe angulations and tortuosity of the aorta and the iliac arteries usually can also led to graft migration with possibile type I endoleaks.

Iliac fixation plays an important role in preventing stentgraft migration. Extension of both iliac limbs to the level of the iliac bifurcation seems to minimize the risk of endograft migration, despite suboptimal neck anatomy.

Type III endoleak is caused mainly by a dislocation of two stentgraft components in a modular stentgraft system (IIIa), generally due to a shortening of the overlapping zones during the procedure. Extreme angulation of the neck or iliac segments may also be a contributing factor. Failure relate to modular disjunction is preventable by ensuring an adequate component overlap during the intervention.

Other causes of type III endoleak are due to a device failure as a consequence of a deficit in the graft fabric (type IIIb).

Patients with type I and III endoleaks have been identified as being at gratest risk of aneurysm rupture. Conventional endoleak management consists in prompt repair of type I and III endoleaks.

Type IV endoleak is determined by an excessive porosity of the stentgraft that appears intact. Since these endoleaks may spontaneously seal, their treatment is not recomended.

Type II endoleak is related to retrograde flow via collaterals, mostly lumbar arteries, hypogastric arteries, inferior mesenteric artery. Although type II endoleak is considered benign, this persistent flow could prevent thrombosis of the aneurysm sac, resulting in a potential risk of continued aneurysm expansion and possibile rupture.

Many early type II endoleak are transient and will resolve spontaneously within six months, but a small minority of patients with untreated endoleak type II may suffer from aneurysm rupture. The treatment of type II endoleaks should considered when it suddenly appears during follow-up or when it persist for more than 6 months without shrinkage of the sac.

Ronsivalle et al [29] have reported the efficacy of the injection of fibrin glue with coils into the aneurysm sac, in addition to the conventional EVAR protocol. The aim of this procedure is to induce clotting of the aneurysm sac, thus reducing the risk of type II endoleaks, potentially leading to late aneurysm rupture.

In our experience, intraoperative intrasac thrombin injection was employed in patients with AAA at high risk of type II endoleaks (absence or modeste intraluminal thrombus, presence of inferior mesenteric artery, lumbar arteries, hypogastric or accessory renal arteries). Early results at follow-up showed a reduction of the incidence of type II endoleak, as well as type I endoleak, since clotting of the aneurysm sac presumably provides also stability of the endograft, so preventing migration of the devices.

Although the high incidence of secondary interventions after EVAR decreased significantly in recent years, largely thanks to devices improvement, the widespread use of the endovascular treatment often leads surgeons to force the indications to EVAR, even in patients with unfavorable anatomy.

Endografts placed outside device guidelines were associated with higher aneurysm-related mortality, reinterventions, graft-related adverse events, indicating that adherence to such guidelines is a foundamental clinical practice.

5. Data from literature

Data from literature about late aneurysm rupture after EVAR and relative mortality were collected. Results are summarized in table 3 and compared with our experience.

The EUROSTAR (European Collaborators on stent-graft techniques for aortic aneurysm repair) registry [4], established in 1996, collected data on the outcome of treatment of patients with infrarenal AAA treated by EVAR, with the purpose to evaluate incidence and risk factors of late rupture, conversion and death. In this large study 2464 patients have been enrolled, with a median follow-up of 12.14 months. Thirteen patients sustained confirmed aneurysm rupture 30 days or more after operation. One rupture occurred in the periopera-

Study (year)	N. late rupture (%)	Overall mortality (%)	N. patients undergoing surgery	Mortality after surgery
Harris (2000) [4]	13/ 2464 (0.52)	8/13 (61.5)	11/13 (84.6)	6/11 (54.54)
Bernhard (2002) [30]	7/3946 (0.17)	4/7 (57)	6/7 (85.7)	3/6 (50)
Hobo (2008) [20]	(1.7)	(4.5)	NR	NR
	(4.5) (*)	(7.4) (*)		
Szmidt (2007) [21]	3/445 (0.67)	0	0	0
Wyss (2010) [22]	22/848 (2.59)	15/22 (68.18)	8/22 (36.36)	1/8 (12.5)
Koole (2011) [23]	26/6337 (0.41)	NR (62)	NR	NR
Metha (2011) [24]	27/1768 (1.52)	4/27 (14.81)	26/27 (96.3)	3/26 (11.5)
Our experience (2011)	22/1500 (1.46)	9/22 (40.9)	22/22 (100)	9/22 (40.9)

(*) presence of concomitant iliac aneurysm

N.R. not reported

Table 3. Incidence and mortality of delayed aneurusysm rupture after EVAR.

tive period (within 30 days). Only those patients with clear signs of rupture (derived from the findings at operation, CT images or autopsy results) were included in the study. Patients who died suddenly before a precise diagnosis could be confirmed (10 patients) were not included. Details of the patients with proved rupture are shown in table 4.

Peak incidence of rupture occurred 18 months after the intervention (range 0-24 months). The annual cumulative rate of rupture approximated to 1% per year (1.4% in the first year, 0.6% in the second year). Twelve patients (85.7%) underwent emergency open surgery, five of whom (41.6%) survived. There were no survivors between the two patients who were not subject to an emergency operation. The overall death rate of late (> 30 days) aneurysm rupture after EVAR was 69.2% (9/13) of the patients.

Proximal type I endoleak, midgraft (type III) endoleak, migration and postoperative kinking of the endograft were proved to be relevant risk factors for rupture. Type II endoleak, distal type I endoleak, endograft stenosis ana thrombosis were present but statistically not significant (table 5).

Persistent endoleak as indicator of failure of the treatment was based on the assumption that the endoleak itself was the cause of the continued expansion and the eventual rupture of the aneurysm sac after EVAR.

Nevertheless, at last three of 10 patients who died suddenly of unknown causes had an aneurysm of a maximum diameter greater than six centimeters before their death. Although there may have been cardiac malfunction or other postoperative causes, rupture was likely to account for some of these 10 deaths.

http://dx.doi.org/10.5772/53415

Serial no.	Time since operation (mo)	Intervention on rupture	Device	Outcome (at 30 d)
1	18	Conversion	Vanguard*	Death
2	24	Conversion	Vanguard*	Death
3	3	Conversion	AneuRx	Death
4	12	Conversion	Stentor*	Survived
5	18	Conversion	Stentor*	Survived
6	6	Conversion	Vanguard*	Death
7	18	Conversion	Vanguard*	Survived
8	18	Nil	Vanguard*	Death
9	6	Conversion	Vanguard*	Survived
10	24	Conversion	Vanguard*	Death
11	3	Nil	Talent	Death
12	18	Conversion	Vanguard*	Death
13	24	Conversion	Vanguard*	Survived
14†	0	Conversion	Talent	Death

*Discontinued model devices.

†One rupture within 30 days of endovascular repair

From: Harris PL, Vallabhaneni SR, Desgranges P, et al. Incidence and risk factors of late rupture, conversion, and death after endovascular repair of infrarenal aortic aneurysms: the EUROSTAR experience. European collaborators on stent/graft techniques for aortic aneurysm repair. J VascSurg 2000;32:739-49

Table 4. Details of patients with a proved rupture of the treated aneurysm.

Moreover, EUROSTAR experience demonstrates that the overall death rate of 64.3% (9/14) for AAA rupture after EVAR is not inferior than the usual expectation of mortality after ruptured AAA repair, as previously reported [31].

The analysis of risk factors for late rupture in the EUROSTAR study confirms the importance of proximal fixation site endoleak, while distal endoleaks seem to have a more benign impact, possibly because of the lower pressure or endotension in the aneurysm sac. Moreover, results of this study seem to confirm that type II endoleak is less important as regard to aneurysm rupture, most of them resolving spontaneously. However, prudence is mandatory because of uncertainty regarding the accuracy of diagnosis of these endoleaks. Kinking of the endovascular devices could also be responsible of the sac rupture as well as stent migration.

Even if the death rate associated with all operations for conversion repair in the EUROSTAR experience was 24.4%, surgeons must realized that the risk of delayed rupture is greater than the risk of conversion.

In 2008 an outcome analysis of EUROSTAR experience compared results following EVAR in patients affected by AAA with (group II) and without (group I) concomitant iliac artery

Adverse factor	Free from rupture and adverse factor (n)	Rupture with adverse factor (n)	Rupture free from adverse factor (n)	Adverse factor free from rupture (n)	P value	Relative hazard ratio (95% CI)
Proximal type I endoleak	2250	3	10	62	.0001	7.59 (2.09-27.62)
Midgraft (type III) endoleak	2224	5	8	88	.0001	8.95 (2.92-27.52)
Stent-graft migration	2248	3	10	64	.0001	4.53 (1.24-16.66)
Kinked endograft	2216	3	10	96	.0001	3.13 (1.40-11.49)
Type II endoleak*	2106	2	11	206	.415*	
Distal type I endoleak*	2177	1	12	135	.776*	
Endograft stenosis*	2275	0	13	37	.646*	
Thrombosed endograft*	2235	0	13	77	.503*	

*Statistically not significant.

From: Harris PL, Vallabhaneni SR, Desgranges P, et al. Incidence and risk factors of late rupture, conversion, and death after endovascular repair of infrarenal aortic aneurysms: the EUROSTAR experience. European collaborators on stent/graft techniques for aortic aneurysm repair. J VascSurg 2000;32:739-49

Table 5. Risk factors for late rupture and their incidence after endovascular repair.

aneurysm [26]. Mortality rates was obtained from the Registry database for the period from October 1996 to November 2006. Group II included more patients classified as ASA III-IV, who were considered more frequently unfit for open surgery, with larger-diameter aneurysms and infrarenal necks, an increased incidence of internal iliac artery occlusion and greater angulation of the aortic neck and iliac artery (Tab. 3).

The 5-year cumulative incidence of distal type I endoleak was higher in group II (9.1%) than in group I (4.3%) as well as the 5-year cumulative incidence of aneurysm rupture (4.5% in group II versus 1.7% in group I; $p = 0.042$) (Fig. 1).

Nevertheless, between the two study groups was not found an aneurysm-related mortality rate significantly different (4.5% in group I and 7.4% in group II). However, this rate could be underestimated because the cause of death was unknown or undefined in a significante number of patients.

In this study distal type I endoleaks was strongly associated ($p < 0.0001$) with the presence of concomitant iliac aneurysms. The greater incidence of these endoleaks appears to be due to a more difficult achievement of an adequate distal seal and fixation of the endograft in the external iliac artery, which is frequently tortuous, angulated or diseased in this area. Distal type I endoleak is probably the cause of the higher incidence of aneurysm rupture observed in these patients.

In 2007 Szmidt et al [21] presented their experience with 445 patients undergoing EVAR between 1998 and 2006. The authors reported three (0.67%) late aneurysm ruptures. In all cases the cause was type I endoleak, due to graft migration in two cases and aneurysm lengthening in the remaining case. All the patients received open aneurysmectomy without any major complications.

	Group I (n=6286)	**Group II (n=1268)**	**p***
Mesasurements			
Infrarenal neck diameter, mm	24.1 +/- 3.3	24.5+/-3.4	<0.001
Infrarenal neck length, mm	26.8+/-11.5	27.7+/-12.6	NS
Maximum aneurysm diameter, mm	60.7+/-10.4	62.3+/-11.2	<0.0001
Common iliac artery, mm	14.8+/-4.7	25.9+/-13.2	<0.0001
Occlusion			
Common or external iliac artery	109 (1.7%)	23 (1.8%)	NS
Hypogastric artery	329 (5.2%)	144 (11.4%)	<0.0001
Angulation			
Aortic neck	1529 (24.3%)	390 (30.8%)	<0.0001
Aneurysm	776 (11.7%)	160 (10.9%)	NS
Iliac artery	2632 (41.9%)	612 (48.3%)	<0.0001

Continuous data are presented as means +/- standard deviation; categorical data are given as counts (percentages).

NS: not significant.

* Univariate analysis.

From: Hobo R, Sybrandy JE, Harris P, Buth J. Endovascular repair of abdominal aortic aneurysms with concomitant iliac artery aneurysm. Outcome analysis of the EUROSTAR experience.J EndovascTher. 2008;15:12-22

Table 6. Aneurysm anatomy of 7554 AAA patients undergoing Endovascular Aneurysm Repair.

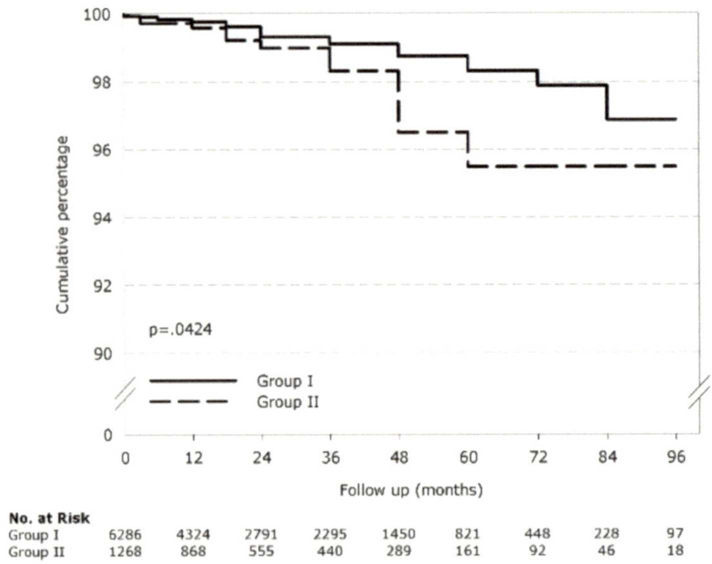

Figure 1. Freedom from aneurysm rupture. *From: Hobo R, Sybrandy JE, Harris P, Buth J. Endovascular repair of abdominal aortic aneurysms with concomitant iliac artery aneurysm. Outcome analysis of the EUROSTAR experience.J EndovascTher. 2008;15:12-22*

However, the late rupture rate in this series is probably underestimated because of a limited follow-up period (mean 30 months) and the dropout of a considerable number of patients.

In a review published in 2009, Schlosser et al [32] identified 270 patients with AAA rupture after EVAR, most of whom occurred within 2-3 years after the operation (Fig. 2).

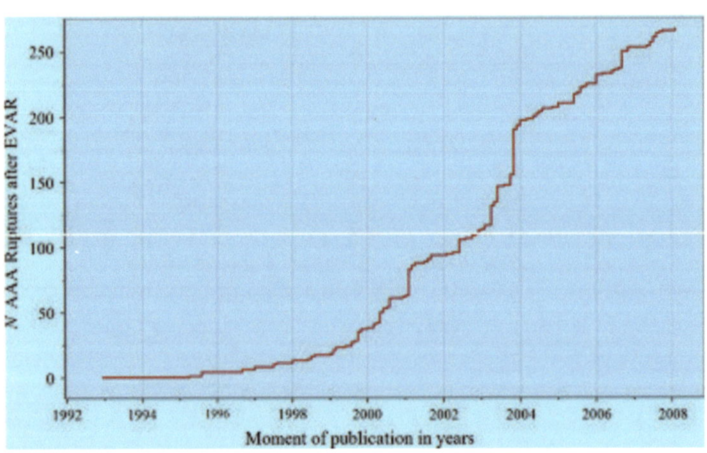

Figure 2. Patients with AAA rupture after aneurysm repair by publication date. From: Schlösser FJV, Gusberg RJ, Dardik A, Lin PH, Verhagen HJM, Moll FL and Muhs BE. Aneurysm rupture after EVAR: can the ultimate failure be predicted? Eur J VascEndovascSurg 37(1):15-22 (2009).

The main cause of rupture was reported for 235 of the 270 patients. Endoleaks were reported in 160 patients (57 type IA, 31 type IB, 23 type II, 26 type III, 0 type IV, 9 endotension, 14 not specified), graft migration in 41, graft disconnection in 11 and infection in 6.

Late ruptures occurred in 164 patients. The mean time interval between the initial procedure and subsequent AAA rupture was 24 +/- 18 months (range 2-96, median 20). 155 out of 202 reported moments of rupture occurred within 27 months after EVAR and their incidence considerably reduced thereafter.

The mean time interval did not differ between men and women in 71 patients in which information about gender and time interval was available. Mean initial AAA diameter was relatively large (65mm).

In 82 patients information about both moments of rupture and AAA diameter was available. Patients with an initial AAA diameter above the mean (> 65mm) had a shorter time interval between EVAR and AAA rupture than patients with smaller-diameters AAA, although this difference was not significant.

The course of AAA diameter during follow-up was described in 101 patients. Growth of the AAA sac occurred in 36, any changes in 39 and shrinkage in 26 patients.

In 41 patients no abnormalities requiring reintervention were found during the follow-up: in 35 no abnormalities (absence of endoleak, stent fractures, migration, graft angulation, insecure fixation, signs of inflammation and sac enlargement) were found at all. In another 6 patients only a small type II endoleak was found and the AAA diameter was stable.

Fifty-six of all patients presented an endoleak during the most recent follow up visits before the rupture occur, 6 of whom were small type II endoleaks without sac enlargement. Other abnormal findings included wire fractures, graft migration or severe graft angulation in 11, insecure fixation in 5, AAA sac inflammation in 1, while AAA rupture itself was diagnosed during a regular follow-up visit in 5 patients.

160 patients underwent open conversion and 26 sustained a redo-EVAR. In 24 patients no repair was performed at all and for 60 no data were available.

AAA ruptures were fatal in about half of the patients (119 out of 231) for whom data about mortality were reported. In patient undergone to endovascular or open repair the results were slightly better: a fatal course occurred in 62 of 138 patients that underwent open conversion and in 7 of 26 patients that were subjected to a redo endovascular ruptured AAA repair.

This study has however some limitations. Because data collection was obtained from the existing literature, informations about many variables could not been avaiable for all patients (e.g. data about neck diameters at the time of EVAR and time of rupture, year of repair, etc.). Another disadvantage is that the determination of the cause of aneurysm rupture was based on the description reported by the authors of the selected articles. Because different authors may have used different criteria to estabilish causes of rupture, this process may have been relatively subjected. Moreover, in 24 of 270 patients, no precise description about diagnostic examinations was provided and no fatal course was described. Theoretically there may have been a possibility that any of these 24 patients had a "symptomatic" AAA instead of a ruptured AAA.

Another disadvantage concerns the limited follow-up period of a significant number of patients, that may partially explain the relatively high number of AAA ruptures in the first 2-3 years after EVAR reported in this study. Indeed, ruptures after 3 years may be underrepresented due to movement of patients to other institutions or due to mortality.

It is interesting to note that a strong association between lager-diameter aneurysm and increased risk of rupture after EVAR has been described by the EUROSTAR registry, Lifeline registry and AneuRx trail [9-15, 33-38].

Increased rupture risk in patients with persistent type II endoleak was reported by Johns et al [39]. Female gender seems to be associated with an increased risk of rupture too [12,13].

Because relatively many ruptures occur between the follow up visits at one and two years after EVAR, an additional follow-up after 18 months may possibly reduce the AAA rupture rate. This may be especially important for patients with early rupture, such as patients with larger AAA diameters, endoleaks or graft migration.

Data from the EVAR trials [16, 40] were analyzed by Wyss et al [22] in order to asses factors associated with AAA rupture after EVAR or open repair. There were no ruptures in the 594 patients undergoing open aneurysmectomy, during a follow-up with average duration of 5.3 years. On the other hand, out of a total of 848 elective EVARs, 27 ruptures occurred during an average follow-up period of 4.8 years (25 in EVAR trial 1 and 2 in EVAR trial 2), with a rate of rupture of 0.8 and 0.2 per 100 patients per year, respectively.

The ruptures were divided into three groups. Group A contains 5 (18.5%) ruptures that occurred in the perioperative period (within 30 days). Group B included 5 (18.5%) patients who sustained rupture more than 30 days after the intervention, without prior complication or signs of failed endovascular treatment. Four of the 5 patients died within 30 days of the rupture. One patient sustained the rupture at home on day 32 and no post-procedural imaging was performed before discharge. Three patients underwent a normal follow-up CT scan within 2 months before rupture, all showing sac shrinkage with any abnormal findings. Another patient showed sac shrinkage and no complications during the first 2 years but he missed the three years follow-up scan. Thus, even if a predischarge scan had been proposed as part of the EVAR trial protocol, three ruptures remained unexplained, despite optimal protocol had been followed.

Group C included 17 (63%) patients with late ruptures with prior complications. Eleven of these patients died within 30 days of the rupture. Sac enlargement had been observed in 15 of 17 patients, with documented endoleaks in 12 of these 15 patients. In the remaining 2 patients, without sac expansion, one sustained graft migration and one presented an endoleak of undfinited origin. Three cases had a type II endoleak as previously described complications. All these patients presented concomitant sac enlargement before rupture. Twelve patients with a prior complication underwent a secondary intervention before rupture.

Surgical repair was performed in 12 out of 27 patients who experienced aneurysm rupture, with an overall surviving rate of 75%. Seven patients (4 in group A and 3 in group C) underwent open repair, 5 of whom survived more than 30 days, while endovascular treatment was performed in 5 patients (1 in group B and 4 in group C), 4 of whom survived more than 30 days. The remaining 15 patients died before aneurysm repair could be attempted.

In this study there was a significant association between rupture and previous detection of complications (type I endoleak, type II endoleak with sac expansion, type III endoleak with migration or kinking of the endograft) and no significant difference in rupture rate between the different kinds of endoprosthesis employed (Cook Zenith, Medtronic Talent, Gore Excluder, others). A risk of rupture doubling for each centimeter increase of top neck diameter was suspected. The analysis also suggested that age was an influential factor, with a risk of rupture increasing with age.

Bernhard et al [30] showed their experience with aneurysm rupture after deployment of Guidant/EVT endograft and reviewed previously reported cases with others devices. The authors collected 47 cases of ruptured AAA after EVAR from 1993 to 2000, seven of whom occurred after the use of Guidant/EVT devices. Causes of rupture are listed in table 7.

Type and source of endoleak	No. of patients
Type I endoleak	27
Proximal attachment	12†
Distal attachment	14
Aorta	10†
Iliac	4
Site not reported	1
Type II endoleak	2
Type III endoleak	11
Modular disconnection	5 (2‡)
Stent erosion through fabric	1
Details not reported	5
Leak present, source not reported	4

†Three patients met criteria for endotension (AAA enlargement in absence of detectable endoleak before AAA rupture). One had proximal leak shown at surgery. Another was classified as proximal leak on basis of known migration at proximal neck; however, no post rupture CT scan, surgery, or autopsy was found to verify this presumption. A third had initial increase in AAA diameter that remained stabile until rupture from distal aortic endoleak. Endoleak was recognized in retrospect.

‡Associated fabric tear in Dacron graft wall and disruption of sutures attaching it to metal frame.

From: Bernhard VM, Mitchell RS, Matsumura JS, Brewster DC, Decker M, Lamparello P, Raithel D, Collin J. Ruptured abdominal aortic aneurysm after endovascular repair.J VascSurg 2002;35:1155-62.

Table 7. Causes of rupture (n = 44 of 47 patients; cause not reported in three patients).

Mortality rate in these cases was 57% (4/7) overall and 50% for surgical repair (3/6). In the 40 additional ruptures related to other devices, for a total of 47, the overall mortality rate for the combined series was 50%, with an operative mortality rate of 41%.

Ruptures after implantation of Guidant/EVT occurred in patients with tube grafts and all were a consequence of a type I endoleak developed at the distal aortic attachment site. Five occurred in 93 patients followed for a mean of 41.8 months and treated with first-generation tube graft, which were prone to develop attachment mechanism fractures. The remaining two ruptures occurred in the subgroup of 166 patients who received second-generation tube endografts.

No ruptures were reported in patients who received bifurcated or unilateral iliac devices, over a mean follow-up of 37.5 months.

Factors contributing to endoleak and postoperative rupture are reported in table 8.

Contributing factors	No. of patients with contributing factors
Loss of endograft integrity	16
Endograft migration	10
Severe angulation of proximal aortic neck	6
Dilatation of distal aortic neck after implant	5
Patient refused intervention for endoleak	5
Delayed or discontinued follow-up	4*
Surgical conversion delayed	4
Poor patient selection	3
Wide distal neck lined with clot	2
Iliac artery attachment site too wide	1
Short proximal aortic neck	2
Error in deployment technique	2
Stiff graft body design	2
Proximal neck thrombus	1
Short distal aortic neck	1
Low graft implantation	1
AAA shrinkage	1
Total	63

*Two patients did not have CT scan for 11 months, although this delay waswithin prescribed time frame of investigational protocol.

Multiple contributing factors were reported in several patients; two in sevenpatients, three in seven patients, and five in two patients.

From: Bernhard VM, Mitchell RS, Matsumura JS, Brewster DC, Decker M, Lamparello P, Raithel D, Collin J. Ruptured abdominal aortic aneurysm after endovascular repair.J VascSurg 2002;35:1155-62.

Table 8. Factors contributing to endoleak and postoperative rupture (information reported for 34 of 47 patients).

http://dx.doi.org/10.5772/53415

In this investigation 9 out of 19 patients in which pre-rupture imaging was available suffered aneurysm rupture despite the absence of aneurysm enlargement. However most of these patients showed other abnormalities that could underlie a rupture.

Authors conclude that (1) the use of tube endografts should be restricted to the rare cases with ideal anatomy, no other alternatives and at high risk for open repair; (2) primary endoleaks have a tendency to early rupture, which entails the need to their treatment without delay; (3) prevention could be possible in some patients if there had been application of strict anatomic criteria for exclusion and rigorous adherence to prestabilited follow-up protocol; (4) outcomes of delayed aneurysm rupture after EVAR are similar to those expected for patients without prior endografts.

A study evaluating the AAA annual rupture risk in patients without detectable endoleak after EVAR (endotension) has been published in 2011 by Koole et al [23]. The basis for this analysis was 6337 patients who were enrolled prospectively in the EUROSTAR database between 1996 and 2006. Perioperative mortality rate of conversion to open AAA repair in these patients was also assessed.

In this study aneurysm enlargement was defined as a diameter increase >/= 8 mm relative to the preoperative diameter measurements. Patients were divided into three groups depending on the degree of shrinkage or enlargement of the aneurysm sac. Group A included patients with > 8 mm aneurysm shrinkage, group B consisted of patients with </= 8 mm shrinkage to </= 8 mm enlargement and group C presented an aneurysm enlargement of > 8 mm. Ruptures occurred in 26 patients: 3/691 (0.4%) patients in group A, 14/5307 (0.32%) patients in group B and 9/339 (2.6%) patients in group C. The median interval to aneurysm rupture after EVAR was 48 months and the mortality rate from rupture was 62%.

The annual rate of rupture in group C was < 1% in the first 4 years but increased to 7.5% up to 13.6% in the years thereafter (table 9), thus suggesting the need for conversion. The mortality rate of elective conversions to open repair was 6.0%. A significant higher conversion rate was observed in group C, compared with group A and B.

Year of FU	Combined FU[a] (years)	Ruptures (n)	Annual rupture rate (%)
1	264	0	0
2	206	1	0.5
3	149	0	0
4	102	0	0
5	67	5	7.5
6	37	0	0
7	22 3	1	3.6

FU, Follow-up; [a]Combined FU years were calculated for each interval.

From: Koole D, Moll FL, Buth J et al. Annual rupture risk of abdominal aortic aneurysm enlargement without detectable endoleak after endovascular abdominal aortic repair. J VascSurg 2011Dec;54(6):1614-22.

Table 9. An overview of the different annual rupture risks in group C.

The authors confirmed the role of aneurysm enlargement without detectable endoleak as an independent factor for conversion. Conventional CT angiography visualizing low-flow endoleaks with a blood-pool contrast agent, dynamic electrocardiographically gated CT angiography or MR angiography are suggested to possibly improve the sensitivity for detecting endoleaks [41-42], thus potentially resulting in a decreased mortality risk from rupture.

Interestingly in this study a large number of patients were lost to follow-up (50% in group A and B; 30% in group C). Consequently, a higher number of ruptures and a higher mortality could be imaginable.

In 2011 Metha et al [24] evaluated the frequency, etiology and outcomes of delayed AAA rupture following EVAR with the aim to estabilish treatment options that facilitated an improvement in survival. Over a mean follow-up of 29 months (range 14-111 months), 27 (1.5%) out of 1768 patients undergoing elective or emergent EVAR sustained delayed AAA rupture and required repair by either open surgical conversion or a redo endovascular treatment. Twenty (74%) patients were lost to follow-up, 17 (63%) patients had type I endoleak with stentgraft migration, 3 (11%) had type I endoleak without stent graft migration, 5 (19%) had type II endoleak and two (7%) experienced aneurysm rupture for undetermined causes. In 15 (55%) patients open surgical repair via retroperitoneal approach was performed, with partial (8 patients, 53%) or complete (7 patients, 47%) stentgraft explantation and aortoiliac reconstruction; 11 (41%) patients underwent a redo-EVAR and one (4%) patient refused treatment and died. Supraceliac aortic clamping was required in three (20%) patients, while supraceliac occlusion balloon was required in two (18%) patients during EVAR. There were three (11%) postoperative deaths: two after open conversion and one following EVAR.

Similar mortality rate are reported by other authors [43-45] despite the use of different techniques (midline vs retroperitoneal approach; supraceliac vs infrarenal vs aortic balloon clamping; complete or partial removal of the graft).

Interesting to note, in 2011 Venermo et al [46] reported that EVAR may reduce the risk of rupture and aneurysm-related mortality despite the presence of persisting proximal type I endoleak, compared to untreated AAA of similar size (11% vs 52%). However this study has some limitations, as it is retrospective, has small cohorts and the two groups are different not having being studied over the same time period or in the same geographic location. Moreover the EVAR group is likely to have received better medical treatment, with tighter blood pressure control and possible use of statins.

Age and sex are also different in this study while having an important impact on EVAR outcome. Suitability for EVAR was found to be associated with a lower rupture rate in unoperated aneurysms [47]. Therefore, knowing the aortic anatomy in the patients not undergoing EVAR would have been interesting.

6. Conclusion

In conclusion: the rupture risk for all EVAR patients is thought to be in the order of 0.5 to 1.2 per 100 patients per years [28,37] and it increases with age. Reasonably this is an underesti-

http://dx.doi.org/10.5772/53415

mated rupture rate as many patients are lost to follow-up and almost a few could have died because of aneurysm rupture.

Moreover, no precise description of the performed diagnostic examinations is provided and no fatal course is described in several publications; consequently, there may have been the possibility that many patients had a "symptomatic" AAA, instead of a ruptured one.

Relatively many ruptures occur between the follow up visits at 1 and 2 years after EVAR. An additional follow-up after 18 months may possibly reduce the AAA rupture rate. However, it is important to note that rupture can occur even for unknown reasons, despite an optimal protocol was followed.

The lesson learned when any major complication is found is that the underlying problem needs to be corrected whenever possible. Particularly, we agree with Chuter's recommendation to treat primary type I endoleaks without delay [48].

Conversion to open repair should be seriously considered, particularly if the complication is not resolved and the patient is fit enough for this intervention.

However, the risk of this approach will need to be evaluated prospectively, as there is a high risk of rupture if patients are left untreated and an uncertain mortality risk by conversion to open repair [4-7,49-52].

Better stentgraft durability and longevity is also required to further reduce this serious complication. Prospective long-term evaluation of specific devices will also be necessary to determine the reliability of endograft exclusion, as well increasing using of statins as protective factors to prevent rupture [47]. Endovascular repair outside manufacturer's instructions for use is associated with an unacceptable risk of proximal type I endoleak, aneurysm-related and all-causes mortality. Actually tube grafts should be limited to patients with ideal anatomy. In all other cases open surgery or use of fenestrated EVAR in short necks should be encouraged.

We strongly agree with Veith that until solution of these problems are found, EVAR will remain an imperfect long-term treatment with mortality rate for conversion in the setting of rupture remaining very high [53].

Author details

Guido Regina[1,4], Domenico Angiletta[1,4], Martinella Fullone[1,4], Davide Marinazzo[1,4], Francesco Talarico[2,3] and Raffaele Pulli[2]

1 Department of Vascular Surgery, University of Bari, Italy

2 Department of Vascular Surgery, University of Florence, Italy

3 Department of Vascular Surgery, Palermo, Italy

4 VASA-MG (Vascular-endovascular Surgery Association of Magna Graecia), Italy

References

[1] *Parodi JC, Palmaz JC, Barone HD.*Transfemoral intraluminal graft implantation for abdominal aortic aneurysms. *Ann VascSurg 1991;5: 491-9.*

[2] *Zarins CK, White RA, Fogarty TJ.* Aneurysm rupture after endovascular repair using the AneuRx stent graft. *J VascSurg 2000;31:960-70.*

[3] *Holzbein TJ, Kretschmer G, Thurnher S, et al.* Midterm durability of abdominal aortic aneurysm endograft repair: a word of caution. *J VascSurg 2001;33(2 Pt 2):46-54.*

[4] *Harris PL, Vallabhaneni SR, Desgranges P, et al.* Incidence and risk factors of late rupture, conversion, and death after endovascular repair of infrarenal aortic aneurysms: the EUROSTAR experience. European collaborators on stent/graft techniques for aortic aneurysm repair. *J VascSurg 2000;32:739-49.*

[5] *Ohki T, Veith FJ, Shaw P, et al.* Increasing incidence of mid and long-term complications after endovascular graft repair of AAAs: a note of caution based on a 9-year experience. *Ann Surg 2001;234:323-34.*

[6] *Brewster DC, Cronenwett JL, Hallett JW Jr, Johnston KW, Krupski WC, Matsumura JS.* Joint Council of the American Association for Vascular Surgery and Society for Vascular Surgery.Guidelines for the treatment of abdominal aortic aneurysms.Report of a subcommittee of the Joint Council of the American Association for Vascular Surgery and Society for Vascular Surgery.*J VascSurg 2003;37:1106-17.*

[7] *Brewster DC, Jones JE, Chung TK, Lamuraglia GM, Kwolek CJ, Watkins MT, et al.* Long-term outcomes after endovascular abdominal aortic aneurysm repair: the first decade. *Ann Surg 2006;244:426-38.*

[8] *Hinnen JW, Koning OHJ, van Bockel JH, Hamming JF.* Aneurysm sac pressure after EVAR: the role of endoleak. *Eur J VascEndovascSurg 2007;34:432-41.*

[9] *Schermerhorn ML, O'Malley AJ, Jhaveri A, Cotterill P, Pomposelli F, Landon BE.* Endovascular vs. open repair of abdominal aortic aneurysm in the Medicare population.*N Engl J Med 2008;358:464e74.*

[10] *Konig GG, Vallabhneni SR, Van Marrewijk CJ, Leurs LJ, Laheij RJ, Buth J.* Procedure-related mortality of endovascular abdominal aortic aneurysm repair using revised reporting standards. *Rev Bras Cir Cardiovasc 2007;22:7e13.*

[11] *Leurs LJ, Buth J, Laheij RJ.* Long-term results of endovascular abdominal aortic aneurysm treatment with the first generation of commercially available stent grafts.*Arch Surg 2007;142: 33e41.*

[12] *Franks SC, Sutton AJ, Bown MJ, Sayers RD.* Systematic review and meta-analysis of 12 years of endovascular abdominal aortic aneurysm repair. *Eur J VascEndovascSurg 2007;33:154e71.*

[13] *Sicard GA, Zwolak RM, Sidawy AN, White RA, Siami FS.* Endovascular abdominal aortic aneurysm repair: long-term outcome measures in patients at high-risk for open surgery. *J VascSurg 2006;44:229e36.*

[14] *Zarins CK.* The US AneuRx Clinical Trial: 6-year clinical update 2002. *J VascSurg 2003;37:904e8.*

[15] *Schermerhorn ML, Finlayson SR, Fillinger MF, Buth J, van Marrewijk C, Cronenwett JL.* Life expectancy after endovascular versus open abdominal aortic aneurysm repair: results of a decision analysis model on the basis of data from EUROSTAR. *J VascSurg 2002;36:1112e20.*

[16] *Greenhalgh RM, Brown LC, Powell JT, et al;* United Kingdom EVAR Trial Investigators.Endovascular versus open repair of abdominal aortic aneurysm. *N Engl J Med. 2010;362(20):1863-71.*

[17] *Prinssen M, Buskens E, Blankensteijn JD.* The Dutch Randomized Endovascular Aneurysm Management (DREAM) trial. Background, design and methods. *J Cardiovasc Surg 2002; 43(3):379-84.*

[18] *Paraskevas KI, Mikhailidis DP, Veith FJ.* Endovascular versus open repair of abdominal aortic aneurysms: interpreting the landmark United Kingdom EVAR-1 results. *J Endovasc Ther 2010; 17(5):599-601.*

[19] *Leurs LJ, Buth J, Harris PL, Blankenstejin JD.* Impact of study design on outcome after endovascular adbominal aneurysm repair. A comparison between the randomized controlled DREAM-trial and the observational EUROSTAR-registry. *Eur J Vasc Endovasc Surg 2007;33(2):172-6*

[20] *Hobo R, Sybrandy JE, Harris P, Buth J.* Endovascular repair of abdominal aortic aneurysms with concomitant iliac artery aneurysm. Outcome analysis of the EUROSTAR experience.*J EndovascTher. 2008;15:12-22.*

[21] *Szmidt J, Galazka Z, Rowinski O, Nazarewski S, Jakimowicz T, Pietrasik K, Grygiel K, Chudzinski W.* Late aneurysm rupture after endovascular abdominal aneurysm repair. *Interact Cardiovasc Thorac Surg. 2007 Aug;6(4):490-4.*

[22] *Wyss TR, Brown LC, Powell JT, Greenhalgh RM.* Rate and predictability of graft rupture after endovascular and open abdominal aortic aneurysm repair: data from the EVAR Trias. *Ann Surg 2010;252(5):805-12.*

[23] *Koole D, Moll FL, Buth J et al.* Annual rupture risk of abdominal aortic aneurysm enlargement without detectable endoleak after endovascular abdominal aortic repair. *J VascSurg 2011Dec;54(6):1614-22.*

[24] *Metha M, Paty PS, Roddy SP et al.* Treatment options for delayed AAA rupture following endovascular repair. *J VascSurg 2011Jan;53(1):14-20.*

[25] *Mehta M, Sternbach Y, Taggert JB, Kreienberg PB, Roddy SP, Paty PS, Ozsvath KJ, Darling RC 3rd.* Long-term outcomes of secondary procedures after endovascular aneurysm repair. *J Vasc Surg. 2010 Dec;52(6):1442-9)*

[26] *De Bruin Jl, Baas AF, Buth J, Prinssen M, Verhoeven EL, Cuypers PW, et al.* DREAM study Group. Long-term outcome of open or endovascular repair of abdominal aortic aneurysm. *N Engl J Med 2010;362:1881-9*

[27] *Moll FL, Powell JT, Fraedrich G, et al.* Management of abdominal aortic aneurysms clinical practice guidelines of the European society for vascular surgery. *Eur J Vasc Endovasc Surg 2011;41(Suppl 1):S1-S58.*

[28] *Conner MS 3rd, Sternbergh WC 3rd, Carter G, Tonnessen BH, Yoselevitz M, Money SR.* Secondary procedures after endovascular aortic aneurysm repair. *J Vasc Surg Nov 2002; 36(5):992-6*

[29] *Ronsivalle S, Faresin F, Franz F, Rettore C, Zanchetta M and Olivieri A.* Aneurysm Sac "Thrombization" and Stabilization in EVAR: A Technique to Reduce the Risk of Type II Endoleak. *J Endovasc Ther. 2010; 17:4, 517-24.*

[30] *Bernhard VM, Mitchell S, Matsumura JS, Brewster DC, Decker M, Lamparello P, Raithel D, Collin J.* Ruptured abdominal aortic aneurysm after endovascular repair. *J Vasc Surg 2002; 35:1155-62.*

[31] *Kantonen I, Lepäntalo M, Brommels M, Luther M, Salenius J-P, Ylönen K.* Mortality in ruptured abdominal aortic aneurysms. The Finnvasc Study Group. *Eur J VascEndovascSurg 1999;17:208-12.*

[32] *Schlösser FJV, Gusberg RJ, Dardik A, Lin PH, Verhagen HJM, Moll FL and Muhs BE.* Aneurysm rupture after EVAR: can the ultimate failure be predicted? *Eur J VascEndovascSurg 2009;37(1):15-22.*

[33] *Acosta S, Ogren M, Bengtsson H, Bergqvist D, Lindblad B, Zdanowski Z.* Increasing incidence of ruptured abdominal aortic aneurysm: a population-basedstudy. *J VascSurg 2006;44:237e43.*

[34] *Wilmink AB, Hubbard CS, Day NE, Quick CR.* The incidence of small abdominal aortic aneurysms and the change in normal infrarenal aortic diameter: implications for screening. *Eur J VascEndovascSurg 2001;21:165e70.*

[35] *Fransen GA, Vallabhaneni SrSR, Van Marrewijk CJ, Laheij RJ, Harris PL, Buth J.* Rupture of infra-renal aortic aneurysm after endovascular repair: a series from EUROSTAR registry. *Eur J VascEndovascSurg 2003;26:487e93.*

[36] *Zarins CK, Crabtree T, Bloch DA, Arko FR, Ouriel K, White RA.* Endovascular aneurysm repair at 5 years: does aneurysm diameter predict outcome? *J VascSurg 2006;44:920e9.*

[37] *Lifeline registry of EVAR publications committee.* Lifeline registry of endovascular aneurysm repair: long-term primary outcome measures. *J VascSurg 2005;42:1e10.*

[38] *Peppelenbosch N, Buth J, Harris PL, van Marrewijk C, Fransen G.* Diameter of abdominal aortic aneurysm and outcome of endovascular aneurysm repair: does size matter? A report from EUROSTAR.*J VascSurg 2004;39:288e97.*

[39] *Jones JE, Atkins MD, Brewster DC, Chung TK, Kwolek CJ, LaMuraglia GM, et al.* Persistent type 2 endoleak after endovascular repair of abdominal aortic aneurysm is associated with adverse late outcomes. *J VascSurg 2007;46:1e8.*

[40] *Greenhalgh RM, Brown LC, Powell JT, et al; United Kingdom EVAR Trial Investigators.* Endovascular repair of aortic aneurysm in patients physically ineligible for open repair. N Eng J Med. 2010;362(20):1872-80.

[41] *Cornelissen SA, Prokop M, Verhagen HJ, Adriaensen ME, Moll FL, Bartels LW.* Detection of occult endoleaks after endovascular treatment of abdominal aortic aneurysm using magnetic resonance imaging with a blood pool contrast agent: preliminary observations. *Invest Radiol 2010;45:548-53.*

[42] *Cornelissen SA, Verhagen HJ, Prokop M, Moll FL, Bartels LW.* Visualizing type IV endoleak using magnetic resonance imaging with a blood pool contrast agent. *J VascSurg 2008;47:861-4.*

[43] *Kelso RL, Lyden SP, Butler B, Greenberg RK, Eagleton MJ, Clair DG.* Late conversion of aortic stent grafts.*J VascSurg 2009;49:589-95.*

[44] *Coppi, G., Gennai, S. &Saitta, G.* Treatment of ruptured abdominal aortic aneurysm after endovascular abdominal aortic repair: A comparison with patients without prior treatment. *J VascSurg 2009;49(3):582-8.*

[45] *Lyden SP, McNamara JM, Sternbach Y et al.* Technical considerations for late removal of aortic endografts. *J VascSurg 2002;36:674-8.*

[46] *Venermo MA, Arko III FR, Salenius JP, Saarinen JP, Zvaigzne A, Zarins CK.* EVAR May Reduce the Risk of Aneurysm Rupture Despite Persisting Type IaEndoleaks. *J EndovascTher. Oct 2011.18(5): 676-682.*

[47] *Powell JT, Brown LC, Greenhalgh RM, et al.* The rupture rate of large abdominal aortic aneurysms: is this modified by anatomical suitability for endovascular repair? *Ann Surg. 2008;247: 173–179.*

[48] *Chuter TAM, Risberg B, Hopkinson BR, Wendt G, Scott AP, Walker PJ, et al.* Clinical experience with a bifurcated endovascular graft for abdominal aortic aneurysm repair.*J Vasc Surg. 1996;24:655–666.*

[49] *Millon A, Deelchand A, Feugier P, et al.* Conversion to open repair after endovascular aneurysm repair: causes and results. A French Multicentric Study.*Eur J VascEndovasc Surg. 2009;38(4):429–434.*

[50] *Pitoulias GA, Schulte S, Donas KP, et al.* Secondary endovascular and conversion procedures for failed endovascular abdominal aortic aneurysm repair: can we still be optimistic? *Vascular 2009;17(1):15–22.*

[51] *Dick F, Greenhalgh RM*. Three-dimensional imaging for EVAR: importance of precise neck length and angulation. *In: Greenhalgh RM, ed. Vascular andEndovascular Controversies Update. London, UK: BIBA Publishing; 2009: 189–195.*

[52] *Brown LC, Greenhalgh RM, Powell JT, et al*. Use of baseline factors to predict complications and re-interventions after endovascular aneurysm repair for abdominal aortic aneurysm. *Br J Surg. 2010;97(8):1207–1217.*

[53] *Veith FJ, Baum RA, Ohki T, Amor M, Adiseshiah M, et al*. Nature and significance of endoleaks and endotension: Summary of opinions expressed at an international conference. *J VascSurg 2002;35(5):1029-35.*

Chapter 8

Endovascular Treatment of Endoleaks Following EVAR

Zaiping Jing, Qingsheng Lu, Jiaxuan Feng and Jian Zhou

Additional information is available at the end of the chapter

http://dx.doi.org/10.5772/54836

1. Introduction

Since the first endovascular aneurysm repair (EVAR) of abdominal aortic aneurysm (AAA) was introduced 20 years ago, work toward reducing the morbidity and mortality has never been halted. Technological advances, as well as increased operator experience, have significantly reduced post-EVAR complications, such as peripheral embolization, postimplantation rupture, graft migration, and contrast-induced nephropathy, et al. However, endoleak — the persistent flow of blood within the aneurysm sac — is one of the major reasons for lifelong imaging surveillance.

Endoleaks are often considered significantly adverse event of EVAR since persistentce of blood flow and pressure in the aneurysm sac. It continues to be a challenge in the endovascular approach to AAA repair. Some of these leaks are related to anatomic factors and patient selection, others are device related, and some (especially type II leaks) seem to be intrinsic to the endovascular procedure. Certain endoleaks require treatment as soon as they are detected to continue to perfuse and pressurize the aneurysm sac, thereby conferring an ongoing risk of aneurysm enlargement and rupture. But the need for treatment of others remains controversial, since the associated increase in intrasac pressure varies depending on the type of endoleak. Using endovascular techniques, the majority of endoleak can be successfully treated, without the need for open surgery. In this chapter, we will introduce the classification, clinical relevance and endovascular management of the endoleaks after EVAR.

2. Definition of endoleak

More than 20 years after the procedure was introduced to treat AAA, it is remarkable that certain aspects of endovascular treatment for AAA remain poorly understood. One major issue is the occurrence and significance of endoleaks. White et al were the first to systematically describe and classify endoleaks, describing five major categories [1]. And these five types of endoleaks have been described by Ad Hoc Committee for standardized reporting practices of EVAR in the Society for Vascular Surgery/ American Association for Vascular Surgery [2]. There were type I to IV endoleaks, and a supplementary category of "endoleaks of undefined origin" which was defined as flow visualized but source undetermined. And there was a separate adjunctive category of "endotension", which was referred to instances of aneurysm expansion after EVAR without detectable flow in aneurysm sac.

- Type I endoleak is defined as a sealing failure at one of the attachment sites of the graft to the vessel wall (proximal leak, type Ia; distal, type Ib; inadequate seal at iliac occlude plug, type Ic). Arterial flow therefore leaks alongside the graft and into the perigraft space.
- Type II endoleak is defined as retrograde flow through collateral vessels (lumbar artery, inferior mesenteric artery, hypogastric artery, and accessory renal artery et al.) into the the aneurysmal sac.
- Type III endoleak is defined as graft failure. Type IIIa endoleak is referred to flow from module disconnection, and type IIIb is flow from fabric disruption.
- Type IV endoleak is from porous fabric of the stent graft.

A more detailed classification of endoleaks and endotension was introduced by an international consensus of experts [3]. The classification included type I to IV endoleaks, and endotension (also recognized as type V endoleak) (see Table 1). As experience has been gained, it is clear that, in some cases, an endoleak can involve more than one mechanism.

Type	Description: source of perigraft flow
I	Attachment site leaks
	Proximal end of endograft
	Distal end of endograft
	Iliac occlude (plug)
II	Branch leaks (without attachment connection)
	Simple or to-and-from (from only 1 patent branch)
	Complex or flow-through (with 2 or more patent branches)
III	Graft defect
	Junction leak or modular disconnection
	Fabric disruption (midgraft hole)
	Minor (<2mm; eg. Suture hole)
	Major (>2mm)
IV Endotension	Graft wall (fabric) porosity; <30days of placement

Type	Description: source of perigraft flow
	Any elevation of intrasac pressure without evidence of endoleak
	Without endoleak
	With sealed endoleak ("virtual endoleak")
	With type I or type III endoleak
	With type II endoleak

Adapted from Veith FJ, Baum RA, Ohki T, Amor M, Adiseshiah M, Blankensteijn JD, et al. Nature and significance of endoleaks and endotension: summary of opinions expressed at an international conference. J Vasc Surg. 2002 May;35(5): 1029-35. With permission.

Table 1. Classification of endoleaks and endotension after endovascular aortic repair.

Besides the cause of perigraft flow, the endoleaks can be classified according to the time of first detection as perioperative (within 24 hours), early (within 90 days after the primary EVAR) and late (more than 3 months after the primary procedure). And endoleaks can also be described as persistent, transient or sealed, recurrent, successfully treated or unsuccessfully treated.

3. Type I endoleak

As this flow is direct and under systemic pressure, it represents a failure in treatment of the aneurysm, which continues to be pressurized and at risk of continued expansion and rupture. Previous study demonstrated that mean pressure index (sac pressure divided by systemic pressure) was varied in the liquid and in the thrombosed sections of the sac after EVAR. They found that type I endoleaks were associated with mean pressure indexes of 93% in the liquid areas and 62% in the thrombus [4]. So it is mandatory to correct type I endoleaks whenever possible, as spontaneous resolution over time cannot be expected.

The incidence of type I endoleak is not low, especially for cases with difficult anatomy situations. The incidence has been reported to be more than 10% of EVAR procedures, with 4.2% at 30 days, 3.5% within 1 year, and 6.7% at 3 year [5].

4. Proximal type I endoleak (type Ia endoleak)

When AAA are with short neck (proximal attachment zones <15 mm), large neck (diameter >32 mm), irregular neck (such as cone-shaped neck), uneven neck (calcification or thrombus) and proximal angulations >60°, the incidence can be higher than the above mentioned [6]. In common circumstances, 20% oversizing of the proximal endograft attachment and deploying the endograft close to the origin of the renal arteries can help to prevent type Ia endoleak and achieve satisfying sealing.

In the pivotal trial period of EVAR, case selection involved adherence to fairly rigorous anatomic criteria, including vessel size, angulation, shape, length of the infrarenal neck, and adequacy of the distal landing zones. With increasing experience and the availability of newer devices, these criteria have been weakened. Nevertheless, there remain certain types of anatomy that are not well suited to EVAR and are best treated with open surgical technique. Proximal attachment zones less than 10 mm, particularly with angulation greater than 60°, present insurmountable problems with the use of currently available devices.

The development of devices more suitable to extreme degrees of angulation, fenestrated and branched devices, and improvement of sealing mechanisms (ie, endovascular stapling) have expanded the use of EVAR. But as the selection criteria of candidates for EVAR have expanded over time, the detection of type Ia endoleak has become more frequent.

The current availability of various proximal extender cuffs (Figure 1) and other modular devices (such as ballooning and bare stent, Figure 2) for dealing with attachment site leaks has allowed most of these leaks to be treated at the time of the initial procedure. Deployment of Palmaz stent (Cordis Endovascular, Johnson and Johnson Co. UK) or sinus-XL Stent (OptiMed, Ettlingen, Germany) to diminish the proximal type I endoleak was introduced [7] (Figure 3).

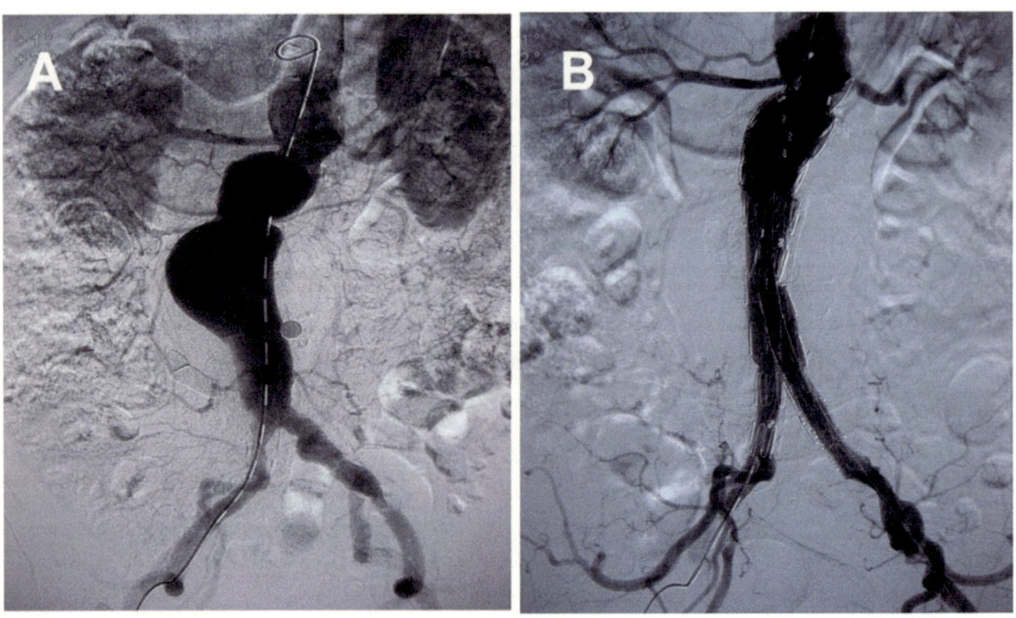

Figure 1. For abdominal aortic aneurysm with saccular neck, adjunctive short-large Cuff is effective to diminish type Ia endoleak, and realize best proximal fixation.

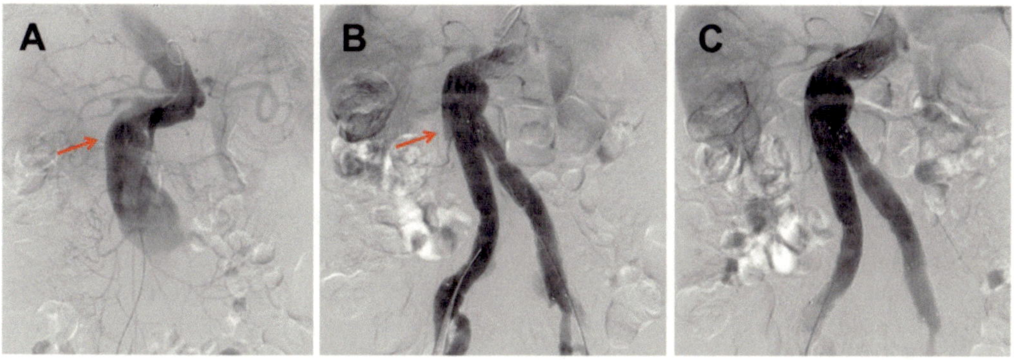

Figure 2. A: Pre-operative angiography revealed the AAA with irregular neck and severe angulation. B: Intra-operative angiography confirmed the significant type Ia endoleak. C: After proximal ballooning, the endoleak was diminished.

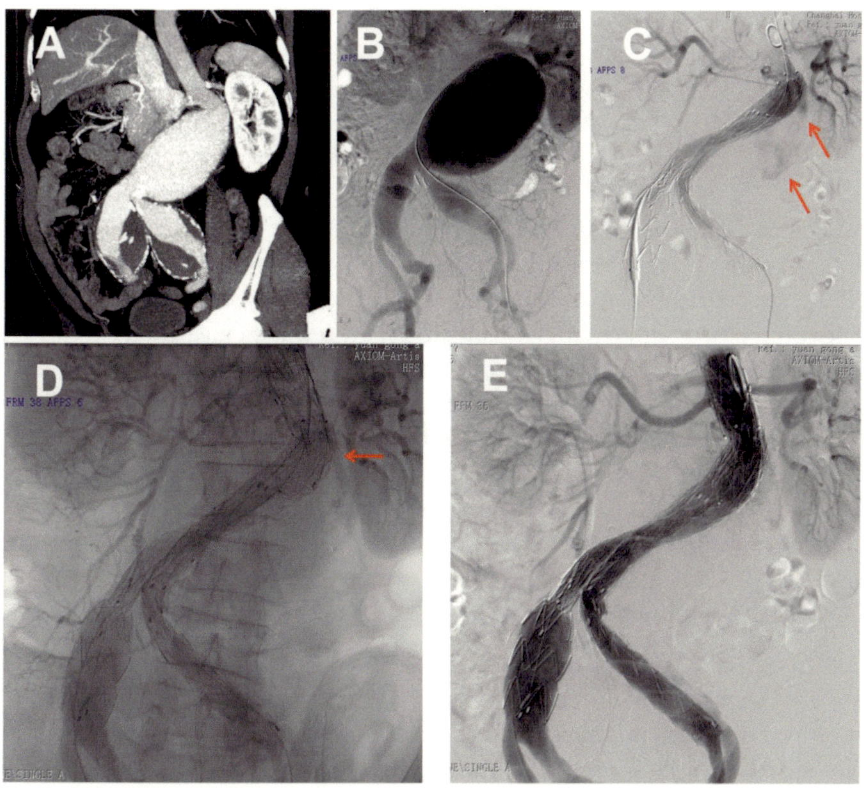

Figure 3. A: Pre-operative CTA revealed AAA, with large aneurism sac (maximal diameter≈90mm) and angulated neck. B: Pre-operative angiography confirmed the large AAA, and bilateral iliac artery aneurysms. C: After the bifurcated endograft and distal extension were deployed, there was remarkable type Ia endoleak. D: After the proximal cuff and ballooning, the type I endoleak was improved, but still significant. E: Proximal bare stent was deployed (sinus-XL Stent, OptiMed, Ettlingen, Germany)), and the final angiography evidenced the diminished endoleak.

However, under some circumstances, such as when the proximal edge of the stent-graft is very close to the renal artery, proximal cuffs cannot further extend the proximal fixation zone. If balloon dilation and additional bare stents cannot eliminate the leak alongside the graft fixation zone, then other practical options are needed to resolve the difficulty endoluminally.

5. Fibrin glue sac embolization to treat type Ia endoleak

Embolization techniques were introduced for treating type I endoleak >10 years ago [8]. The use of microcoils, n-butyl 2-cyanoacrylate adhesive, or other embolic agents (such as Onyx) have been utilized to treat type I endoleaks, but their effectiveness is still unproven [6,9,10]. Studies of fibrin glue embolization of endoleak are few and primarily focused on the prevention of type II endoleak [11-13]. So we examined our 5-year experience using fibrin glue to assess the technique's feasibility, safety, and effectiveness in treating type I endoleaks in the intraoperative setting.

6. Methods

6.1. EVAR procedure

Between August 2002 to February 2009, 783 patients with AAA underwent EVAR at our institution. All patients were evaluated preoperatively with computed tomographic angiography (CTA); appropriate reconstructions from the CT datasets were analyzed on a workstation (Leonardo; Siemens, Erlangen, Germany) to obtain pertinent measurements for endograft sizing (20% oversizing typically used). During the EVAR procedure, endoleaks were identified by angiography and classified as delineated in the current reporting standards [2]. According to our policy, type I endoleaks were treated at the time of diagnosis. If a type I endoleak was still present after proximal balloon dilation and cuff placement, or if a proximal cuff could not be placed because of a short landing zone, a standard procedure was employed to embolize the aneurysm sac using fibrin glue.

6.2. Embolization technique

According to our standard EVAR protocol, a 0.035-inch guidewire was positioned in the aneurysm sac before the main body of the stent-graft was deployed. In patients with a persistent type I endoleak after initial closure procedures failed, a 23-mm-long 5-F Brite Tip introducer sheath (Cordis Europe, Roden, The Netherlands) was advanced along the preloaded guidewire into the aneurysm sac. An aneurysmogram was performed to demonstrate the patency of the aneurysm and the flow direction in the aortic branches, such as the lumbar and hypogastric arteries. If no other source of the leak could be found, such as an accessory renal artery arising from the aneurysm or combined types I and II endoleaks, a pressure transducer (Edwards Lifesciences, Irvine, CA, USA) was connected to the 5-F catheter [14]. The intrasac pressure was measured by placing the catheter tip at 3 different locations around the nidus of the endoleak. The mean of the 3 pressures was recorded, as were the systolic, diastolic, and mean systemic pressures and the pulse pressure. The mean pressure indexes (MPI, sac pressure divided by systemic pressure) were calculated.

Next, a 25-cm-long, double-lumen Duplocath catheter (Baxter/Hyland Immuno AG, Vienna, Austria) connected to a Duploject Y-connector was introduced into the Brite Tip sheath. To block proximal blood flow when the glue was injected, a balloon was positioned in the proximal native aorta. The 5-mL aprotinin and thrombin solutions (Bei Xiu Biotech Co. Ltd., Guangzhou, PR China) were injected into the aneurysm sac through the 2 syringes of the Duploject Y-connector; the components synthesized fibrin glue in the sac as they mixed. Blocking proximal blood at this time facilitates formation of the clot. After the fibrin glue injection, the intrasac pressure was again recorded to monitor the change caused by embolization. The embolization procedure was repeated until the type I endoleak was eliminated, as evidenced by stable contrast inside the sac, a decrease in the intrasac pressure, and angiography (Figure 4).

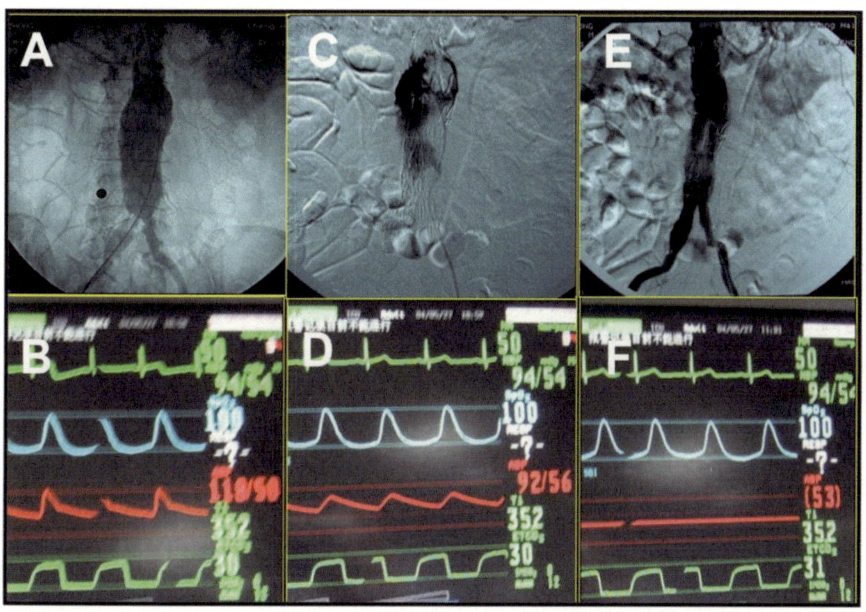

Figure 4. A: Abdominal aortic aneurysm with severe calcified neck. B: The system pressure was revealed by the red wave and number: 118/50mmHg. C: The intra-operative angiography after the first endografting revealed type Ia endoleak. Proximal cuff and ballooning could not eliminate the endoleak. D: The Intra-sac Pressure was measured by pre-placed intrasac catheter. The sac pressure was 92/56 mmHg. E: After intra-sac jel coagulation, the endoleak was eliminated. F: The intra-sac pressure decreased. The amplitude of the systolic-diastolic waveform was reduced significantly after the fibrin glue embolization, which was considered as a sign of diminish of endoleak.

In follow-up, CTA was performed at 3, 6, and 12 months and annually thereafter. Maximum aneurysm diameter and the presence of endoleaks were recorded. A >2-mm decrease in sac diameter was considered significant. The endpoints of follow-up were death and severe ischemic events, such as paraplegia, ischemic intestinal obstruction, renal artery occlusion, and lower limb ischemia.

6.3. Patient sample

A retrospective review of records and our department's vascular database was conducted to identify all patients who underwent fibrin glue sac embolization for type I endoleak. The search found 42 (5.4%) patients (37 men; mean age 73±8 years, range 51–88) who had persistent type I endoleaks treated intraoperatively with intrasac fibrin glue injection. Patient and aneurysm characteristics are given in Table 1. The mean maximal aneurysm diameter was 59.5±14.7 mm (range 41–100). The mean diameter of the proximal neck was 21.4±4.5 mm, and the mean length was 22.7±14.7 mm; notably, 16 (38.1%) patients had proximal necks <10 mm long. Five (11.9%) patients had proximal neck angulation >60°.

Patient characteristics	
Age, y	73.31±8.35
Men	37 (88.1%)
Comorbidities	38 (90.5%)
Hypertension	28 (66.7%)
Hyperlipidemia	8 (19.0%)
Diabetes	3 (7.1%)
Urinary system diseases*	8 (19.0%)
Coronary heart disease	8 (19.0%)
Pulmonary disease†	7 (16.7%)
Tobacco use ("/>20 years)	27 (62.3%)
Aneurysm characteristics	
Maximal aneurysm diameter, mm	59.5±14.7
Aneurysm length, mm	84.1±30.4
Proximal neck diameter, mm	21.4±4.5
Proximal neck length, mm	22.7±14.7
Proximal neck length <10 mm	16 (38.1%)
Proximal neck angulation	38.5±30.7
Proximal neck angle "/>60°	5 (11.9%)

Continuous data are presented as means ± standard deviation; categorical data are given as counts (percentages).

*Chronic renal failure, cyst, urinary stone, renal artery stenosis.

†Chronic obstructive pulmonary disease, tuberculosis.

Table 2. Patient and Aneurysm Characteristics

The most commonly used stent-graft was the Talent model (Medtronic Vascular, Santa Rosa, CA, USA) in 32 (76.2%) patients, following by the Zenith (Cook Inc., Bloomington, IN, USA) in 6 (14.3%), and the Aegis (MicroPort Medical, Shanghai, People's Republic of China) in 4 (9.5%). Twenty (47.6%) patients had more than 1 stent-graft deployed to exclude the aneurysm. The mean oversizing rate was 21.2%±12.0% in this cohort.

6.4. Statistical analysis

Parametric data are presented as mean ± standard deviation; nonparametric data (e.g., follow-up time) are given as median and range. Survival analysis was performed using the Kaplan-Meier method; comparisons were examined using a paired sample *t* test. A threshold of 0.05 was used for statistical significance.

7. Results

In the 42 patients with type I endoleak resistant to first-line procedures (balloon dilation and stent/cuff placement), 22 additional devices (8 stents, 14 cuffs) were placed in the initial attempts to resolve the endoleak. After fibrin glue injection, 41 (97.6%) of the 42 endoleaks were resolved with a mean 15±10 ml of glue. Nearly half of the patients (20, 47.6%) received ≤10 mL of glue; 5 (11.9%) patients needed >30 ml. One endoleak persisted despite proximal cuff implantation and the use of 30 ml of glue.

Systolic, diastolic, mean, and pulse pressures and the MPI were all significantly decreased after fibrin glue embolization, especially the pulse pressure (Table 2). The amplitude of the systolic-diastolic waveforms of the 41 successfully treated patients were reduced significantly after the fibrin glue embolization, which was considered as a sign of diminish of endoleak.

Pressure	Pre-embolization		Post-embolization		Decrease	
	Sac Pressure, mmHg	MPI, %	Sac Pressure, mmHg	MPI, %	Sac Pressure, mmHg	MPI, %
Systolic	119.3±18.6	92.2±5.3	44.7±9.4	34.1±6.2	74.5±12.1*	57.9±4.2*
Diastolic	70.3±9.3	79.5±7.6	38.7±5.9	43.2±6.7	31.7±5.7*	27.0±5.1*
Mean	86.6±12.2	87.8±4.4	40.7±6.9	35.6±6.4	46.0±7.5*	51.2±3.2*
Pulse	48.8±10.3	124.1±8.4	6.0±4.0	15.3±9.5	42.8±8.0*	108.5±6.2*

Data are presented as means ± standard deviation.

MPI: mean pressure index.

*p<0.05.

Table 3. Comparison Between Pre- and Post-embolization Intrasac Pressures

No patient exhibited an allergic response to fibrin glue injection, but 1 (2.4%) patient developed right lower extremity ischemia, which was related to wire/catheter manipulations rather than the fibrin glue treatment itself. The 80-year-old patient who had a failed fibrin glue attempt was converted to open surgery; he died in the Intensive Care Unit 2 months later from multiorgan dysfunction syndrome. Two patients who were successfully treated by fibrin glue injection succumbed to myocardial infarction within 5 days of the EVAR procedure (30-day mortality 4.8%).

Over a median follow-up of 39.9 months (range 10–88), the surviving patients complied with the surveillance protocol without loss to follow-up. Three patients died; 1 death was due to progression of an untreated AAA and the others to causes unrelated to aortic aneurysm disease. Cumulative survival was 90.5% at 1 year, 87.0% at 3 years, 82.6% at 5 years.

The mean maximal aneurysm diameter at the latest follow-up visit in 39 patients was 49.0±11.6 mm, significantly different from the 59.5±14.7 mm preoperative maximal aneurysm diameter ($p<0.001$). Postoperative maximal aneurysm diameters decreased in 25 patients and were stable in 10 patients. Of the 4 patients with increased aneurysm diameter detected during follow-up, a 73-year-old patient had a 22-mm increase after 44 months owing to a type IV endoleak; this patient was converted to open surgery. Two other patients (81 and 77 years of age) had diameter increases of 23 mm after 4 months and 6 mm after 34 months, respectively, but no blood flow within the aneurysm sac was found by CTA. Considering their advanced age, these patients are being closely followed. The last patient had a 20-mm increase after 4 months; he died of renal failure brought on by renal artery compression from the enlarged aneurysm, but no endoleak could be found. No stent-graft dislocation, fracture, or other complication was found in the follow-up period; in particular, no recurrence of type I endoleak was revealed by follow-up CTA.

8. Discussion

Various proximal extender cuffs and other adjuncts, such as balloon molding and bare stents, can deal with most of type I endoleaks once detected. However, when no sufficient landing zone is available proximally, the potential to occlude the renal arteries precludes the deployment of a proximal cuff. In some cases, even proximal balloon dilation and extension cuff implantation cannot resolve the type I endoleak. Under these circumstances, catheter-based procedures, including glue and/or coil deposition, can be performed [9,10]. Maldonado et al. reported the success rates for several methods of treating type I endoleaks: n-butyl cyanoacrylate 92.3%, extender cuffs 80%, and coils with or without thrombin 75%. Microcoil embolization can be laborious and time-consuming. Moreover, when numerous coils are deployed, the financial burden is too great for our patients without medical insurance, so we employed fibrin glue. In our study, which had a larger sample and longer follow-up, 98% of the type I endoleaks were eliminated by transcatheter fibrin glue embolotherapy, superior to the other methods tested so far.

http://dx.doi.org/10.5772/54836

Fibrin glue is a non-cytotoxic, fully resorbable biological adhesive matrix. The 2 main components are a fibrinogen solution containing plasmatic proteins and factor XIII and a thrombin solution with calcium chloride and an antifibrinolytic agent, such as aprotinin. The fibrinogen component, when mixed with thrombin, is converted into polymerizing fibrin monomers. Factor XIII is activated by thrombin in the presence of calcium ions, and the premature lysis of the clot is prevented by aprotinin. Mixing fibrinogen and thrombin simulates the environment of the last stages of the natural coagulation cascade to form a structured fibrin clot similar to a physiological clot, which may be naturally degraded by proteolytic enzymes from the fibrinolytic system, such as plasmin. As a result of its hemostatic and adhesive properties, fibrin glue has been extensively used in Europe in most surgical specialties for over 3 decades to reduce postoperative bleeding, to increase tissue plane adherence, for drug delivery, and in regenerative medicine or tissue engineering [15]. In animal experiments, Pacanowski et al. showed that fibrin glue injection could reduce the strain and pressure transmitted to the aortic aneurysm wall after endovascular exclusion, similar to fresh thrombus [16].

Several studies have reported the safety and effectiveness of fibrin glue for preventing/treating type II endoleaks by the transarterial or direct sac puncture method [11-13,17]. However, the application of fibrin glue to treat type I endoleak has evoked several concerns, namely, the possibility of outflow vessel embolization (such as inferior mesenteric artery and lumbar artery), which may cause ischemia or infarction; the potential for aneurysm thrombosis under systematic pressure; and endoleak recurrence in the long term.

To counter these concerns, we performed angiography to rule out collateral circulation, so all of our patients had pure type I endoleaks. Second, before the injection of fibrin glue, blood flow in the proximal native aorta was blocked by a balloon so that the glue mixture could form a structured fibrin clot and achieve aneurysm sac thrombosis. This procedure prevented embolic clot runoff into a collateral channel. Third, fibrin glue injection in our hands was highly effective in eliminating type I endoleaks, with sustained resolution through a mean 40 months of follow-up. During that time, the mean maximal aneurysm diameter decreased significantly by 9 mm, a strong indicator of durable aneurysm exclusion [18]. Moreover, no fibrin glue–related complication or mortality was encountered in follow-up.

To monitor the effects of glue injection, intrasac pressure and MPI were measured routinely in our patients. Type I endoleaks were associated with elevated MPI in the majority of cases, which was similar to the data from Dias et al [4]. According to the physical theory $Tc = pR/2$, tension (Tc) in the aneurysm wall rises with increased intrasac pressure (p) [19]. Comparing pre- and post-embolization intrasac pressures, we found significant pressure reductions after embolization, especially in the pulse pressure, reflecting diminished radial tension in the aneurysm wall.

Intrasac pressure monitoring is still a controversial issue. Some studies have discussed the relationship between intrasac pressure and endoleak changes [14, 20], citing these variables as markers of successful embolization. Dias et al. found that the pressure varied in different areas of the perigraft space and according to the content within the aneurysm sac, which brought into question the accuracy of the intrasac pressure monitoring [4]. So, for every pressure measurement, we placed the catheter tip at 3 different locations around the endoleak. Moreover, the intrasac pressures, especially the pulse pressure, did indeed decrease in the same measurement location after fibrin glue embolization. Thus, the intrasac pressure measurement, accompanied by final angiography, provided reliable proof of endoleak elimination.

9. Conclusion of the fibrin glue embolization to treat type I endoleak

Fibrin glue sac embolization to eliminate type I endoleak after EVAR yielded optimal results in our study, with nearly all the type I endoleaks resolved and no recurrence in follow-up. We believe that fibrin glue embolization may be an ideal option for treating type I endoleak in patients with unfavorable proximal neck anatomy and an alternative to cuff extension with chimney graft rescue of covered renal arteries [21]. Balloon occlusion of the proximal aorta must be done during glue injection to block proximal flow and facilitate formation of a structured fibrin clot. Intrasac pressure monitoring, as well as aortography, appear to be reliable methods of evaluating the effectiveness of fibrin glue sac embolization.

As to prevent the type Ia endoleak on unfavorable aneurysm neck, branched stent-graft, fenestrated stent-graft, or chimney techniques can extend the proximal sealing zone. We believe that this is the trend to decrease the incidence of type Ia endoleak. So in this way, in the last 3 years, the frequency of fibrin glue sac embolization has been significantly reduced.

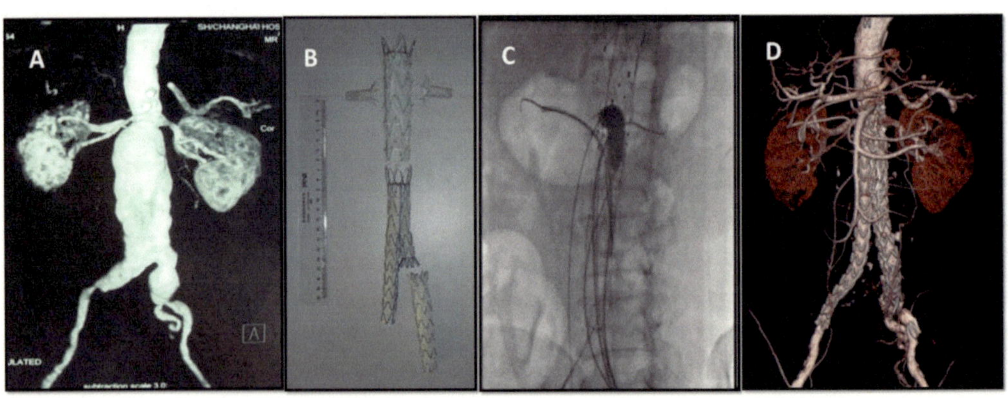

Figure 5. A. Juxta-renal AAA. B. Home-made fenestrated stent-graft of vascular surgery department, Changhai hospital, Shanghai, China. C. Intra-operative alignment. D: 2-year follow-up CTA showed complete exclusion of the AAA, and patent RA and SMA.

http://dx.doi.org/10.5772/54836

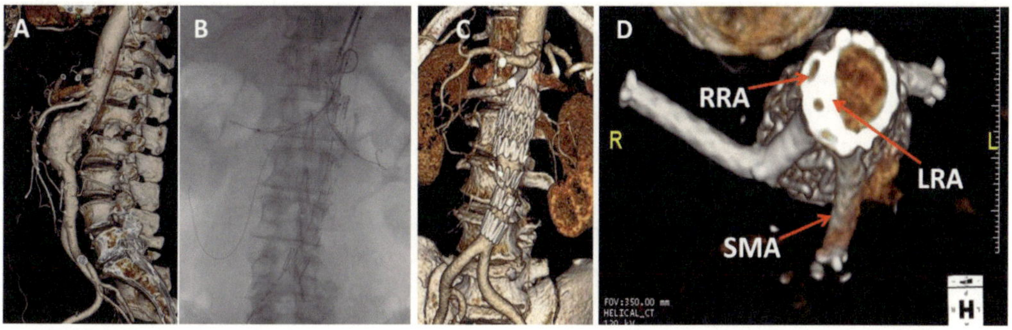

Figure 6. A. Juxta-renal AAA. B. Stenting the RA and SMA before the endografting. C and D: 1-year follow-up demonstrated complete exclusion of the aneurysm and patent branch arteries.

10. Distal type I endoleak (type Ib endoleak)

The type Ib endoleak is more common in patients with dilated, calcified, short and tortuous iliac arteries. This can occur when the limb of the graft is too short or migrates upwards due to sac retraction and aortic distortion. Sometimes, when the common iliac artery is short, and the hypogastric artery need to be preserved, distal bare stent can be used to prevent upwards migrates of the iliac extension (Figure 7).

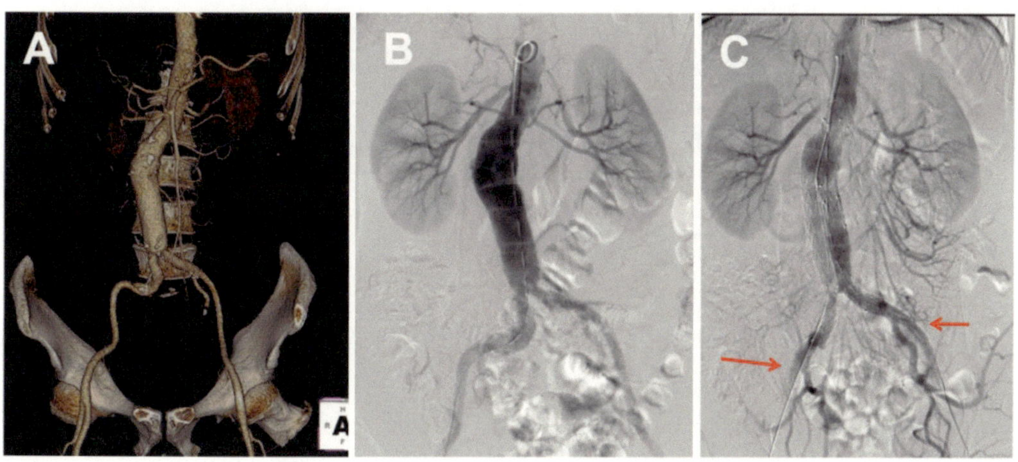

Figure 7. A: 3D reconstruction of pre-operative CTA revealed AAA. The bilateral iliac arteries were in normal diameter. And the common iliac arteries are short. B to C: Distal bare stents were deployed and overlapped with distal extension endograft, to prevent upwards migrates of the iliac extension.

If both sides of hypogastric arteries are involved by the iliac aneurysm, Iliac Branched Device (IBD) or the Sandwich technique with external iliac artery and internal iliac artery stent-grafting can be used to preserve the one hypogastric artery. And the other one could be occluded. These techniques are proven to be feasible to prevent pelvic ischemic complications and type Ib endoleak (Figure 8).

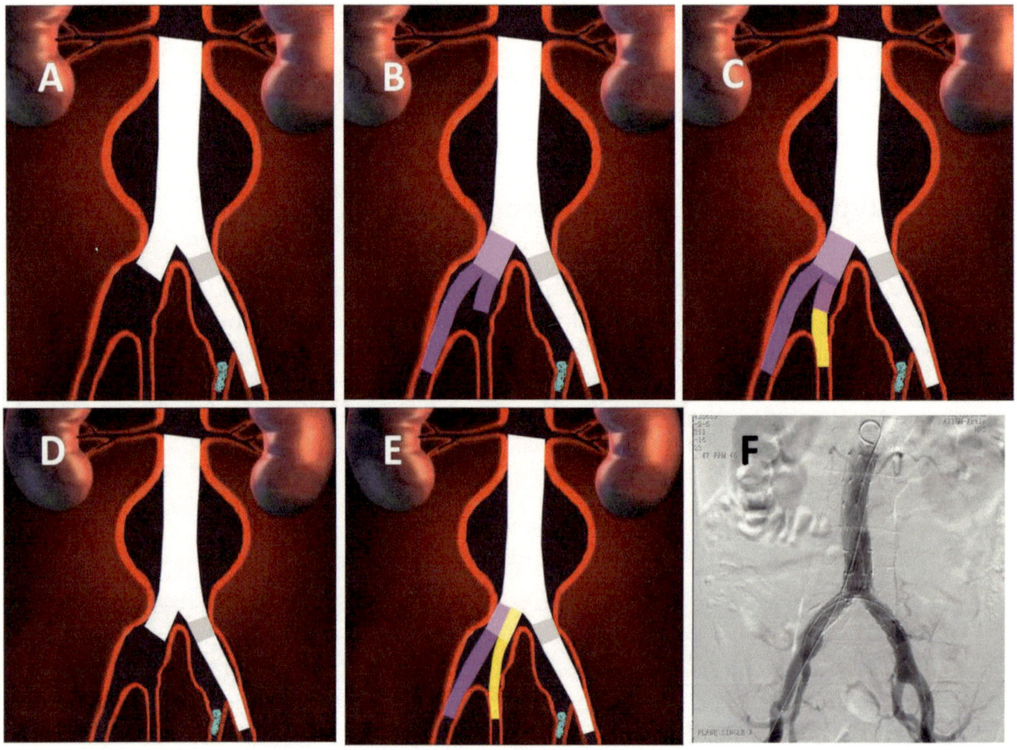

Figure 8. A to C: Iliac Branched Device (IBD) with extension into internal iliac artery. D to F: the Sandwich technique with separated external iliac artery limb and internal iliac artery limb.

Type Ib endoleak is usually treated by distal extension, while distal embolization with microcatheters and glues is less often required as a result of the variety of extender limbs and covered stents available as effective tools. However, sometimes, hypogastric arteries need to be preserved. If required, distal embolization is easier to perform than proximal embolization, as the leak is readily located with a simple curved catheter (Figure 9).

http://dx.doi.org/10.5772/54836

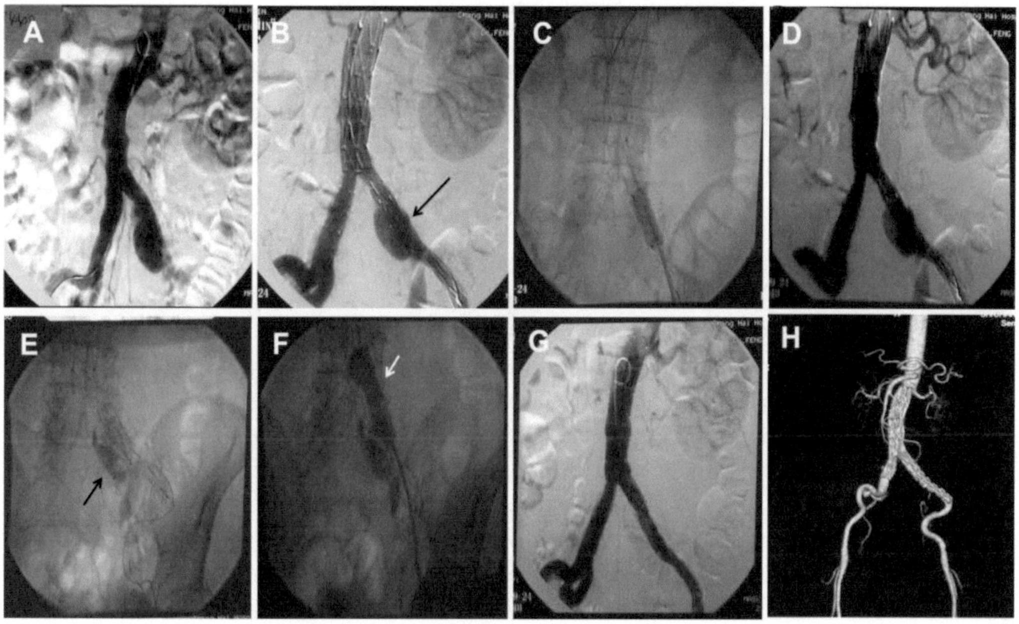

Figure 9. A: Pre-operative angiography revealed AAA (thrombosed) and left common iliac artery aneurysm. B: After bifurcated endografting with left extention were deployed, the type Ib endoleak was noted (as black arrow showed). C to D: Ballooning could not diminish the endoleak. E: The distal edge of the extension was probed from the ipsilateral femoral artery. After the tip of the simple curved catheter engaged the channel of leak, a smooth microcatheter could be advanced into this channel. As the black arrow showed, it is essential to pass the microcatheter into the perigraft space and perform angiography to rue out a combined type I and type II endoleak, which is quite common. F: The white arrow showed the proximal ballooning before the embolic agent was injected. G: Final angiography confirmed the satisfying exclusion of the AAA. H: One year follow-up CTA showed no endoleak existed, and the aneurysm was completely excluded.

11. Type II endoleaks

Type II endoleak is the most commonly encountered endoleak, and it is much more controversial than type I endoleak. Defined as retrograde flow through collateral vessels into the perigraft space, type II endoleaks prevent thrombosis of the sac and create a potential risk of continued aneurysm expansion and possible rupture. They do not appear to be related to the specific design or material of the endograft used and may appear immediately at the time of graft implantation, at the time of the first follow-up imaging study, or in a delayed fashion months or years after the EVAR procedure [22]. These leaks have also been noted to show resolution and then reappear on subsequent studies. The significance of type II leaks has long been debated, as have appropriate methods of follow-up and determination of the need for intervention. Because at least some of these endoleaks will persist and be associated with aneurysm expansion, there is a need for repeated follow-up imaging studies, which add to the expense of the endovascular approach. There is also the issue of the anxiety engendered in the patient who is uncertain whether his or her aneurysm has been adequately treated.

The best indicator of hemodynamic significance of a type II endoeak is the associated change in the aneurysm sac: if the sac increases in size, higher pressure and a relatively higher risk of long-term rupture are implied. If the sac is stable or decreasing in size, the risk is likely to be less. An analysis of a large EVAR series found that intervention was necessary only when the sac expanded and that persistent type II endoleaks in the absence of sac expansion could be safely observed [23]. These data are consistent with the earlier recommendations from the EUROSTAR study [5].

After a type II endoleak has been identified on imaging studies, aortography above and within the endograft usually permits exclusion of a type I endoleak and sometimes demonstrates the type II endoleak, particularly on late-phase images. Flush aortography is the starting point but is clearly inadequate to investigate an endoleak, as the majority will not be demonstrated without selective angiography. If the flush study does not show a leak that is present on the imaging study, selective angiography of the superior mesenteric artery and at least one hypogastric artery is performed with prolonged imaging to identify collateral pathways. Specific findings on the imaging study are often suggestive of the source of the leak (eg, left anterolateral blush from the IMA or posterolateral blush for lumbar artery), but may be misleading. The superior mesenteric artery will sometimes fill an IMA endoleak via the middle colic and marginal arteries, but the actual leak may not be demonstrated on main superior mesenteric artery injection. A microcatheter placed superselectively in the marginal artery will be more definitive, showing retrograde filling of the native origin of the IMA with filling of the leak if present. If the marginal artery is of adequate diameter and it is not excessively tortuous, it may be possible to pass the microcatheter back to the origin of the vessel and into the perigraft space. Angiography will then demonstrate the actual size of the leak and demonstrate the direction of flow. Embolization can then be carried out with use of NBCA adhesive, coils, or Onyx co- polymer (Micro Therapeutics, Irvine, California) [24]. Transvascular embolization in the IMA distribution should not be performed if the origin of the vessel cannot be reached, as there is a significant risk of creating colonic ischemia. If a transvascular approach is not possible, the leak can be approached directly by the sac puncture technique described later in the present report. Clipping of the IMA via a laparoscopic approach has also been reported [25].

If the endoleak cannot be reached by transvascular methods, direct puncture of the aneurysm sac with CT, fluoroscopic, or US guidance can be performed [26]. Proper positioning of the catheter in the endoleak cavity is signaled by pulsatile return of blood and opacification of lumbar arteries or IMA on manual injection of contrast. Coils, glue, or thrombin are then deployed until there is no further blood return. There also have been promising results using transcaval embolization for the treatment of type II endoleak. The success rate was reported to be 83% after one year [27].

12. Type III endoleaks

Type III endoleaks arise from inadequate or ineffective seal at the graft junction points between overlapped graft segments or from disconnections and separation of components. Less often they are the result of fabric erosion related to material fatigue (Figure 10). Type III endoleak are infrequent, and the incidence was reported to be 4% after 1 year [28]. Because either of these problems results in arterial flow directly into the perigraft space, they are similar to a type I endoleak and always require intervention. Some failures related to modular dysjunction are preventable by the operator in terms of ensuring adequate overlap of graft components, a parameter that is generally specified by the manufacturer. Extreme angulation of the neck or iliac segments may also be a contributing factor, and may also increase the risk of device migration. Most fabric failures are associated with specific graft materials and designs that have been subsequently modified or withdrawn from the market. Type III endoleaks can generally be treated with deployment of additional stent graft components.

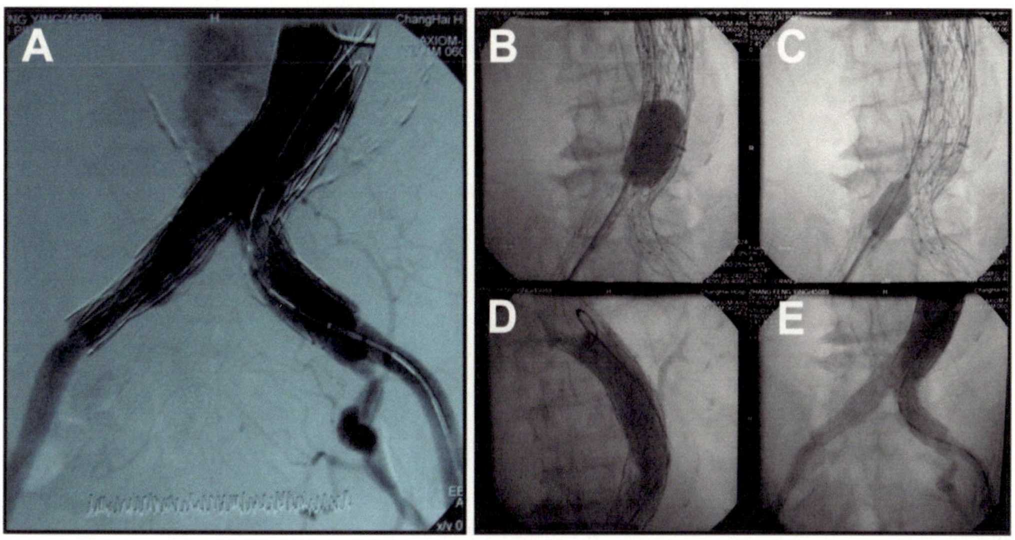

Figure 10. A: Six years after primary EVAR, type III endoleak was identified by routine follow-up CTA. The pre-operative angiography confirmed the graft erosion. B to C: A new one-piece bifurcated endograft was deployed in the previous one,and ballooning was performed. D to E: Aortography above and within the endograft was then performed to confirm the successful exclusion of the endoleak.

13. Type IV and type V endoleaks

Type IV endoleaks are not true leaks but represent passage of blood through the graft fabric as a result of porosity. Typically this type of endoleak is transient and only noted at the time of repair appearing as a blush on the post-deployment angiogram, when patients are often fully anticoagulated, and resolve spontaneously after the withdrawal of anticoagulation [29]. This type of endoleak has been eliminated by changes in graft porosity.

Type V "endoleak" is defined as continued aneurysm sac expansion without a demonstrable leak on any imaging modality. Also referred to as "endotension," this phenomenon remains poorly understood, but is likely caused by pulsation of the graft wall, with transmission of the pulse wave through the perigraft space to the native aneurysm wall. It is therefore likely to be related to the graft design, including stent structure and fabric compliance. But we observed persistent pressurization of an aneurysm sac with slow blood flow (slow flow endoleak), which is below the sensitivity limits for detection with current imaging technology. A considerable ultrafiltrate across a microporous fabric can fill the aneurysm and increase the pressure. Endotension seemed more common with expanded ePTFE fabric grafts rather than a woven polyester fabric [30].

Since the source of endotension can be difficult to detect, treatment strategies must be individualized. Relining devices with different low porosity endografts may abolish sac growth or induce sac shrinkage. Occasionally, endograft explantation and conversion to open surgery may be required when no clear cause of endotension can be detected, and endoleak cannot be ruled out (Figure 11).

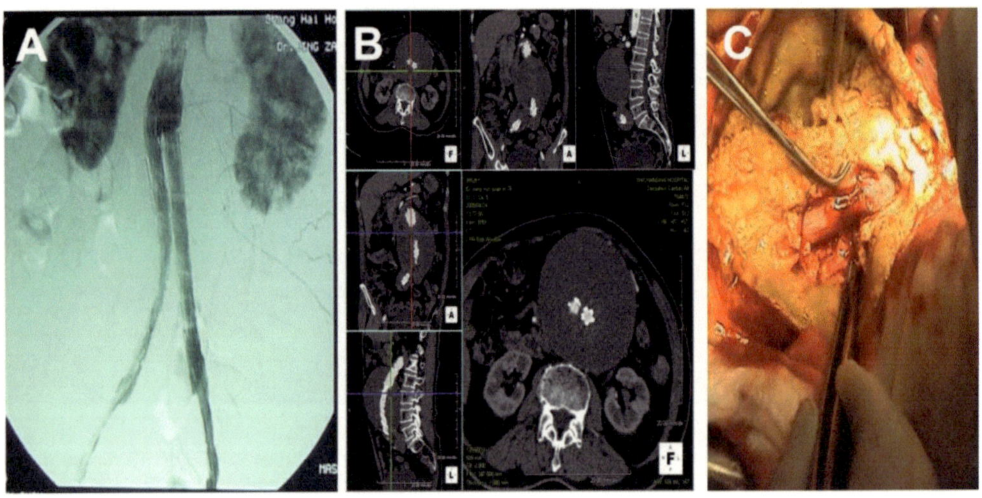

Figure 11. A: Post-operative angiography indicated the successful exclusion of the AAA. B: Four years after the primary EVAR, the aneurysm sac increased in size, without visible endoleak. C: Type V Endoleak was found during the secondary open surgery. The seepage flow and graft erosion was found. When the previous graft was removed and the infra-renal abdominal aorta was reconstructed by a new prosthesis, this patient was successfully treated.

14. Conclusion words

Endoleaks continue to be a challenge in the endovascular approach to aneurysm repair. Some of these leaks are device-related and their occurrence has been reduced with continuously improving graft design, whereas type II endoleaks appear to be an intrinsic risk of the endovascular approach. According to our experience, the vast majority of these endoleaks can be treated endoluminally, without resorting to open surgical repair.

http://dx.doi.org/10.5772/54836

Fibrin glue sac embolization to eliminate type I endoleak after EVAR yielded optimal results in our study. We believe that fibrin glue embolization may be an ideal option for treating type I endoleak in patients with unfavorable proximal neck anatomy and an alternative to cuff extension with chimney graft rescue of covered renal arteries. It is our hope that successful embolization of endoleaks can eliminate or at least reduce the need for lifelong follow-up imaging studies, an important goal in improving patient satisfaction and the economics of the endovascular approach to aneurysm repair. In recent years, the fenestrated stent-graft, branched stent-graft, chimney technique, sandwich technique and Iliac Branched Device, et al, significantly expanded the indication of EVAR, and remarkably reduced the incidence of type I endoleak. We believe that new devices and techniques are the trend to prevent the occurrence of type I endoleak, and finally diminish the usage of glue embolization technique.

In some studies, type II endoleak was aggressively evaluated and treated: if they persist beyond the 6-month study unless there has been shrinkage of the aneurysm sac. But we hold conservative attitude. Persistent type II endoleaks, in the absence of sac expansion, could be safely observed.

Author details

Zaiping Jing*, Qingsheng Lu, Jiaxuan Feng and Jian Zhou

*Address all correspondence to: xueguanky@163.net

From the Department of Vascular Surgery, Changhai Hospital, Second Military Medical University, Shanghai, China

References

[1] White, G. H, Yu, W, May, J, et al. Endoleak as a complication of endoluminal grafting of abdominal aortic aneurysms: classification, incidence, diagnosis, and management. J Endovasc Surg. (1997). , 4, 152-168.

[2] Chaikof, E. L, Blankensteijn, J. D, Harris, P. L, et al. Reporting standards for endovascular aortic aneurysm repair. J Vasc Surg. (2002). , 35, 1048-1060.

[3] Veith, F. J, Baum, R. A, Ohki, T, et al. Nature and significance of endoleaks and endotension: summary of opinions expressed at an international conference. J Vasc Surg. (2002). , 35, 1029-1038.

[4] Dias, N. V, Ivancev, K, Resch, T. A, et al. Endoleaks after endovascular aneurysm repair lead to nonuniform intra-aneurysm sac pressure. J Vasc Surg. (2007). , 46, 197-203.

[5] Van Marrewijk, C, Buth, J, Harris, P. L, et al. Significance of endoleaks after endovascular repair of abdominal aortic aneurysm: the EUROSTAR experience. J Vasc Surg. (2002). , 35, 461-473.

[6] Rosen, R. J, & Green, R. M. Endoleak management following endovascular aneurysm repair. J Vasc Interv Radiol. (2008). , 19, 37-43.

[7] Faries, P. L, Cadot, H, Agarwal, G, et al. Management of endoleak after endovascular aneurysm repair: cuffs, coils, and conversion. J Vasc Surg. (2003). , 37, 1155-1161.

[8] Kato, N, Semba, C. P, & Dake, M. D. Embolization of perigraft leaks after endovascular stent-graft treatment of aortic aneurysms. J Vasc Interv Radiol. (1996). , 7, 805-811.

[9] Maldonado, T. S, Rosen, R. J, Rockman, C. B, et al. Initial successful management of type I endoleak after endovascular aortic aneurysm repair with n-butyl cyanoacrylate adhesive. J Vasc Surg. (2003). , 38, 664-670.

[10] Grisafi, J. L, Boiteau, G, Detschelt, E, et al. Endoluminal treatment of type IA endoleak with Onyx. J Vasc Surg. (2010). , 52, 1346-9.

[11] Zanchetta, M, Faresin, F, Pedon, L, et al. Fibrin glue aneurysm sac embolization at the time of endografting. J Endovasc Ther. (2005). , 12, 579-582.

[12] Pilon, F, Tosato, F, Danieli, D, et al. Intrasac fibrin glue injection after platinum coils placement: the efficacy of a simple intraoperative procedure in preventing type II endoleak after endovascular aneurysm repair. Interact Cardiovasc Thorac Surg. (2010). , 11, 78-82.

[13] Meyer, F, Ricke, J, Pech, M, et al. Impressive closure of a sustaining periprosthetic endoleak (type II) using fibrin glue application after former endovascular placement of an infrarenal aortic prosthesis. Int J Surg. (2009). , 7, 84-86.

[14] Baum, R. A, Carpenter, J. P, Cope, C, et al. Aneurysm sac pressure measurements after endovascular repair of abdominal aortic aneurysms. J Vasc Surg. (2001). , 33, 32-41.

[15] Clark, R. A. Fibrin glue for wound repair: facts and fancy. Thromb Haemost. (2003). , 90, 1003-1006.

[16] Pacanowski, J. P, Stevens, S. L, Freeman, M. B, et al. Endotension distribution and the role of thrombus following endovascular AAA exclusion. J Endovasc Ther. (2002). , 9, 639-651.

[17] Ronsivalle, S, Faresin, F, Franz, F, Rettore, C, Zanchetta, M, & Olivieri, A. Aneurysm sac "thrombization" and stabilization in EVAR: a technique to reduce the risk of type II endoleak. J Endovasc Ther. (2010). , 17, 517-24.

[18] Houbballah, R, Majewski, M, & Becquemin, J. P. Significant sac retraction after endovascular aneurysm repair is a robust indicator of durable treatment success. J Vasc Surg. (2010). , 52, 878-83.

[19] Baxendale, B. R, Baker, D. M, Hutchinson, A, et al. Haemodynamic and metabolic response to endovascular repair of infrarenal aortic aneurysms. Br J Anaesth. (1996)., 77, 581-585.

[20] Mehta, M, Veith, F. J, Ohki, T, et al. Significance of endotension, endoleak, and aneurysm pulsatility after endovascular repair. J Vasc Surg. (2003)., 37, 842-846.

[21] Ohrlander, T, Sonesson, B, Ivancev, K, et al. The chimney graft: a technique for preserving or rescuing aortic branch vessels in stent-graft sealing zones. J Endovasc Ther. (2008)., 15, 427-432.

[22] Sheehan, M. K, Ouriel, K, Greenberg, R, et al. Are type II endoleaks after endovascular aneurysm repair endograft dependent? J Vasc Surg. (2006)., 43, 657-61.

[23] Bernhard, V. M, Mitchell, R. S, Matsumura, J. S, et al. Ruptured abdominal aortic aneurysm after endovascular repair. J Vasc Surg. (2002)., 35, 1155-62.

[24] Martin, M. L, Dolmatch, B. L, Fry, P. D, & Machan, L. S. Treatment of type II endoleaks with Onyx. J Vasc Interv Radiol. (2001)., 12, 629-32.

[25] Zhou, W, Lumsden, A. B, & Li, J. IMA clipping for a type ii endoleak: combined laparoscopic and endovascular approach. Surg Laparosc Endosc Percutan Tech. (2006)., 16, 272-5.

[26] Baum, R. A, Carpenter, J. P, Golden, M. A, et al. Treatment of type 2 endoleaks after endovascular repair of abdominal aortic aneurysms: comparison of transarterial and translumbar techniques. J Vasc Surg. (2002)., 35, 23-9.

[27] Mansueto, G, Cenzi, D, Scuro, A, et al. Treatment of type II endoleak with a transcatheter transcaval approach: results at 1-year follow-up. J Vasc Surg. (2007)., 45, 1120-7.

[28] Wilt, T. J, Lederle, F. A, Macdonald, R, et al. Comparison of endovascular and open surgical repairs for abdominal aortic aneurysm. Evid Rep Technol Assess. (2006)., 144, 1-113.

[29] Kanaoka, Y, Ohki, T, Huang, J, et al. A comparison between standard and high density Resilient AneuRx in reducing aneurysm sac pressure in a chronic canine model. J Vasc Surg. (2009)., 49, 1021-8.

[30] Haider, S. E, Najjar, S. F, Cho, J. S, et al. Sac behavior after aneurysm treatment with the Gore Excluder low-permeability aortic endoprosthesis: 12-month comparison to the original Excluder device. J Vasc Surg. (2006)., 44, 694-700.

Chapter 9

Extended Aortic Replacement Via Median Sternotomy with Left Anterolateral Thoracotomy

Satoshi Yamashiro, Yukio Kuniyoshi,
Hitoshi Inafuku, Yuya Kise and Ryoko Arakaki

Additional information is available at the end of the chapter

http://dx.doi.org/10.5772/50809

1. Objective

Prevention of cerebral injury is an important consideration during repair of an aortic arch aneurysm, and a major goal of cerebral protection techniques. We describe extended thoracic aortic aneurysms treated using our surgical strategy.

2. Patients and methods

Between January 2001 and December 2011, 31 patients (22 men and 9 women; mean age, of 68.9 ± 9.5 y) underwent total replacement of the arch and descending aorta. Seven patients underwent emergency surgery (22.6%). At that time, a median sternotomy with left anterolateral thoracotomy provided a good visual field and bilateral axillary arteries were preferentially used for systemic as well as selective cerebral perfusion.

3. Results

Two patients died in hospital (hospital mortality, 6.5%). Mechanical ventilation was required after surgery for 6.3 ± 7.4 days. Permanent neurological dysfunction developed in 1 (3.2 %) patient who died of sepsis 2 years after the operation. Although prolonged mechanical ventilation support was necessary, all patients recovered uneventfully.

4. Conclusion

Our results suggested that total arch replacement through a median sternotomy plus left anterolateral thoracotomy seems to be helpful for extended replacement of the thoracic aorta, as well as a distal re-operation for dissecting type A. Moreover, our results suggested that perfusion from the bilateral axillary arteries can help prevent cerebral damage.

Despite advances in surgical techniques such as management of anesthesia and cardiopulmonary bypass (CPB)[1,5], brain injury after aortic arch surgery remains an important source of morbidity and mortality because of the advanced age of the patients and the presence of severe comorbidities [6]. Extended thoracic aortic aneurysms involving the ascending aorta, arch, and descending aorta are often approached in staged operations [7]. However, a single-stage replacement of the aortic arch and descending aorta might be a preferable surgical option for specific types of atherosclerotic aneurysm, such as chronic type A or B dissection. We describe our experience with extended aortic replacement through a median sternotomy with left anterolateral thoracotomy using our current strategy.

5. Patients and methods

Between January 2001 and December 2011, 31 consecutive patients with extended thoracic aortic aneurysms underwent total replacement of the arch and descending aorta at our institution.

Total number of patients	31
Age	68.9 +/- 9.5 years (56 - 83)
Gender (M/F)	22/9
Diagnosis	
Atherosclerotic	11 (35.5%)
Chronic type B dissection	7 (22.6%)
Chronic type A dissection	7 (22.6%)
Acute type A dissection	3 (9.7%)
Infectious	3 (9.7%)
Emergency	6 (19.4%)
Rupture (impending)	3 (9.7%)
Acute type A dissection	3 (9.7%)
Previous operative history	9 (34.8%)
Ascending aorta or Arch replacement	7 (22.6%)
AVR + CABG	1 (3.2%)
CABG	1 (3.2%)
Y graft replacement for AAA	2 (6.5%)

http://dx.doi.org/10.5772/50809

Total number of patients	31
Underlying dysorders	
HT	23 (74.2%)
DM	11 (35.5%)
HL	18 (58.1%)
Concomitant operation	5 (16.1%)
CABG	2 (6.5%)
AVR	1 (3.2%)
AVR+MVR+CABG	1 (3.2%)
Bentall operation with CABG	1 (3.2%)

Table 1. Characteristics of patients who underwent total arch with descending aortic replacement for extended thoracic aortic aneurysm between January 2001 and December 2011 at our institution. M, male; F, female; AVR, aortic valve replacement; CABG, coronary artery bypass grafting; AAA, abdominal aortic aneurysm; HT, hypertension; DM, diabetes mellitus; HL, hyperlipidemia; MVR, mitral valve replacement.

Table 1 shows the characteristics of the 22 male and 9 female patients (mean age, of 68.9 ± 9.5 y; range, 56 to 83 y). Eleven had atherosclerotic distal arch aneurysms, 7 had chronic type B dissection, 7 had chronic type A dissection after graft replacement of the ascending aorta or aortic arch, 3 had acute type A dissection, and 3 had infectious arch aneurysms. Three patients had a ruptured or impending ruptured aneurysm of the arch aorta, and three patients had acute type A dissection that required emergency surgery (22.6%). Coronary angiography was also performed before surgery for all patients except for those in emergency. Seven patients had undergone a previous graft replacement of the ascending aorta, 1 had aortic valve replacement (AVR), and 1 had a coronary artery bypass graft (CABG). Five patients underwent concomitant cardiac procedures, namely CABG in 2, AVR in 1, AVR and mitral valve replacement (MVR) with CABG in 1 and the Bentall procedure with CABG in 1.

6. Surgical technique

Patients were endotracheally intubated with a double-lumen tube to deflate the lungs and then positioned on an operating table with the chest rotated 60 degrees from supine towards the right. A 5- to 6-cm transverse skin incision was made before the median sternotomy at about 1 cm below the middle and lateral part of the clavicle. The axillary and right femoral arteries (FA) were exposed, and the heart, ascending aorta, aortic arch, and arch vessels were exposed through a median sternotomy with a sternum transection plus a left fourth intercostal thoracotomy (the "Door open" method). This combined approach was applied if the predicted level of the distal anastomosis was below the sixth vertebra, and it provided a good visual field of the whole heart as well as of the entire aorta. The perfusion site was selected based on preoperative computed tomographic scans. Bilateral or right axillary arteries (bilateral in 17, right in 13) with or without the right FA were used as the perfusion site for all except 1 patient for whom the ascending aorta was used with the right femoral artery.

When using the axillary artery, an 8-mm-diameter graft was anastomosed to the bilateral or right axillary arteries for systemic arterial cannulation after systemic heparinization. These grafts were used for antegrade selective cerebral perfusion (SCP) after deep hypothermic circulatory arrest (HCA). Antegrade SCP was established through vascular grafts anastomosed to the bilateral axillary arteries and a perfusion catheter placed directly into the left carotid artery. Moreover, the left common carotid artery was directly cannulated as described [9], to prevent cerebral thromboembolization in two patients. Figure 1 shows a schema of the surgical approach and cerebral protection. Distal anastomosis proceeded under cross-clamping of the distal descending aorta with distal perfusion through FA in 18 patients to prevent visceral ischemia. The remaining 14 patients underwent open distal anastomosis, after the completion of which, the graft was drawn anteriorly into the isolated residual distal arch aorta. Meanwhile the left phrenic and left recurrent laryngeal nerves were identified, mobilized with the aneurysmal wall, and protected. Antegrade SCP was terminated after reconstruction of the arch vessels, and then the proximal side of arch graft was sutured to the stump of the ascending aorta. The root of the left subclavian artery was ligated when an 8-mm-diameter graft was anastomosed to the left axillary artery, and reconstructed by graft-graft anastomosis using a 5-0 polypropylene running suture.

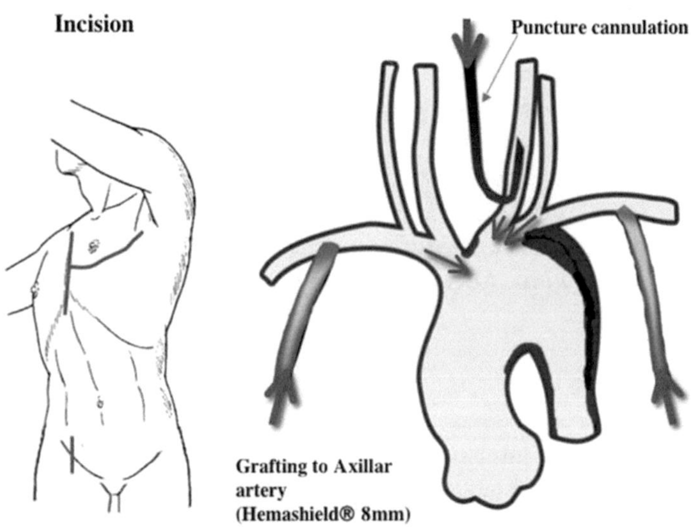

Figure 1. Schema of surgical approach and cerebral protection.

7. Results

Table 2 shows that the durations of surgery, total cardiopulmonary bypass (CPB), cardiac ischemia, HCA and SCP were 669.6 ± 191.7, 247.9 ± 79.6, 163.0 ± 71.3, 55.6 ± 20.9 and 117.4

http://dx.doi.org/10.5772/50809

±32.5 minutes, respectively. None of these values significantly differed between patients after total arch replacement through a median sternotomy and those who also had a left anterolateral thoracotomy (data not shown).

Surgical duration	669.6+/- 191.7 minutes
Total CPB time	247.9 +/- 79.6 minutes
Cardiac arrest time	163.0 +/- 71.3 minutes
SCP time	117.4 +/- 32.5 minutes
HCA time (13 patients)	55.6 +/- 20.9 minutes
Hospital death	2 (6.5%)
Mechanical ventilation duration	6.3 +/- 7.4 days
Complication	
Respiratory failure	22 (71.0%)
Cerebral infarction	1 (3.2%)
Acute renal failure	2 (6.5%)
Hospitalization after surgery	35.3 +/- 6.7 days
Late death	1 (3.3%)
Follow-up duration	58.1 +/- 26.1 months

Table 2. Operative results. CPB, cardiopulmonary bypass; SCP, selective cerebral perfusion; HCA, hypothermic circulatory arrest.

Two patients died in hospital (hospital mortality, 6.5%). One patient with a ruptured arch aneurysm died of multiple organ failure (MOF) on postoperative day 70. He had undergone emergency surgery due to aneurysmal rupture and was in a state of preoperative shock. The other patient had a distal pseudoaneurysm after arch replacement for type A dissection, and required simultaneous AVR and MVR with CABG. He died of MOF on postoperative day 17. However, neither of these patients was complicated with cerebral damage.

Early morbidity in 22 patients comprised pulmonary failure, defined as requiring respiratory support for > 48 hours. Mechanical ventilation was required after surgery for 6.3 ± 7.4 days. Two patients who had preoperative left recurrent laryngeal nerve palsy developed persistent hoarseness after the operation. No new phrenic or left recurrent laryngeal nerve palsies developed as a result of surgery. Permanent neurological dysfunction, defined as permanent neurological deficits with localizing neurological signs and corresponding new defects on CT images, occurred in 1 (3.2%) patient, who died of sepsis 2 years after the operation. The length of the hospital stay after surgery was 35.3 ± 6.7 days. The actuarial survival rate at 5 years after surgery was 90.1% (Figure 2), and the patients were followed up after surgery for 58.1 ± 26.1 months.

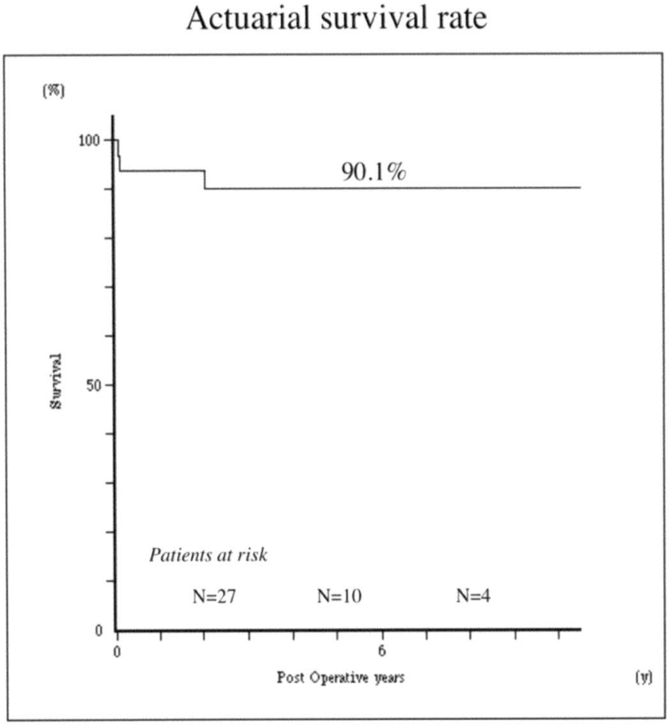

Figure 2. Actuarial survival rates among 31 patients with extensive replacement of the thoracic aorta.

8. Discussion

Indications for approaches in patients with arch aneurysms are controversial, because the surgical results of extended arch replacement are suboptimal. The combined surgical approach (median sternotomy with left anterolateral thoracotomy) to treating thoracic aortic aneurysms has been considered too invasive [3]. We found in our series that the durations of surgery and of relative mechanical circulation were significantly elongated. Therefore, 17 patients required respiratory support for > 72 h, although they gradually recovered without complications. Mechanical ventilation was required after surgery for 7.3 ± 8.4 days. All of the surviving patients recovered uneventfully except for those who became complicated with cerebral infarction. The combined approach seemed to be too invasive for respiratory function. On the other hand, Ohata et al. [2] found no significant differences in respiratory function or in the inflammatory response between patients who underwent total arch replacement through a median sternotomy and those who also had a left anterolateral thoracotomy. Especially in the distal reoperative situation for dissecting type A, the retrosternal space can be easily excised from a left thoracotomy, although adhesion due to previous surgeries can be moderate or severe. The cannulae are conveniently situated anteriorly away from the main operative field, which improves access to the aortic arch and descending thoracic aorta. Moreover, the ability to

http://dx.doi.org/10.5772/50809

visualize and protect the phrenic and recurrent laryngeal nerves contributes to extending the recovery of patients with impaired respiratory function.

The prevention of cerebral embolism is an important consideration during repair of an aortic arch or ascending aortic aneurysm, and is a major goal of cerebral protection techniques. Selection of the arterial cannulation site for CPB is critical o achieve this. The ascending aorta or FA is usually selected as an arterial cannulation site [1, 5]. However, cerebral embolism can occur in both cannulation sites, because of severe atherosclerotic changes in the ascending aorta near the arch aneurysm or retrograde perfusion via the femoral artery [3, 11]. The important variables that are considered to influence the occurrence of postoperative stroke following aortic arch repair, and which might be affected by the method of cannulation, include the presence of clots and atheromas in the aorta, and dissection as the etiology of aneurysms. Svenson et al. [8] started to use subclavian or axillary artery cannulation strategy with HCA and antegrade brain perfusion 1995, and found it to be a safe approach for aortic arch surgery as the stroke risk was < 2%. The theoretical advantages of using the subclavian or axillary artery site for inflow for complex cardiac and cardioaortic operations have recently become apparent [8, 9]. These possible advantages include a decreased likelihood of stroke from embolic material, less likely malperfusion with aortic dissection, reduced disruption of atheroma or calcified plaques, and the ability to administer antegrade brain perfusion. Only one patient in our series who had undergone ascending aortic perfusion developed cerebral infarction. We suspected that the infarction was due to embolism from an atheroma in the arch aorta. Since 2000, we have preferentially used axillary arteries for perfusion with total arch replacement except for this patient. No other patients have developed neurologic injury since then.

Ergin et al. [10] reported that temporary neurological dysfunction was a clinical marker of an insidious but significant neurological injury associated with measurable long-term deficits in cerebral function. Therefore, we have used only SCP in aortic arch repair because of the extended duration of cerebral safety and the low incidence of temporary neurological dysfunction. However, atheromatous emboli traveling to the brain, which is considered to be a main cause of permanent neurological dysfunction, remains a serious major concern during SCP. Antegrade SCP is physiological and the time taken to ensure cerebral safety should be much longer. However, arch-vessel cannulation is required for this maneuver, which carries a risk of cerebral embolization. Many embolic sources are caused by systemic CPB perfusion via the ascending aorta across the arch aneurysm, or otherwise, retrograde CPB perfusion via the FA, or cannulation to the arch vessels for SCP. The need to cannulate arterial vessels and to manipulate often severely atherosclerotic aneurysms enhances the potential for embolization into the cerebral circulation, resulting in focal lesions and neurological injury. Svenson and colleague [9] described that when using the subclavian or axillary arteries for inflow, direct cannulation is associated with a greater risk of local complications, including dissection of the artery, inadequate flow, abutment of the cannula tip against the carotid artery wall, and tears that are difficult to repair because arterial tissue is fragile and often traumatized. We then switched arterial inflow to a side graft sewn to the vessels, and a delicate and sometimes difficult repair of the artery was not required at the end of the operation. Instead, the side graft could simply be over-sewn and tied off or clipped. We doubt whether whole brain perfusion is sufficient with only right axillary artery perfusion. The best approach for cerebral protection during these procedures remains a matter of controversy. Although the procedures are continually undergoing refinement with improved results, associated brain injury can still arise despite the application of all cerebral protection techniques suitable for these operations. Thus, left-side brain perfusion was added. Therefore, bilateral axillaries were routinely used as the perfusion site in current 17 patients. Moreover, vertebral perfusion via the left axillary artery is important for spinal as well as cerebral protection. Simultaneously sewing a graft to a bilateral axillary artery takes about 20 to 30 minutes. The axillary artery always has less atherosclerotic change than the ascending aorta or the FA, and it can easily be exposed [12-14]. During reconstruction of the left subclavian artery, a side graft could simply be sewn onto a graft that was anastomosed to the left axillary artery beforehand.

Recently, several reports of total endovascular treatment of aortic arch with branched stent graft or fenestrated device demonstrated feasible results [15]. Kawaguchi et al [16] described that thoracic endovascular repair (TEVAR) tends to have a lower rate of serious complications than open surgery. They reported that cerebral infarction rate in patients who received a fenestrated device was 5.5%. Actually, TEVAR does not require extracorporeal circulation; therefore, patients do not have low cerebral perfusion during the procedure. Certainly, we agree to endovascular treatment of pathologies affecting the ascending aorta and aortic arch is feasible in limited patients. Although, TEVAR cannot be considered a well-established treatment method just yet, especially in aortic arch. Technical difficulties with graft design and deployment persist [17]. Therefore, we thought extensive surgery have not been avoidable in this series, especially in dissection and patients who required concomitant procedures.

We believe that extensive reimplantation of the thoracic aorta accompanied by adequate distal aortic perfusion under distal clamping to avoid hypothermic circulatory arrest are effective. Our results suggested that total arch replacement through a median sternotomy plus left anterolateral thoracotomy allowed expeditious and extended replacement of the thoracic aorta and distal re-operation for dissecting type A aneurysms. This experience with median sternotomy together with left anterolateral thoracotomy approach and cannulation illustrates that our method is safe and effective. This study is limited by the relatively small size. However the analysis of our results may have practical implications in going evolution in these severe cases.

Author details

Satoshi Yamashiro*, Yukio Kuniyoshi, Hitoshi Inafuku, Yuya Kise and Ryoko Arakaki

*Address all correspondence to: y3104@med.u-ryukyu.ac.jp

Department of Thoracic and Cardiovascular Surgery, Graduate school of Medicine, University of the Ryukyus, Okinawa, Japan

http://dx.doi.org/10.5772/50809

References

[1] Crawford, E. S., Kirklin, J. W., Naftel, D. C., Svensson, L. G., Coselli, J. S., & Safi, H. J. (1992). Surgery for acute dissection of ascending aorta: should the arch be included? *J Thorac Cardiovasc Surg*, 104, 46-59.

[2] Kuniyoshi, Y., Koja, K., Miyagi, K., Uezu, T., Yamashiro, S., Arakaki, K., Mabuni, K., & Senaha, S. (2004). Direct cannulation of the common carotid artery during the ascending aortic or aortic arch replacement. *Jpn J Thorac Cardiovasc Surg*, 52, 247-253.

[3] Wesatby, S., & Katsumata, T. (1998). Proximal aortic perfusion for complex arch and descending aortic disease. *J Thorac Cardiovasc Surg*, 115, 162-167.

[4] Ohata, T., Sakakibara, T., Takano, H., & Ishizaka, T. (2003). Total arch replacement for thoracic aortic aneurysm via median sternotomy with or without left anterolateral thoracotomy. *Ann Thorac Surg*, 75, 1792-1796.

[5] Kazui, T., Washiyama, N., Bashar, A. H. M., Terada, H., Suzuki, T., Ohkura, K., & Yamashita, K. (2002). Surgical outcome of acute type A aortic dissection: analysis of risk factors. *Ann Thorac Surg*, 74, 75-82.

[6] Okita, Y., Ando, M., Minatoya, K., Kitamura, S., Takamoto, S., & Nakajima, N. (1999). Predictive factors for mortality and cerebral complications in atherosclerotic aneurysm of the aortic arch. *Ann Thorac Surg*, 67, 72-78.

[7] Borst, H. G., & Frank, G. (1988). Treatment of extensive aortic aneurysms by a new multiple-stage approach. *J Thorac Surg*, 95, 11-13.

[8] Svenson, L. G., Nadolny, E. M., Penney, D. L., Jacobson, J., Kimmel, W. A., Entrup, M. H., & D'Agostino, R. S. (2001). Prospective randomized neurocognitive and S-100 study of hypothermic circulatory arrest, retrograde brain perfusion, and antegrade brain perfusion for aortic arch operations. *Ann Thorac Surg*, 71, 1905-1912.

[9] Svenson, L. G., Blackstone, E. H., Rajeswaran, J., Sabik, J. F., Lytle, B. W., Gonzalez-Stawinski, G., Varvitsiotis, P., Banbury, M. K., Mc Carthy, P. M., Pettersson, G. B., & Cosgrove, D. M. (2004). Does the arterial cannulation site for circulatory arrest influence stroke risk? *Ann Thorac Surg*, 78, 1274-1284.

[10] Ergin, M. A., Uysal, S., Reich, D. L., Apaydin, A., Lansman, S. L., Mc Cullough, J. N., & Griepp, R. B. (1999). Temporary neurological dysfunction after deep hypothermic circulatory arrest: a clinical marker of long term functional deficit. *Ann Thorac Surg*, 67, 1887-1890.

[11] Numata, S., Ogino, H., Sasaki, H., Hanafusa, Y., Hirata, M., Ando, M., & Kitamura, S. (2003). Total arch replacement using antegrade selective cerebral perfusion with right axillary artery perfusion. *Eur J Cardiothorac Surg*, 23, 771-775.

[12] Strauch, J. T., Spielvogel, D., Lauten, A., Lansman, S. L., Mc Murtry, K., & Bodian, Griepp. R. B. (2004). Axillary artery cannulation: routine use in ascending aorta and aortic arch replacement. *Ann Thorac Surg*, 78, 103-108.

[13] Kurisu, K., Ochiai, Y., Hisahara, M., Tanaka, K., Onzuka, T., & Tominaga, R. (2006). Bilateral axillary arterial perfusion in surgery on thoracic aorta. *Asian Cardiovasc Thorac Ann*, 14, 145-149.

[14] Shimazaki, Y., Watanabe, T., Uchida, T., Takeda, F., Uesho, K., Koshika, M., Nakashima, K., & Inui, K. (2003). Outcome of aortic arch surgery in patients aged 70 years or older: axillary artery cannulation and selective cerebral perfusion supports. *J Cardiol*, 41, 7-12.

[15] Melissano, G., Civilini, E., Bertoglio, L., Calliari, F., Setacci, F., Calori, G., & Chiesa, R. (2007). Results of endografting of the aortic arch in different landing zones. *Euro J Vasc Endovasc Surg*, 33, 561-566.

[16] Kawaguchi, S., Yokoi, Y., Shimazaki, T., Koide, K., Matsumoto, M., & Shigematsu, H. (2008). Thoracic endovascular aneurysm repair in Japan: Experience with fenestrated stent grafts in the treatment of distal arch aneurysms. *J Vasc Surg*, 48, 24S-29S.

[17] Brar, R., Ali, T., Morgan, R., Laftus, I., & Thompson, M. (2008). Endovascular repair of an aortic arch aneurysm using a branched-stent graft. *Eur J Vasc Endovasc Surg*, 36, 545-549.

Chapter 10

A Novel Treatment Strategy for Infected Abdominal Aortic Aneurysms

Osamu Yamashita, Koichi Yoshimura,
Noriyasu Morikage, Akira Furutani and
Kimikazu Hamano

Additional information is available at the end of the chapter

http://dx.doi.org/10.5772/52813

1. Introduction

Infected abdominal aortic aneurysms are rare, but the symptoms are prone to become severe during the clinical course, and the prognosis is poor, with a high rate of rupture [1]. There are 2 objectives in the treatment of infected aortic aneurysms: prevention of aneurysm rupture and infection control. However, it is not easy to achieve both. No guideline has been established yet, and many issues such as diagnostic method, the method of administering antibiotics before and after operation, timing of the operation, and operative procedure remain to be improved. Regarding operative procedures, approaches such as the use of a rifampicin-soaked prosthetic graft, covering the prosthetic graft with the greater omentum, and anatomical reconstruction have been reported in recent years [1]. Nevertheless, postoperative infection control is never easy, and the treatment results of infected aneurysms are still unsatisfactory. Therefore, we have devised a treatment policy to control local infection in a stricter manner by introducing the pulse-irrigation method that uses a pulsatile irrigation device and a temporary abdominal wall closure method that uses the vacuum-assisted closure (VAC) technique in patients with strong intraperitoneal contamination in addition to conventional operative procedures. In this study, we retrospectively verified the usefulness of our unique treatment strategy featuring the addition of these 2 new ideas using the treatment results of infected abdominal aortic aneurysms from the past 10 years.

2. Patients and methods

The subjects were 12 patients who had been treated for infected abdominal aortic aneurysms in our institution between January 2002 and December 2011. In total, 390 patients underwent the abdominal aortic aneurysm operation during the same period, and these 12 subjects accounted for 3.1% of them.

Patient	Age/Sex	Symptom	CRP (mg/dL) on admission	Risk factor
1	66/M	Fever	40.2	Untreated DM
2	84/F	Fever, pain	14.2	Malnutrition
3	64/M	Fever, pain	14.2	Untreated DM
4	74/M	Fever, pain	14.9	Colon cancer
5	52/F	Fever, pain	20.0	-
6	65/M	Fever, pain	8.3	-
7	71/M	Fever, pain	13.5	Alcoholic LC
8	80/M	Fever, pain	7.1	Alcoholic LC
9	66/M	-	0.0	-
10	60/M	Fever, pain	6.5	-
11	64/M	Fever, pain	8.8	-
12	60/M	Fever	26.9	Steroid therapy

Table 1. Patient characteristics. CRP, C-reactive protein; DM, diabetes mellitus; LC, liver cirrhosis

The subjects were 10 men and 2 women who were 52–84 years of age (mean, 67.1 ± 8.9 years) (Table 1). In accordance with a report by Hsu et al. [2], patients with abdominal aortic aneurysm were diagnosed with infected abdominal aortic aneurysm when they exhibited physical symptoms such as abdominal pain and back pain, inflammatory findings such as fever and increased white blood cell count and C-reactive protein (CRP), rapid enlargement of the aneurysm by contrast-enhanced computed tomography (CT), formation of pseudo-, saccular, or lobular aneurysms, or periaortic stranding [3]. For patients whose diagnoses were difficult, fluorodeoxyglucose-positron emission tomography/CT (FDG-PET/CT) was performed to aid diagnosis. The basic treatment policy dictated that patients were considered to have infected aortic aneurysm if they had any of the abovementioned physical symptoms, inflammatory findings, or CT findings in addition to the presence of an aneurysm, following which treatment with antibiotics was immediately started, and surgical procedures were performed after the inflammatory findings improved, in principle. On the other hand, emergency surgery was selected for patients who continued to exhibit symptoms or inflammatory findings even after antibiotic treatment, or who were suspected of having aneurysm rupture or impending rupture.

In principle, the operative procedure involved the following 5 steps.

1. Total resection of the aneurysm wall and surrounding infected tissue by laparotomy;
2. sufficient pulse irrigation with 10 L or more saline using a pulsatile irrigation device (SurgiLav® Plus Irrigation System, Stryker);
3. anatomical reconstruction using a gelatin-coated Dacron graft (Gelweave™, Terumo) soaked in 0.5% rifampicin (Sandoz) [4]; and
4. covering the prosthetic graft with the pedicled omental flap. Furthermore,
5. for patients with severe intraperitoneal contamination, temporary abdominal wall closure using the VAC technique was performed.

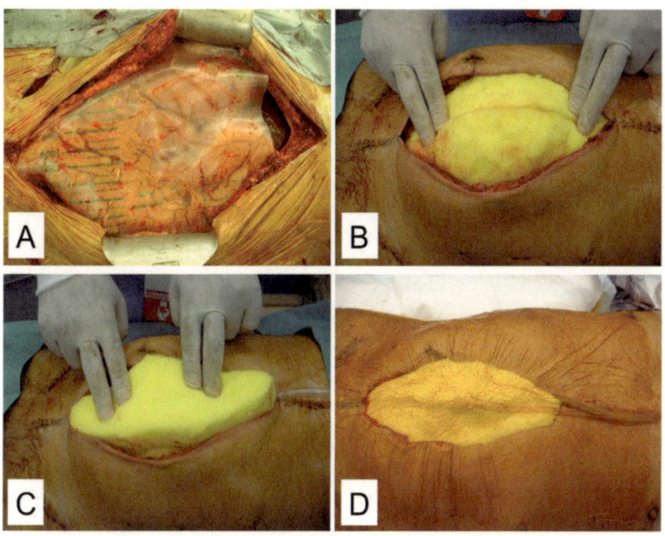

Figure 1. Temporary abdominal wall closure using the vacuum-assisted closure (VAC) technique. A, Placement of a vinyl sheet with slits in the abdominal cavity. B, Placement of polyurethane foam sponges over the sheet. C, Placement of a drainage tube on the sponges and coverage with other sponges. D, Draping and suction. (Modified from [7])

In this study, the amounts of bacteria in the operative fields were measured before and after the pulse irrigation and were used to verify the efficacy of the pulse-irrigation method. More specifically, the operative surface was wiped with sterilized cotton swabs before resection of the aneurysm wall and surrounding tissue, and was wiped with sterilized cotton swabs again after resection and irrigation. We then performed bacteria culture tests using these sterilized cotton swabs as samples. Regarding temporary abdominal wall closure using the VAC technique after abdominal aortic aneurysm resection, others and we have reported its use in preventing abdominal compartment syndrome in patients with non-infected aneurysm rupture [5-7]. Pursuant to our previous method [7], we performed temporary abdominal wall closure using the VAC technique to drain infectious peritoneal effusion. More specifically, a vinyl chloride sheet with slits of ca. 2-cm long at 1- to 2-cm intervals was placed directly in the abdominal cavity, after which sterilized polyurethane foam sponges were placed over the sheet and a drainage tube was placed on them, which was again covered with sponges and draped (Ioban™ 2 Special Incise Draip, 3M Healthcare) (Figure 1). The drainage tube was continuously suctioned using 140–150 mmHg suction pressure. The sponges were changed every 2 days, and secondary abdominal wall closure was performed after negative bacteria cultures of these sponges were confirmed twice.

After the operation, antibiotics were administered until inflammatory findings became negative. Even in early disappearance of inflammatory findings, intravenous injection was administered for a minimum of 14 days, in principle, followed by a minimum 14-day oral administration.

3. Results

The physical symptoms observed at the time of hospital visit were 11 cases of fever, 9 cases of abdominal pain or back pain, and 1 case of diarrhea (Table 1). All but 1 patient exhibited high CRP values. For risk factors of infection, 2 patients had untreated diabetes, 2 patients had alcoholic liver cirrhosis, 1 patient was malnourished, 1 patient had cancer, and 1 patient was undergoing steroid therapy. Blood cultures were performed for all but 1 patient, and only 2 patients (18%) were positive (Table 2). The possible source of infection was identified in 6 patients: fasciitis of the leg, intraperitoneal abscess, radicular abscess, bacterial endocarditis, bacterial enteritis, and multiple iliopsoas abscesses with infectious spondylitis.

Patient	Blood culture	Infection source	Bacteria cultured from blood or specimen
1	ND	Fasciitis of the leg	Group A *Streptococcus*
2	Negative	Unknown	-
3	Positive	Unknown	*Listeria*
4	Negative	Abdominal abscess	*Enterococcus*
5	Negative	Unknown	*Salmonella*
6	Negative	Unknown	Group A *Streptococcus*
7	Negative	Unknown	-
8	Negative	Unknown	*Listeria*
9	Negative	Radicular abscess	-
10	Negative	Bacterial endocarditis	-
11	Negative	Bacterial enteritis	-
12	Positive	Multiple abscess	MRSA

Table 2. Infection sources and pathogenic bacteria. ND, not done; MRSA, methicillin-resistant *Staphylococcus aureus*

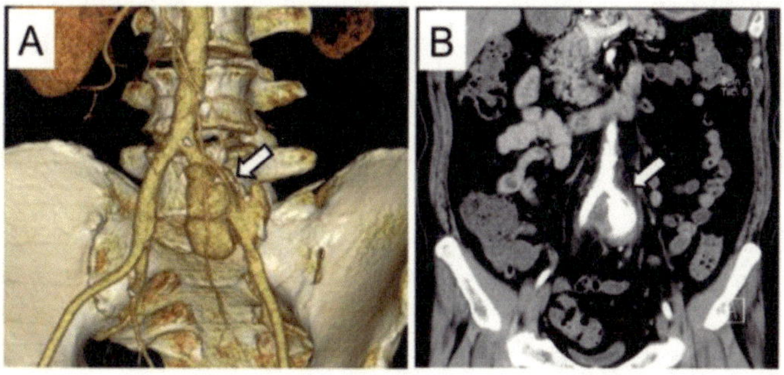

Figure 2. Reconstructed and coronal images of contrast-enhanced computed tomography (CT). A, Volume-rendering CT image of the left common iliac artery revealing a saccular and lobular aneurysm (arrow). B, Coronal CT image of the left common iliac artery revealing an aneurysm with periaortic infiltration and stranding (arrow). (Modified from [18])

Contrast-enhanced CT revealed rupture in 2 patients, while 8 patients had saccular or lobular aneurysms. Of these, 7 had increased tissue concentration surrounding the aneurysm (periaortic stranding) (Figure 2). Two patients had their CT images captured multiple times during the course, and rapid enlargement of the aneurysm was observed in both. As a result of the FDG-PET/CT being performed in 4 patients, their maximum standard uptake value (SUVmax) was found to exceed 5.0, proving that FDG-PET/CT is useful in aiding the diagnosis of infected aortic aneurysm (Figure 3).

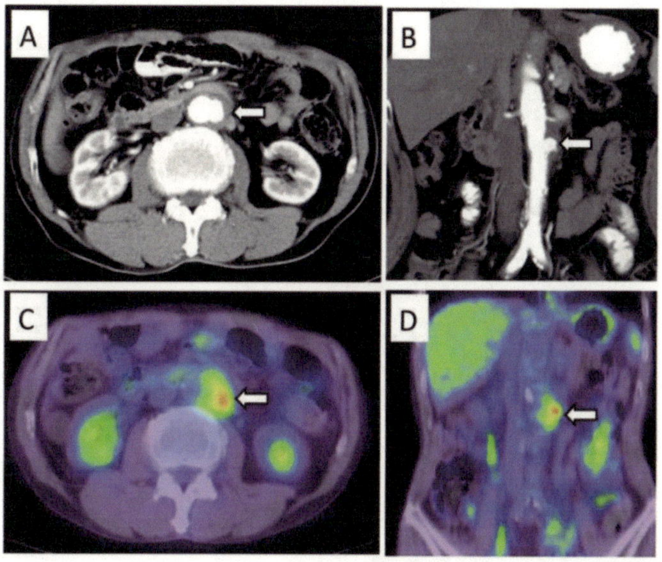

Figure 3. Images of contrast-enhanced computed tomography (CT) and fluorodeoxyglucose-positron emission tomography (FDG-PET)/CT. A and B, Axial and coronal CT images of the infrarenal aorta revealing a saccular aneurysm (arrows). C and D, Axial and coronal FDG-PET/CT images revealing abnormal FDG hypermetabolism with maximum standard uptake value (SUVmax) of 6.2 in the abdominal aorta wall and periaortic space (arrows). (Modified from [18])

Patient	Period from admission to operation (days)	Surgical procedure	Postoperative administration of antibiotics, div/po (days)	Period from operation to discharge (days)	Outcome (months)
1	26	R, O	23/60	30	Alive (105)
2	0	V, O	20/14	20	Dead (6)
3	1	R, O	19/14	26	Alive (68)
4	0	R, V, O	20/14	23	Alive (66)
5	0	R, O	14/14	25	Alive (61)
6	2	R, O	41/14	46	Alive (47)
7	0	O	14/14	38	Alive (47)
8	4	R	42/14	43	Alive (43)
9	8	R, O	14/14	15	Alive (26)
10	8	R, O	14/150	41	Alive (26)
11	10	R, O	14/14	14	Alive (24)
12	48	R, O	14/14	35	Alive (23)

Table 3. Surgical procedures and results. R, rifampicin-soaked graft; V, vacuum-assisted closure technique; O, wrapping by omental flap; div, drip infusion of vein; po, per os

Regarding operation timing, 4 patients were each diagnosed with rupture or impending rupture, and they underwent emergency surgery (Table 3). Three patients who maintained their physical conditions without improvement underwent urgent surgery, and the remaining 5 patients underwent elective surgery after the inflammatory symptoms improved. The mean period from admission to surgery was 8.9 ± 14.3 days (0–48 days).

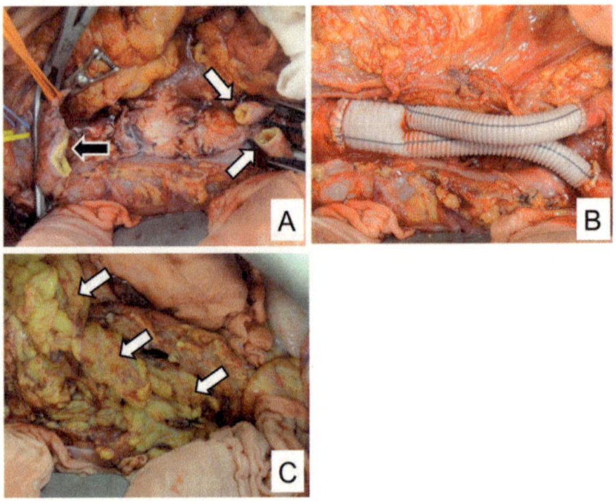

Figure 4. Conventional operative procedures. A, Operative photograph after resection of the aneurysm wall and surrounding infected tissue. Black and white arrows indicate the aortic stump and the common iliac artery stumps, respectively. B, Anatomical reconstruction using rifampicin-soaked Dacron graft. C, Pedicled omental flap wrapping the graft (arrows).

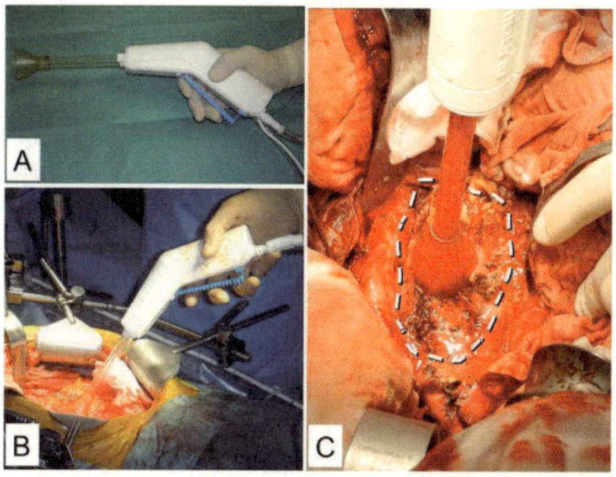

Figure 5. Pulse irrigation using the pulsatile irrigation device. A, SurgiLav® Plus Irrigation System (Stryker), comprising a handpiece assembly with irrigation tubing and a multi-orifice tip with soft cone splash shield. B and C, Operative photographs demonstrating the use of the pulsatile irrigation device, which enables users to clean contaminated areas using high-pressure pulsatile lavage. White dotted line indicates the area from which the aneurysm wall and surrounding infected tissue have been removed.

Regarding operative procedure, infected tissue, including the aneurysm wall, was wholly removed from all patients (Figure 4A), and followed by pulse irrigation using the pulsatile irrigation device (Figure 5) and anatomical reconstruction (Figure 4B). Regarding the grafts, rifampicin-soaked grafts were used in 10 patients, whereas rifampicin could not be prepared for 2 patients due to emergency surgery (Table 3). In the patient with concurrent colon cancer with formation of intraperitoneal abscess and the patient with aneurysm rupture who had widely extended retroperitoneal hemorrhage, the abdominal wall was temporarily closed using the VAC technique before it was closed in a secondary operation after intraperitoneal infection was controlled. In 11 patients in whom the greater omentum could be used, the graft was covered using the pedicled omental flap (Figure 4C, Table 3). Of the 12 patients in this study, pathogenic bacteria were identified in the operative field in 5 patients before irrigation. By contrast, the amount of bacteria in these patients was markedly reduced after the pulse irrigation (Table 4). In addition, pathogenic bacteria were eventually identified in 7 of the 12 patients: group A *Streptococcus* in 2 patients, *Listeria* in 2 patients, *Enterococcus* in 1 patient, *Salmonella* in 1 patient, and methicillin-resistant *Staphylococcus aureus* (MRSA) in 1 patient (Table 2).

The mean period of postoperative intravenous antibiotics administration was 20.7 ± 10.1 days and the mean period of oral administration was 29.1 ± 40.2 days (Table 3). It was noteworthy that in 10 of 12 patients (83.3%), antibiotics administration was ended relatively early, i.e., after 14 days. The mean period of hospitalization from surgery until discharge was 33.8 ± 10.8 days. For postoperative complications, ileus and sepsis resulting from urinary tract infection were observed each in 1 patient. However, both improved within a short time. Eleven patients were discharged and sent home, and the remaining patient was transferred to another hospital for rehabilitation, meaning no patient died during hospitalization

(Table 3). Although 1 patient died from an unrelated cause 6 months after operation, the remaining 11 patients had no reinfection until now and are still alive.

Patient	Bacteria cultured from aneurysm	Bacterial volume, pre-/post-irrigation
1	Group A *Streptococcus*	+/-
2	-	
3	*Listeria*	+++/Few
4	*Enterococcus*	+++/Few
5	*Salmonella*	+/-
6	Group A *Streptococcus*	+/-
7	-	
8	-	
9	-	
10	-	
11	-	
12	-	

Table 4. Effect of pulse irrigation. +++, Bacteria were detected throughout the whole medium; +, Bacteria were detected in only part of the smear; Few, Less than 5 bacteria colonies were detected; -, Bacteria were not detected

4. Discussion

Infected abdominal aortic aneurysm is a rare disease, and its incidence is said to be 0.6%–3.0% [2,8-10]. Despite the advances in antibiotics and surgical materials, mortality is reported to be 11%–36%, and the prognosis of the disease is still poor [2,8,11,12]. Reduced immunity of the patient is considered a risk factor for infected aneurysm. Specifically, diabetes, malignant tumors, immunodeficiency, trauma, alcohol poisoning, and steroid administration have been reported [8,10,12]. Seven of our 12 patients had these risk factors. Moreover, Oderich et al. reported that 93% of 43 patients with infected aneurysm were symptomatic, and fever and pain were observed in 77% and 65% of patients, respectively [12]. As most of our patients were also symptomatic, patients with abdominal aortic aneurysm that exhibit inflammatory symptoms should be managed based on the suspicion of infected aneurysm.

Traditionally, diagnosis of infected aortic aneurysm dictated that patients must have bacteria detected from the aortic aneurysm wall, surrounding tissue, or blood, as well as clinical findings associated with inflammation [8]. However, in not a few patients who were given antibiotics by former physicians, pathogenic bacteria could not be detected or inflammatory findings were poor. In fact, the probability of detecting bacteria in the wall of the aneurysm or in blood culture has been reported to be around 10%–40% [10,13], and the positive rate for preoperative blood culture in this study was only 18.1%. Practically, it is difficult to detect bacteria from blood culture before operation in many cases, especially in patients with rupture or impending rupture, as there is insufficient time for bacteria detection. Meanwhile, a potent basis for diagnosis should be considered when contrast-enhanced CT reveals characteristic findings such as multilobular or saccular aneurysms and increased concentration in the surrounding tissue, or aneurysm diameter that rapidly enlarges in a short time. Macedo et al. reported that the CT findings of infected aneurysms most commonly revealed saccular and lobular aneurysms, accounting for 93% of all cases, followed by increased concentration in the tissue surrounding the aneurysm accounting for 48% of cases [3]. Considering the results of this study, in which physical symptoms, inflammatory findings, and characteristic CT findings were observed in 92%, 92%, and 100% of patients, respectively, infected aneurysm is a reasonable diagnosis if a patient exhibits the physical or inflammatory symptoms along with characteristic findings by contrast-enhanced CT [2,14].

However, it may be difficult to arrive at a diagnosis of infected aneurysm if patients are asymptomatic, have poor inflammatory findings, or have concurrent infection at other sites in addition to an uninfected aneurysm. The usefulness of FDG PET/CT has recently been reported as a diagnostic aid in such patients [15-17]. The patient in Figure 3 exhibited no physical symptoms or inflammatory findings during the course, only revealing a rapidly enlarging saccular aneurysm that was not present 1 year ago. We then performed FDG-PET/CT in this patient under the suspicion of infected aneurysm from the CT findings and observed FDG accumulation (SUVmax, 6.2) conforming to the aneurysm. Therefore, treatment for infected aneurysm was started immediately, producing favorable results. This patient was eventually diagnosed with infected aneurysm by a postoperative pathological test of the aneurysm wall. Recently, we evaluated the usefulness of FDG-PET/CT diagnosis in 4 patients with infected aneurysm against 8 patients as control, and reported 100% sensitivity and 100% specificity at an SUVmax cutoff value of 3.97 [18]. Although our previous report represents a preliminary evaluation involving a small number of patients, FDG-PET/CT could be a useful test for the diagnosis of infected aortic aneurysm through the evaluation of many patients and for the definition of an appropriate SUVmax cutoff value.

Regarding operation timing, onset is acute and the risk of rupture is high, thus it is considered desirable to perform the operation as early as possible, whereas some are of the opinion that the operation should be performed after the infection is resolved with antibiotics [2,9]. The biggest and potentially fatal postoperative complication is infection of the graft, and its prevention can influence the outcome [9]. More specifically, emergency surgery without promising infection control will never achieve good results. Therefore, our policy is to treat the patient with antibiotics as adequately as possible preoperatively and improve physical symptoms and inflammatory findings before performing the operation. Of course, prompt surgery should be considered for patients with rupture or continuous pain, or if the form of an aneurysm changes rapidly on imaging. However, in principle, it is recommended that surgery be performed after infection is controlled as much as possible.

Regarding operative procedure, non-anatomical bypass surgery in a clean operative field was once recommended after resection of the infected aneurysm wall and debridement of the surrounding tissue [19]. In contrast, many have reported that favorable results were obtained with in situ anatomical reconstruction [12,20,21]. In fact, the mortality of non-anatomical reconstruction is reported to be 25%–42%, whereas that of anatomical reconstruction is around 10%–33%, which still indicates high mortality even though anatomical reconstruction appears to be a superior method of reconstruction [8,9,12]. As mentioned earlier, the prevention of graft infection is considered important for improving the surgical results of infected aortic aneurysm, thus ideas such as the use of rifampicin-soaked grafts and covering the graft with the greater omentum have been implemented. Despite this, mortality remains considerably high; therefore, further ideas are required. Although endovascular treatment using a stent-graft has been reported [22,23], the premise for endovascular treatment is the remnant of aneurysm tissue. Even though its usefulness in patients in whom preoperative infection control was favorable has been reported, an important issue remains regarding its application to patients in whom infection control by antibiotics cannot be expected [24].

Graft infection is a rare complication in aneurysm operations in non-infected patients, where graft replacement is performed in a clean field. This means that the key to preventing graft infection in an infected aneurysm must be complete removal of infected tissue from the operative field and in close proximity to a clean field. As infected tissue is strongly adhered to its surroundings, it is very difficult to remove it completely by conventional dissection or resection. Therefore, the role of the irrigation procedure, which is to dilute the remaining bacteria in the operative field as much as possible and to reduce the opportunities for infection, is considered important. In this study, we performed pulse irrigation using a pulsatile irrigation device to remove the bacteria remaining after resection of the aneurysm and surrounding tissue. Pulse irrigation can aid in cleaning contaminated areas with high water pressure and high water volume using irrigation solutions such as saline. As a result, contaminants can be removed in a short time by thorough irrigation as compared with conventional irrigation using a syringe, etc. Currently, this pulse-irrigation method is used in the field of orthopedic surgery [25]. Hargrove et al. reported that it was useful in preventing artificial joint infection after artificial hip joint replacement [26]. However, no report to date has described the usefulness of pulse irrigation in the field of vascular surgery, including in infected aneurysm. In this study, we evaluated the changes in the amounts of bacteria before and after irrigation, and clearly demonstrated that the amount of bacteria in all patients markedly decreased after pulse irrigation. Although a comparison of the surgical outcomes between before and after the introduction of pulse irrigation has not been performed, none of the 12 patients who underwent pulse irrigation had postoperative reinfection, indicating that the pulse irrigation method is highly useful in the elimination of bacteria. Of the several pulse irrigation systems that are currently available, we used the SurgiLav® Plus Irrigation System (Stryker) in this study. This model has a built-in battery, thus can be used as is without requiring a connection to a power source. In addition, the hand-control set contains an outflow nozzle and a suction tube for irrigation solutions, making it possible to perform irrigation and suction simultaneously. With several nozzle tips to choose from, the outflow nozzle can be changed depending on the irrigation site and purpose. As the amount of irrigation increases, there will be substantial splashing of the discharged irrigation solution. Therefore, tips that are better for local irrigation should be used to prevent bacteria from scattering. The maximum perfusion volume of this model is ca. 1500 mL/min, permitting large-volume irrigation in a short time; thus, we believe that it could lead to reductions in aortic clamp time and surgical time.

As far as ideas for the treatment of infected aortic aneurysm go, measures such as the type of antibiotics and the period of use, the use of antibiotic-bonded grafts, and reconstruction methods have been considered. Nevertheless, discussions on irrigation methods have been limited so far. In practice, there remains room for discussion of the amount and content of irrigation solutions. However, based on the results of this study, we consider pulse irrigation an indispensable technique in the operative procedure for infected aneurysm, and it should be highly recommended. We also believe that there are many areas where it can be useful, i.e., not only in infected aneurysm, but also in peripheral artery bypass surgery in contaminated operative fields, graft infection, etc.

In infected abdominal aortic aneurysms, there have been cases where the entire abdominal cavity was contaminated, such as in patients with concurrent intraperitoneal abscess and rupture. As we acknowledge that infection cannot be controlled sufficiently in such patients even if pulse irrigation were used, we carried out temporary abdominal wall closure using the VAC technique in this study. The use of the VAC technique not only permits the drainage of bacteria that cannot be eliminated by retroperitoneum pulse irrigation and thus are spread in the abdominal cavity, but is also expected to prevent abdominal compartment syndrome in patients with rupture [5-7]. In fact, the VAC technique of our group has already produced favorable therapeutic results in patients with mediastinitis after cardiovascular surgery [27]. Taken together, and despite the small number of patients in this study, we believe that the VAC technique is useful in controlling infection spread in the entire abdominal cavity.

There is no definite view as yet regarding postoperative administration of antimicrobial agents. Some have reported that the administration period is 6 or 8 weeks [2,11,19], while others have reported lifetime administration [8,28]. In principle, we administer antibiotics intravenously until postoperative inflammatory findings (fever, white blood cell count, and CRP) improve, followed by the minimum 14-day oral antibiotics administration. As a result, oral administration ended within 14 days in 10 of 12 patients; furthermore, no patient has had recurrence of infection thus far. This period of antibiotics administration appears brief in comparison with that of previous reports [2,8,11,19,28], and this may be the benefit of successful infection control resulting from the efficient reduction of bacteria by intraoperative pulse irrigation and the VAC technique.

5. Conclusions

This study is the first report demonstrating the usefulness of pulse irrigation and the VAC technique in patients with infected abdominal aortic aneurysm. To treat patients with infected aortic aneurysm, we have introduced the pulse-irrigation method using a pulsatile irrigation device into the conventional surgical procedures, which include resection of the aneurysm wall and infected tissue, anatomical reconstruction using a rifampicin-soaked graft, and covering the graft with a pedicled omental flap. Furthermore, we performed temporary abdominal wall closure using the VAC technique concurrently in patients with severe intraperitoneal contamination. As a result of the introduction of these new methods to enhance intra- and postoperative infection control, the lives of all 12 patients were successfully saved. Consequently, this novel treatment strategy for infected abdominal aortic aneurysms is likely to be useful and can be recommended.

Acknowledgements

This work was supported by a Grant-in-Aid for Scientific Research (KAKENHI) from the Japan Society for the Promotion of Science (to K.Y.), the Takeda Science Foundation (to K.Y.), and the SENSHIN Medical Research Foundation (to K.Y.).

Author details

Osamu Yamashita, Koichi Yoshimura*, Noriyasu Morikage, Akira Furutani and Kimikazu Hamano

*Address all correspondence to: yoshimko@yamaguchi-u.ac.jp

Department of Surgery and Clinical Science, Yamaguchi University Graduate School of Medicine, Ube, Japan

References

[1] Weaver, M. R., & Reddy, D. J. (2010). Infected Aneurysm. *In: Cronenwett J.L., Johnston K.W. (eds.) Vascular Surgery. Philadelphia: Saunders*, 2156-2167.

[2] Hsu, R. B., Chen, R. J., Wang, S. S., & Chu, S. H. (2004). Infected aortic aneurysms: clinical outcome and risk factor analysis. *Journal of Vascular Surgery*, 40(1), 30-35.

[3] Macedo, T. A., Stanson, A. W., Oderich, G. S., Johnson, C. M., Panneton, J. M., & Tie, M. L. (2004). Infected aortic aneurysms: imaging findings. *Radiology*, 231(1), 250-257.

[4] Chaikof, E. L., Brewster, D. C., Dalman, R. L., Makaroun, M. S., Illig, K. A., Sicard, G. A., et al. (2009). The care of patients with an abdominal aortic aneurysm: the Society for Vascular Surgery practice guidelines. *Journal of Vascular Surgery*, 50(4), S2-S49.

[5] Rasmussen, T. E., Hallett, J. W. Jr, Noel, AA, Jenkins, G., Bower, T. C., Cherry, K. J. Jr, et al. (2002). Early abdominal closure with mesh reduces multiple organ failure after

ruptured abdominal aortic aneurysm repair: guidelines from a 10-year case-control study. *Journal of Vascular Surgery*, 35(2), 246-253.

[6] Mayer, D., Rancic, Z., Meier, C., Pfammatter, T., Veith, F. J., & Lachat, M. (2009). Open abdomen treatment following endovascular repair of ruptured abdominal aortic aneurysms. *Journal of Vascular Surgery*, 50(1), 1-7.

[7] Morikage, N., Onoda, M., Nomura, S., Yoshimura, K., Furutani, A., & Hamano, K. (2009). Surgical strategy for ruptured abdominal aortic aneurysms in cases of severe shock. *Japanese Journal of Vascular Surgery (in Japanese)*, 18(1), 1-8.

[8] Muller, B. T., Wegener, O. R., Grabitz, K., Pillny, M., Thomas, L., & Sandmann, W. (2001). Mycotic aneurysms of the thoracic and abdominal aorta and iliac arteries: experience with anatomic and extra-anatomic repair in 33 cases. *Journal of Vascular Surgery*, 33(1), 106-113.

[9] Sessa, C., Farah, I., Voirin, L., Magne, J. L., Brion, J. P., & Guidicelli, H. (1997). Infected aneurysms of the infrarenal abdominal aorta: diagnostic criteria and therapeutic strategy. *Annals of Vascular Surgery*, 11(5), 453-463.

[10] Gomes, M. N., Choyke, P. L., & Wallace, R. B. (1992). Infected aortic aneurysms. A changing entity. *Annals of Surgery*, 215(5), 435-442.

[11] Moneta, G. L., Taylor, L. M. Jr, Yeager, R. A., Edwards, J. M., Nicoloff, A. D., Mc Connell, D. B., et al. (1998). Surgical treatment of infected aortic aneurysm. *American Journal of Surgery*, 175(5), 396-369.

[12] Oderich, G. S., Panneton, J. M., Bower, T. C., Cherry, K. J. Jr , Rowland, C. M., Noel, A. A., et al. (2001). Infected aortic aneurysms: aggressive presentation, complicated early outcome, but durable results. *Journal of Vascular Surgery*, 34(5), 900-908.

[13] Ernst, C. B., Campbell, H. C. Jr, Daugherty, ME, Sachatello, C. R., & Griffen, W. O. Jr. (1977). Incidence and significance of intra-operative bacterial cultures during abdominal aortic aneurysmectomy. *Annals of Surgery*, 185(6), 626-633.

[14] Maeda, H., Umezawa, H., Goshima, M., Hattori, T., Nakamura, T., Umeda, T., et al. (2011). Primary infected abdominal aortic aneurysm: surgical procedures, early mortality rates, and a survey of the prevalence of infectious organisms over a 30-year period. *Surgery Today*, 41(3), 346-351.

[15] van der Vaart, M. G., Meerwaldt, R., Slart, R. H., van Dam, G. M., Tio, R. A., & Zeebregts, C. J. (2008). Application of PET/SPECT imaging in vascular disease. *European Journal of Vascular and Endovascular Surgery*, 35(5), 507-513.

[16] Choi, S.J, Lee, J.S, Cheong, M.H, Byun, S.S, & Hyun, I.Y. (2008). F-18 FDG PET/CT in the management of infected abdominal aortic aneurysm due to Salmonella. *Clinical Nuclear Medicine*, 33(7), 492-495.

[17] Davison, J. M., Montilla-Soler, J. L., Broussard, E., Wilson, R., Cap, A., & Allen, T. (2005). F-18 FDG PET-CT imaging of a mycotic aneurysm. *Clinical Nuclear Medicine,* 30(7), 483-487.

[18] Yamashita, O., Morikage, N., Okazaki, Y., Suehiro, K., Yoshimura, K., Suga, K., et al. (2011). Positron emission tomography and computed tomography in the diagnosis of an infected aneurysm. *The Journal of Japanese College of Angiology (in Japanese),* 51(4), 473-479.

[19] Takano, H., Taniguchi, K., Kuki, S., Nakamura, T., Miyagawa, S., & Masai, T. (2003). Mycotic aneurysm of the infrarenal abdominal aorta infected by Clostridium septicum: a case report of surgical management and review of the literature. *Journal of Vascular Surgery,* 38(4), 847-851.

[20] Hsu, R. B., Tsay, Y. G., Wang, S. S., & Chu, S. H. (2002). Surgical treatment for primary infected aneurysm of the descending thoracic aorta, abdominal aorta, and iliac arteries. *Journal of Vascular Surgery,* 36(4), 746-750.

[21] Robinson, J. A., & Johansen, K. (1991). Aortic sepsis: is there a role for in situ graft reconstruction? Journal of Vascular Surgery discussion 82-84., 13(5), 677-682.

[22] Lee, K. H., Won, J. Y., Lee, do Y., Choi, D., Shim, W. H., Chang, B. C., et al. (2006). Stent-graft treatment of infected aortic and arterial aneurysms. *Journal of Endovascular Therapy,* 13(3), 338-345.

[23] Hartman, V., Jiang, H., & Thomas, B. (2009). Succesful [Successful] endovascular repair of an abdominal mycotic aneurysm. A case report. *Acta Chirurgica Belgica,* 109(6), 788-790.

[24] Kan, C. D., Yen, H. T., Kan, C. B., & Yang, Y. J. (2012). The feasibility of endovascular aortic repair strategy in treating infected aortic aneurysms. *Journal of Vascular Surgery,* 55(1), 55-60.

[25] Flow-Investigators. (2010). Fluid lavage of open wounds (FLOW): design and rationale for a large, multicenter collaborative 2 x 3 factorial trial of irrigating pressures and solutions in patients with open fractures. *BMC Musculoskeletal Disorders,* 85 EOF, http://www.biomedcentral.com/1471-2474/11/85, (accessed 04 May 2012).

[26] Hargrove, R., Ridgeway, S., Russell, R., Norris, M., Packham, I., & Levy, B. (2006). Does pulse lavage reduce hip hemiarthroplasty infection rates? *The Journal of Hospital Infection,* 62(4), 446-449.

[27] Kobayashi, T., Mikamo, A., Kurazumi, H., Suzuki, R., Shirasawa, B., & Hamano, K. (2011). Secondary omental and pectoralis major double flap reconstruction following aggressive sternectomy for deep sternal wound infections after cardiac surgery. *Journal of Cardiothoracic Surgery,* 6, 56.

[28] Abdel, Azim. T. A. (2005). Infected aortic aneurysms. *Acta Chirurgica Belgica,* 105(5), 482-486.

Chapter 11

A Proposal for Redesigning Aortofemoral Prosthetic Y Graft for Treating Abdominal Aortic Aneurysms

Tetsuo Fujimoto, Hiroshi Iwamura,
Yasuyuki Shiraishi, Tomoyuki Yambe,
Kiyotaka Iwasaki and Mitsuo Umezu

Additional information is available at the end of the chapter

http://dx.doi.org/10.5772/ 52979

1. Introduction

Aortofemoral Y grafts are applied commonly in the treatment on those abdominal aortic aneurysms which are at a high risk of rupture. Typically in these Y grafts, the diameter of the stem conduit is 16mm and that of the branch conduit is 8 mm. The ratio of the stem to the branch is different from that of the natural anatomical bifurcation: the branch diameter is small in comparison with that of the natural vessel. It is supposed that the branch diameter is too small to allow these graft implants to work effectively. Consequently, new grafts with a 9-mm branch diameter have been recently implemented in clinical applications as shown in Fig. 1 [1]. However, it has not been discussed fully from the viewpoint of hemodynamics whether this difference of scale at the bifurcation has an actual influence on the blood flow. Many prosthetic devices, including the Y grafts that are discussed here, are currently being used in clinical applications. Although some of these devices should be redesigned in order to improve their properties, methodologies for redesigning them have not been established. In this study, Y grafts have been selected as a subject of study; however, it is not that a completely newly-designed product is introduced, but that a new concept, by which a new product can be developed or redesigned, is presented. At first, the effect of bifurcation on pressure loss in the Y graft is explored by experiments conducted under conditions of steady flow. This is done in order to understand basically the characteristics of bifurcation flow, such as that which is found in a Y graft. Secondly, additional experiments were conducted in order to demonstrate the effects of an incremental increase in branch diameter in a newly designed aortofemoral Y graft under conditions of pulsatile flow.

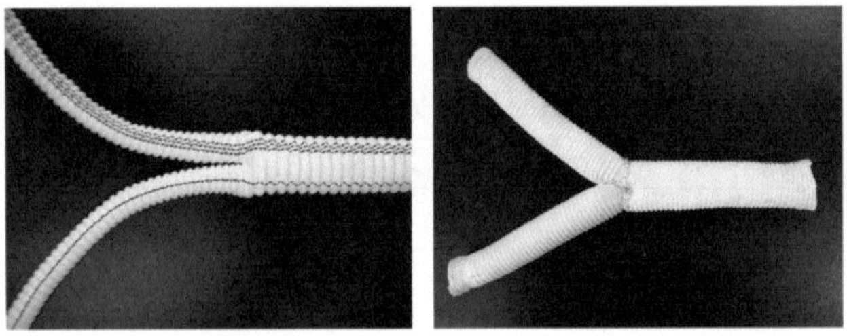

(a) Conventional graft (b) Newer graft

Figure 1. Photographs of aortofemoral Y grafts

2. Effect of bifurcation on pressure loss in aortofemoral prosthetic Y grafts

2.1. Purpose of steady flow experiments

The flow of fluid such as blood in a circular tube with a constant inner diameter causes pressure to drop due to energy loss. If there is a bifurcation in the circular tube, generally change in the flow causes additional energy loss. It is important to understand how the bifurcation has an influence on the flow from the viewpoint of hydrodynamics in order to design Y grafts. Therefore, the experiments were conducted to attempt to indicate the effect of bifurcation on flow under a steady flow condition.

2.2. Method of steady flow experiments

2.2.1. Bifurcation model

Three types of fluid models of rigid aortofemoral Y grafts were made as shown in Fig. 2 [1][2][3]. Epoxy was used as the material of the models that were produced by the lost wax method.

First of all, the mold, whose outer shape replicates the inner shape of the Y graft, is made from wax. The wax mold is immersed in melted liquid-state epoxy which solidifies in several hours. Secondly, after the material becomes a solid epoxy block, it is heated up and the wax in the block runs out. Finally, from the above process, the epoxy block, in which the flow channel that replicates the inner shape of the Y graft is formed, with a smooth inner surface, becomes the fluid model of the Y graft for experiments.

There are an inlet and two outlets in the bifurcation models. Correspondingly, the conduit of the inlet end is called the stem and the conduits of the outlet ends are called the branches. The first model, in which the diameter of the stem is 16 mm and that of the branches is 8 mm, replicates conventional grafts. In the second model, which replicates the newer graft, the branch diameter is 9 mm and the stem diameter is the same as that of the conventional

http://dx.doi.org/10.5772/ 52979

graft. In the third model, which replicates yet another style of newer graft, the branch diameter is 12 mm and the stem diameter is the same as those of the other two models.

In all models, the structure is symmetrical along the long axis of the stem conduit, the angle between the branch conduits is 60 degrees, and the lengths of the stem and branch conduits are 195 mm and 170 or 190 mm respectively. In order to measure the pressure in the flow, the ports are set in the models along the flow channels.

2.2.2. *Test circuit for steady flow experiments*

A fluid test circuit was set up in order to conduct experiments for these three bifurcation models as shown in Fig. 3 [1]. The circuit consists of a higher overflow tank, a lower overflow tank, a valve for regulating flow rate, and manometers for measuring pressure in these bifurcation models.

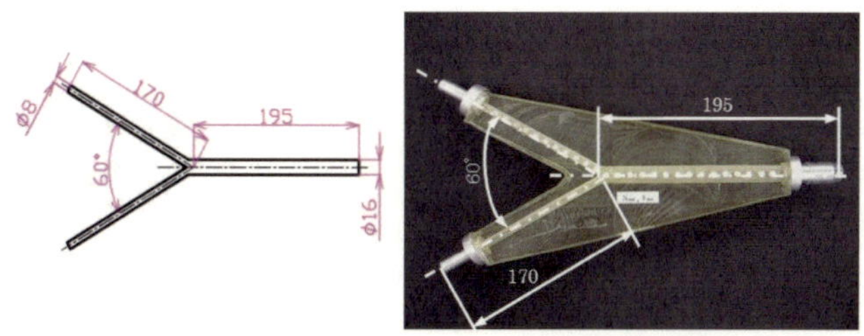

(a) Conventional model (Stem diameter: 16 mm, Branch diameter: 8 mm)

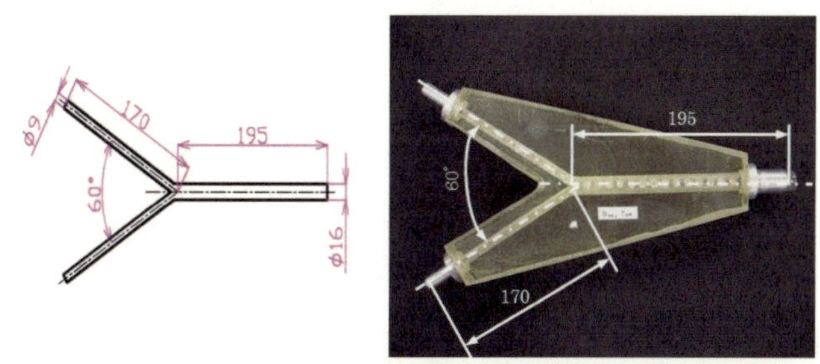

(b) Newer model (Stem diameter: 16 mm, Branch diameter: 9 mm)

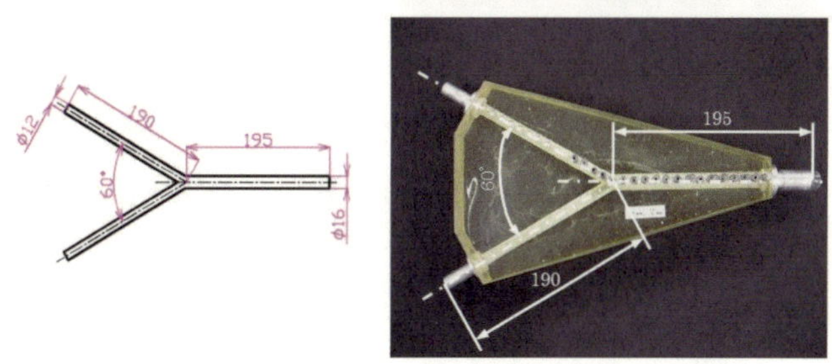

(c) Newer model (Stem diameter: 16 mm, Branch diameter: 12 mm)

Figure 2. Three types of models of rigid aortofemoral Y grafts

Each model is installed between the higher and the lower overflow tank in the test circuit, in which tap water is used as the fluid. The height of the water in the manometer is called water head, which indicates static pressure in the flow channel. The higher tank loads the inlet of the bifurcation model with constant 1000 mm water head, or pressure, through the regulating valve and the lower tank loads the outlets of the model with constant 300 mm water head. The fluid in the circuit is driven by the constant pressure gradient between these two tanks and thus has a condition of steady flow.

The manometers are connected to the ports on the model to measure the pressures of the flow, and the flow rate is measured by weighing the water overflowed from the lower tank.

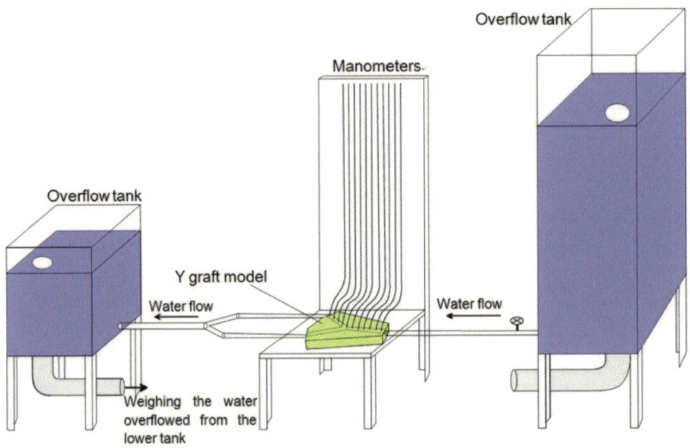

Figure 3. Test circuit used for steady flow study

2.3. Effect of bifurcation under condition of steady flow

The results from the conducted experiments were analyzed to explore the relationships between pressure and flow rate in the bifurcation model under the condition of steady flow.

Energy loss due to fluid flow through the bifurcation causes a reduction in the pressure of the flow (that is, the pressure gradient along the flow stream). At first, it is simply confirmed how the pressure gradient between the inlet and the outlet of the bifurcation model changes when the flow rate increases. The flow rate is shown here in the form of a Reynolds number as a dimensionless parameter to enable discussion of these flow properties generally.

In Fig. 4, it is shown that the pressure gradients change to Reynolds numbers that range from 2000 to 5000 [1][2][3]. These Reynolds numbers might be supposed to be large in comparison with those in the natural abdominal aorta, but these numbers were settled in order to figure out the characteristics of the bifurcation flow from the view point of hydrodynamics rather than the flow of the natural aorta.

Pressure gradients increase as Reynolds number increases in all bifurcation models; however, changes in these pressure gradients differ in degree among these models. An increase in

http://dx.doi.org/10.5772/ 52979

the branch diameter is accompanied by a decrease in the pressure gradient. In fact, the pressure gradient between the inlet and the outlets was only 1 mmHg in the case of a 12 mm branch, which was 4 mmHg less than that of the 8 mm branch at Reynolds number 5000. As mentioned above, the effect, that an increase in the branch diameter causes a decrease in the pressure gradient, grows in accord with increase in the Reynolds number.

The pressure gradient discussed above is caused by flow resistance in the stem conduit, the branch conduit, and the bifurcation itself. In other words, summation of the energy loss in the fluid flow at the stem conduit, the branch conduit, and the bifurcation is estimated as the pressure gradient. Next, it is important to discuss whether the difference in the structure of the bifurcation has an essential influence on the pressure gradient.

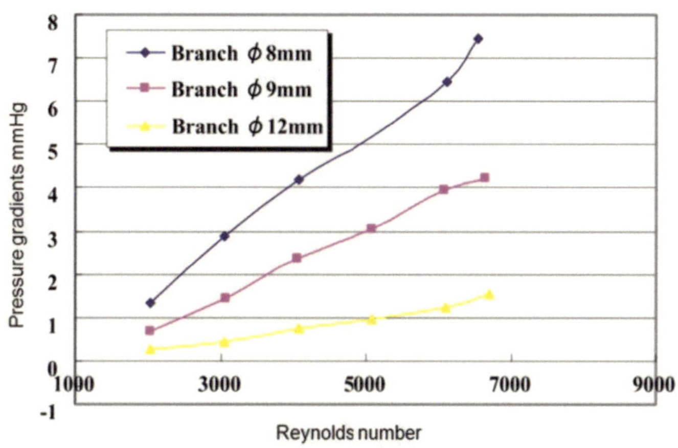

Figure 4. Pressure gradients at each Reynolds number

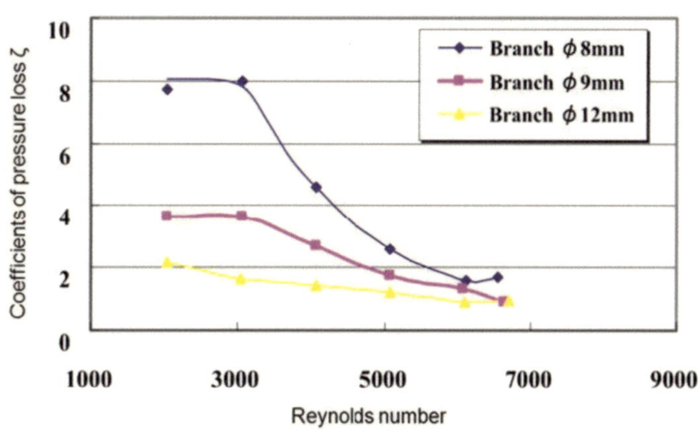

Figure 5. Coefficients of pressure loss at each Reynolds number

In order to evaluate the effect of the bifurcation not including the stem and the branch conduits, we focus on the flow at the bifurcation in itself.

When it is supposed that the pressure loss due to the bifurcation is proportional to the kinetic energy of the flow through it, the pressure loss ΔP is presented as

$$\Delta P = \zeta \rho V^2 / 2 \tag{1}$$

where ζ is the coefficient of pressure loss, ϱ is density of the fluid, and V is the flow velocity.

From the measured pressures in the stem and the branch conduits, the pressure loss ΔP due to the bifurcation in itself is calculated. Furthermore, the coefficient of pressure loss ζ, by which the flow resistance can be compared among the different bifurcations, is calculated from the above formula based on the flow rate measurements.

In Fig. 5, the relations of the calculated coefficient of pressure loss ζ to the Reynolds number are shown. In the 12 mm branch, the coefficient of pressure loss due to bifurcation is less than half of that in the 8 mm branch.

Summing up the results of these experiments, in which variation in the branch diameter in the bifurcation model was evaluated from the standpoint of hydrodynamics in epoxy-based models, it was revealed that in the bifurcations an incremental increase of only 4 mm in branch diameter affects hydrodynamic characteristics drastically under steady flow conditions.

3. Characteristics of a newly designed aortofemoral prosthetic Y graft under pulsatile flow conditions

3.1. Purpose of pulsatile flow experiments

In the experiments on steady flow mentioned above, flow in bifurcations was studied. The results showed that an increase in the branch diameter of the bifurcation is accompanied by a decrease in the pressure gradient and that the size of the bifurcation has an essential influence on the flow through it. From these results, it might be suggested that a larger conduit branch for a Y graft would be more efficient, because there is a potential for an increase in downstream flow from implanted Y grafts. However, there are many differences between the experimental conditions in the test circuit and those in the natural aorta, of which the most notable is the condition of the flow, which was steady in the experiment but is pulsatile in the aorta. In pulsatile flow, other effects not confirmed in the steady flow experiments may occur. Thus, it is not clear whether the results obtained under the condition of steady flow can be applied directly to the natural aorta.

Additional study is necessary to evaluate the effects of the new graft model in the setting of the natural aorta, and there are several possible methods for this study. For instance, experiments either in an animal or in a mock circuit simulating the natural blood circulation are

http://dx.doi.org/10.5772/ 52979

employed typically. In the former, natural pulsatile flow conditions can be obtained, but it is difficult to measure stable hemodynamic conditions repeatedly. However, in the latter, it is not difficult to measure pressure and flow, but it is necessary to confirm whether it actually simulates the natural setting.

In this study, a mock circulatory system was set up to conduct experiments under pulsatile flow condition.

The mock circulatory system, in which bifurcation models replicating Y grafts are installed and fluid is fed through the grafts, simulates the left ventricle, the aorta, and the peripheral vessels. The structures of the bifurcation models and the mock system, as well as the reason that the mock system can be used to mimic hemodynamics in the aorta, are explained first. After that, the results obtained from the experiments are described.

3.2. Method of pulsatile flow experiments

3.2.1. Bifurcation models used for experiments

In the pulsatile flow experiments, three models of rigid aortofemoral Y grafts, essentially the same as those used in the experiments of steady flow, were used as shown in Fig. 2. The type of epoxy, model material, and methods used in this experiment were the same as those in the steady flow experiments.

In all models, the diameter of the stem conduit is 16 mm. The diameters of the branch conduits in the first, the second and the third model are 8, 9, and 12 mm respectively; the first model corresponds to a conventional Y graft, and the second and the third models to newer grafts. The length of each conduit and the angle between the branch conduits are the same as those of the models used in the steady flow experiments.

3.2.2. Mock circulatory system for pulsatile flow experiments

A mock circulatory system was constructed as shown in Fig. 6 to conduct experiments under conditions similar to those in the natural blood circulatory system [1][4][5]. The mock system consisted of a pulsatile pump, valves for flow resistance, compliance units, and overflow tanks.

The pulsatile pump, which was driven by a pulse motor, had an inlet and an outlet port. The inlet port and the outlet port were connected to an overflow tank and a compliance unit respectively. The outlet port was also connected to another downstream-side overflow tank in order to regulate pressure and flow rate. The pump, which functionally simulated the left ventricle, could output as much fluid volume as was set preliminarily and could create given flow patterns.

Three valves were installed upstream from the overflow tanks to regulate flow resistance. When the resistance was increased by the valve, the flow rate into the overflow tank decreased. Thus, an increase in the resistance corresponded to constriction of vessels in the blood circulatory system. On the other hand, a decrease in the resistance corresponded to dilatation of blood vessels. By operating these valves, changes in flow resistance of the mock system represented changes in the diameters of actual blood vessels.

Three compliance units were installed in the mock system. Each compliance unit had a casing made from acryl into which an elastic membrane and a spring were built. Pressure in the fluid was changed through contact with the membrane, which in turn was pressed by the spring. Owing to the restoring force of the spring built in the unit, the unit achieved the effect changing pressure in accordance with changes in the fluid volume. As fluid volume in the unit increased, so did the restoring force of the spring, and thus pressure intensified. In the contrasting situation, an increment in pressure attenuated in the case of a decrease in the restoring force of the spring. Blood vessels in the natural circulatory system are supposed to consist of elements of resistance and compliance from the viewpoint of dynamics. The element of compliance is caused mainly by the elasticity of the vessel wall. A stronger restoring force in the spring indicated higher elasticity, comparatively. On the other hand, a weaker force indicated that the elasticity was lower. Therefore, through inclusion of the compliance unit, the mock system could simulate the elasticity of the vessel wall.

By combination of the valve as a resistance element and the compliance unit as an elasticity element, input impedance of the vessel could be regulated, as will be discussed later.

Each bifurcation model was installed in the mock system and physiological saline was fed through the fluid circuit. Pressure and flow rate at the inlet and the outlet of each model were measured under conditions of pulsatile flow by pressure transducers and electromagnetic flow meters.

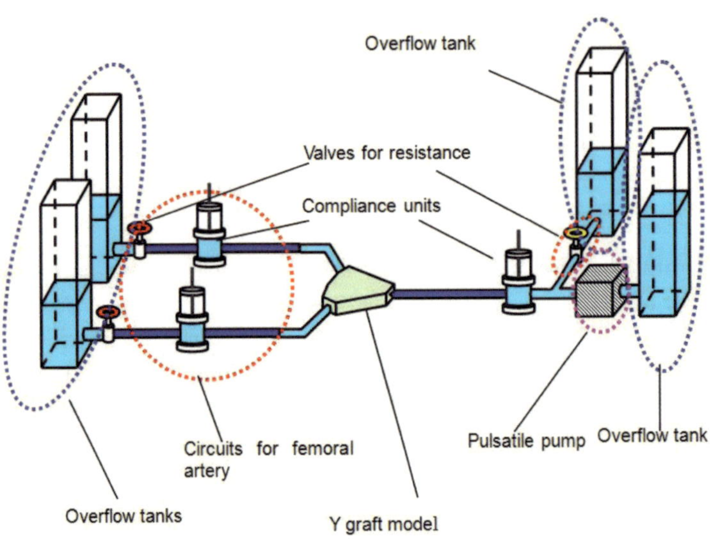

Figure 6. Mock circulatory system for pulsatile flow experiments

http://dx.doi.org/10.5772/ 52979

3.2.3. *Experimental conditions*

Experiments were conducted in the mock system described above to evaluate the newer Y graft under conditions of pulsatile flow. However, the question of whether or not the constructed mock system simulates effectively the natural blood circulatory system must be answered. How can the question be answered? In steady flow in a circular tube, pressure and flow rate are constant with time. Therefore, a property of flow is presented simply by a ratio of pressure divided by flow rate or velocity as a flow resistance.

In pulsatile flow such as blood flow in the artery, a property of flow is indicated generally as the input impedance instead of as the flow resistance as mentioned above [6][7]. It is difficult to evaluate the characteristics of pulsatile flow, in which pressure and flow rate change constantly with time; however, pressure and flow rate are periodic signals that are generally represented as an expanded series.

Next, a basic explanation about the input impedance is shown. Pressure *P(t)* and flow rate *Q(t)* are expanded in Fourier series as follows [5][8][9],

$$P(t) = P_0 + \sum_{n=1}^{\infty} P_n \cos(2\pi n f_1 t - \alpha_n) \tag{2}$$

$$Q(t) = Q_0 + \sum_{n=1}^{\infty} Q_n \cos(2\pi n f_1 t - \beta_n) \tag{3}$$

where P_0 and Q_0 are time averages of *P(t)* and *Q(t)*, P_n and Q_n are amplitudes of n-order harmonic, f_1 is fundamental frequency, and α_n and β_n are phases of n-order harmonic.

Input impedance is represented as modulus Z_n and phase Ψ_n as follows,

$$Z_n = \frac{P_n}{Q_n} \tag{4}$$

$$\psi_n = \beta_n - \alpha_n \tag{5}$$

We conducted an animal experiment, in which a goat weighing 51 kg was used, in order to estimate the input impedance at the femoral artery [5]. The input impedance was calculated by the above process from the measured pressure and flow rate in the femoral artery of the animal. Some examples of the results are shown in Figs. 7 and 8. In Fig. 7 (a) and (b), the modulus and the phase are plotted corresponding to frequencies under a control condition. An increase in the frequency is accompanied by a decrease in the modulus and the phase changes from negative to positive with an increase in the frequency. They are typical changes in the input impedance of the artery. In Fig. 8, changes in the input impedance are shown when a vasoconstrictor was injected into the experimental animal. The tendency is same in both cases; however, the modulus in the case of vasoconstriction is higher than that in the control condition. This indicates that change in the vessel can be represented quantitatively. The modulus at a frequency of 0 Hz indicates an average resistance of the artery system and is an especially important value. The value of the modulus increases from 1.0 x10^4 to 3.4 x 10^4 dyne·sec/cm^3 when the vessel is constricted.

We assumed that a mock system can simulate the natural system in terms of evaluating the Y grafts from the view point of hydrodynamics, when the modulus of the mock system at the femoral artery approximates that of the natural system, because the branch conduits of a Y graft are connected to the femoral arteries.

In the mock system, by regulating the valves as resistance elements and the compliance units as elasticity elements, the mean flow rate at the inlet of the bifurcation model could be made to be 1.0 liter/min with the conditions of the input impedance in the femoral artery being 1.0 x10^4 and 3.4 x 10^4 dyne·sec/cm^3 at 0 Hz as shown in Fig. 9. Each modulus obtained from the mock system was similar to those from the animal experiment.

3.3. Characteristics of newly designed Y graft under condition of pulsatile flow

From the above discussion, the efficacy of the newly designed Y grafts, that is those with an increased diameter of the branch conduit, can be evaluated in the mock system, in which the input impedance in the femoral artery approximates that in the natural system. To do this, it was important to set suitable conditions by regulating the valves and the compliance units. In the experiments, suitable conditions were those in which the mean flow rate at the inlet of the bifurcation model was 1.0 liter/min and the input impedance of the femoral artery was 1.0 x10^4 dyne·sec/cm^3 at 0 Hz in the mock system as above mentioned.

The results of experiments obtained under these conditions are shown in Fig. 10 [1][5][10]. The pressure and the flow rate were measured at the inlet of the bifurcation model by a pressure transducer and an electromagnetic flow meter. The mean pressures were equivalent to 66 mmHg in all models, but the flow rates changed due to the diameter of the branch conduit, as shown in Fig. 10 (a) and (b). The mean flow rate was 1.0 l/min in both the 8 mm and the 9 mm branch. However, in the 12mm branch, the mean flow rate was increased by 0.2 liter/min under the same conditions. An increase in the branch diameter caused an increase in the flow through the branch even if the input impedance in the femoral artery was the same across different branch diameters.

http://dx.doi.org/10.5772/ 52979

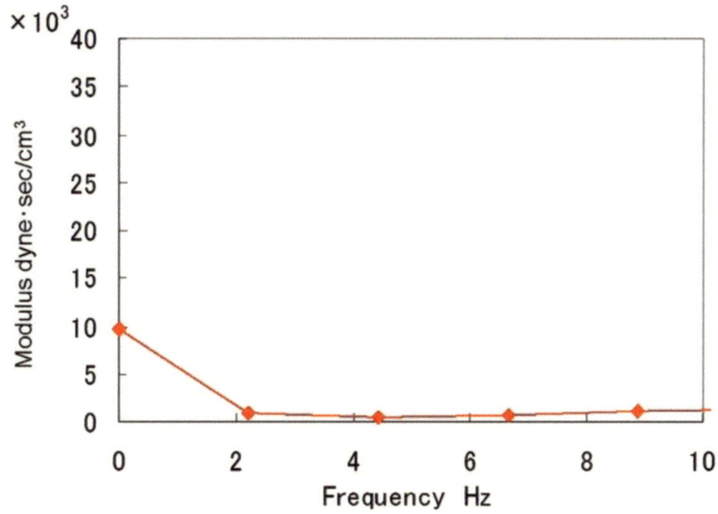

(a) Modulus of input impedance

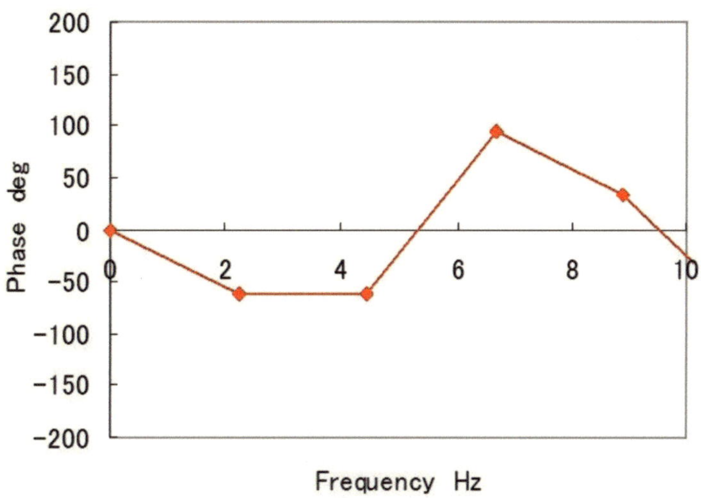

(b) Phase of input impedance

Figure 7. Input impedance in the femoral artery obtained in an animal experment under control condition

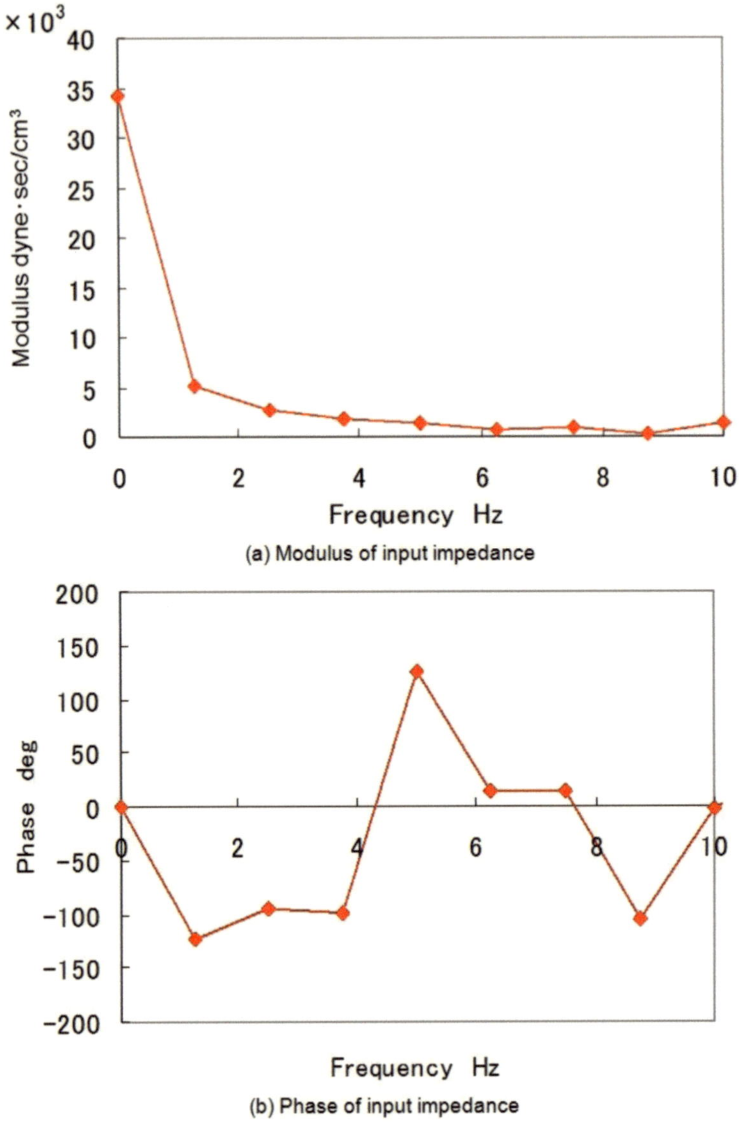

Figure 8. Input impedance in the femoral artery obtained in an animal experment under vasoconstrictive condition

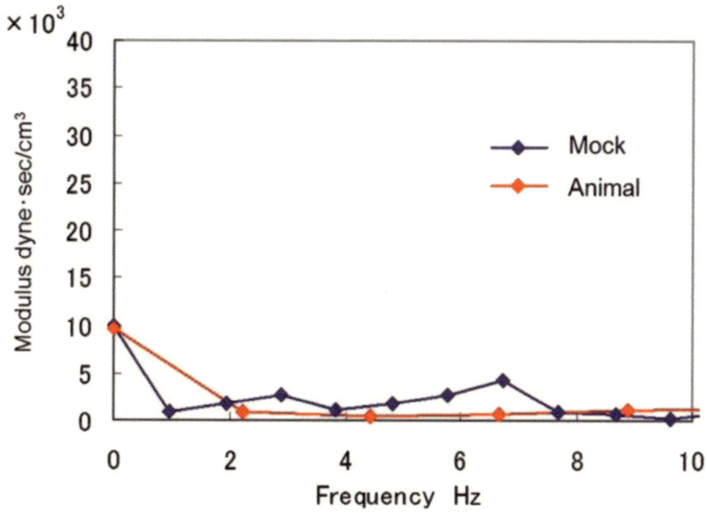

(a) Modulus obtained under control condition

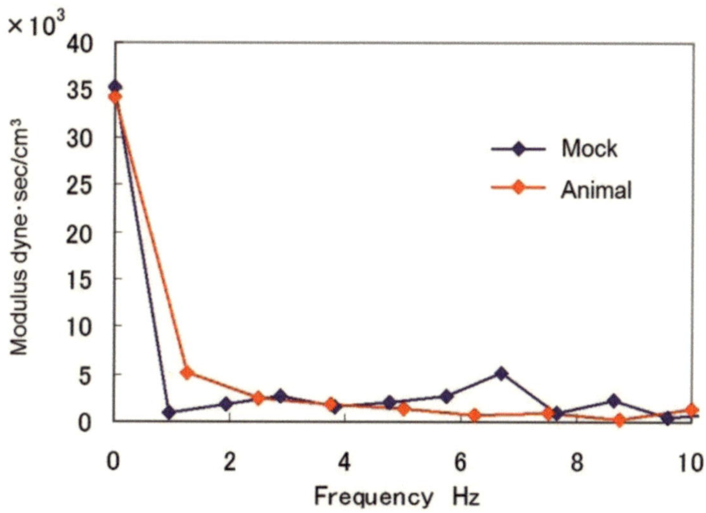

(b) Modulus obtained under vasoconstrictive condition

Figure 9. Comparison of input impedance in the femoral artery obtained in the mock circulatory system with that in an animal experiment. Mock and Animal indicate experimental results in the mock circulatory system and the experimental animal respectively.

When the mean flow rates were equivalent to 1.2 l/min across all models, the pressures changed due to the diameter of the branch conduit as shown in Fig. 11 (a) and (b). The mean pressure was 85 mmHg in the 8 mm branch; however, the mean pressure decreased by 19 mmHg in the 12mm branch under the same conditions.

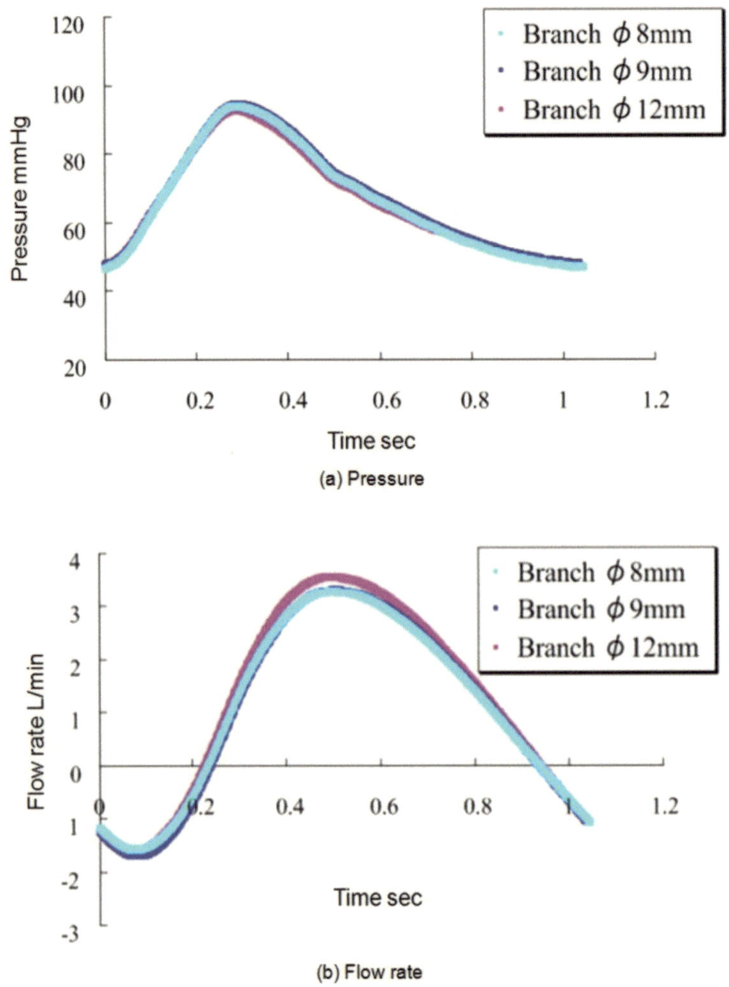

Figure 10. Results of pulsatile flow experiments under condition of constant mean pressure

In addition, when the input impedance was increased up to 3.0 x 10^4 dyne·sec/cm^3 at 0 Hz by regulating the resistant unit in the mock circuit, the results were found to be the same as those in which the impedance was 1.0 x10^4 dyne·sec/cm^3 [5].

Summing up the results of these experiments, a newly designed aortofemoral Y graft was compared with a conventional graft from the standpoint of hydrodynamics using epoxy-based models under pulsatile flow conditions. As a result, it was revealed that an incremental increase in the branch diameter increases definitely the flow rate through the graft.

http://dx.doi.org/10.5772/ 52979

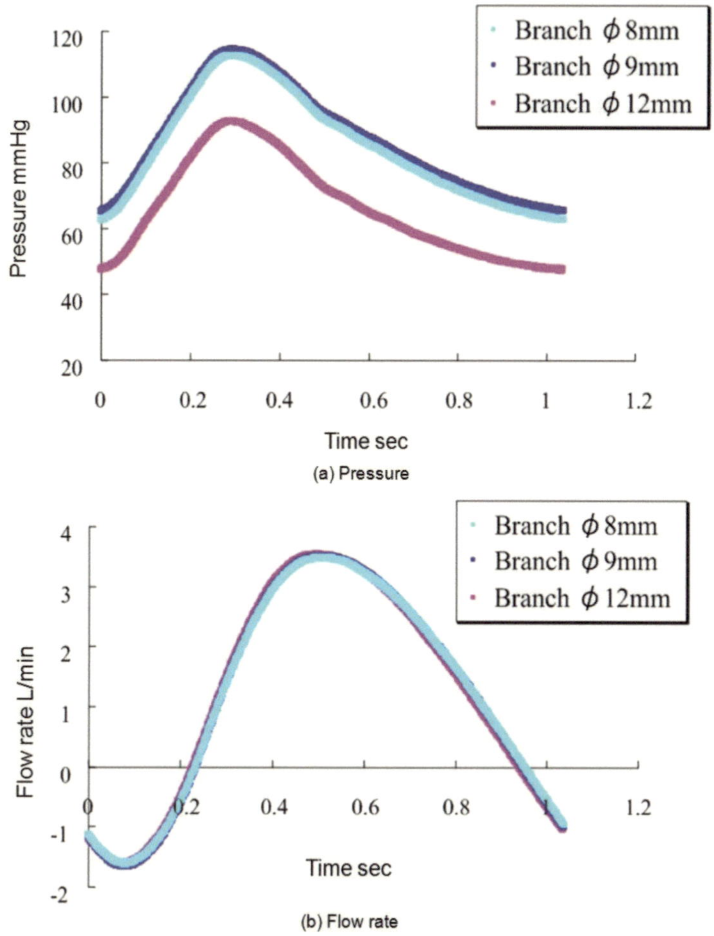

Figure 11. Results of pulsatile flow experiments under condition of constant mean flow rate

4. Conclusion

In aortofemoral Y grafts for treating abdominal aortic aneurysms, the ratio of the stem conduit to the branch conduit is different from that in the native bifurcation anatomically. Because the branch diameter is small compared with that of the natural vessel, it is supposed that the difference of scale at the bifurcation in Y grafts has an influence on the blood flow. Thus, variation in the branch diameter in aortofemoral Y grafts was discussed from the standpoint of hydrodynamics.

First, a basic evaluation of the effect of variation in the branch diameter in the bifurcation was executed using epoxy-based models. As a result, it was revealed that in the bifurcations an incremental increase of only 4 mm in branch diameter affects hydrodynamic characteristics drastically under steady flow conditions.

Secondly, using epoxy-based models, a newly designed Y graft with 12 mm branches was compared with a conventional graft with an 8 mm branch under pulsatile flow conditions in a mock circulatory system that simulated the natural system. The result revealed that an increase in the branch diameter undoubtedly increases the flow rate through the graft even under the same input impedance in the femoral artery.

These results are suggested to be useful for a proposal concerning the redesign of aortofemoral prosthetic Y graft for treating abdominal aortic aneurysms. In this study, Y grafts are selected as a subject of study. However, it is not that a completely newly-designed product is introduced so much as a new concept, by which a new product can be developed or redesigned, is presented.

Author details

Tetsuo Fujimoto[1*], Hiroshi Iwamura[2], Yasuyuki Shiraishi[3], Tomoyuki Yambe[3], Kiyotaka Iwasaki[1] and Mitsuo Umezu[1]

*Address all correspondence to: fujimoto@aoni.waseda.jp

1 Waseda University, Japan

2 Owari General Hospital, Japan

3 Tohoku University, Japan

References

[1] Fujimoto, T., Nakano, S., Iwamura, H., Shiraishi, Y., Yambe, T., & Umezu, M. (2008). A study on a newly designed aortofemoral prosthetic Y graft. *Biocybernetics and Biomedical Engineering*, 28(1), 59-63.

[2] Hayafumi, Ohashi. (2004). Fundamental study on development of a newly designed aortofemoral Y graft. *Master degree thesis. Shibaura Institute of Technology*.

[3] Fujimoto, T., Ohashi, H., Arai, K., Okamoto, K., Iwamura, H., Shiraishi, Y., & Umezu, M. (2003). Effect of bifurcation on pressure loss in aortofemoral prosthetic Y grafts. *Int J Artif Organs*, 26(7), 629.

[4] Fujimoto, T., Kawaguchi, D., Shiraishi, Y., Iwasaki, K., Arita, M., & Umezu, M. (2003). Evaluation of freestyle bioprosthesis behavior in mechanical circulatory system. *Biocybernetics and Biomedical Engineering*, 23(2), 51-55.

[5] Shunsuke, Shimizu. (2006). A study on relation between shape of Y grafts and hemodynamics in the aorta. *Master degree thesis. Shibaura Institute of Technology.*

[6] Nichols, W. W., & O'Rourke, M. F. (1997). McDonald's Blood Flow in Arteries(4th ed.). *London: Arnold.*

[7] Li-J, J. K. (2004). Dynamics of the vascular system. *Singapore: World Scientific.*

[8] Fujimoto, T., Katou, Y., Naemura, K., Fujimasu, H., & Umezu, M. (1995). Calculation of input impedance to reproduce the aorta in mechanical circulatory system. *Jpn J Artif Organs*, 24(1), 221-225.

[9] Fujimoto, T., Shiraishu, Y., & Umezu, M. (1996). An experiment on aortic pressure wave in a mechanical circulatory system. *Jpn J Artif Organs*, 25(1), 31-34.

[10] Fujimoto, T., Nakano, S., Iwamura, H., Shiraishi, Y., Yambe, T., & Umezu, M. (2006). Characteristics of a newly designed aortofemoral prosthetic Y graft under pulsatile flow conditions. *Int J Artif Organs*, 29(5), 546.

Chapter 12

Numerical Simulation in Ulcer-Like Projection due to Type B Aortic Dissection with Complete Thrombosis Type

Futoshi Mori, Hiroshi Ohtake, Go Watanabe and Teruo Matsuzawa

Additional information is available at the end of the chapter

http://dx.doi.org/10.5772/52559

1. Introduction

The aging society has rapidly progressed worldwide and the mortality and morbidity rates of aortic diseases are increasing. In particular, aortic aneurysm and aortic dissection are serious disorders. These may be fatal if their diagnosis and treatment are delayed. In 2006, guideline for the diagnosis and treatment of aortic aneurysm and aortic dissection was established in Japan [1]. In 2010, a guideline for the diagnosis and management of patients with thoracic aortic diseasewas established in the United States[2]. These guidelines pay particular attention to the diagnosis and treatment of aortic diseases. We investigated the possibility of estimating time-dependent changes in these diseases using Computational Fluid Dynamics (CFD) simulation. This chapter describes the numerical simulations used for ulcer-like projections due to aortic dissections with complete thrombosis. By combining the results of CFD and diagnostic imaging, we can anticipate future improvements in diagnosis.

1.1. Definition and classifications of aortic dissection

A blood vessel wall comprises three layers: the intima (inner layer), the media (middle layer), and the adventitia (outer layer). The pathogenesis of an aortic dissection involves an intimal tear or damage to the aortic wall. This condition is characterized by the rapid development of an intimal flap that separates the true lumen from the false lumen [3]. Intimal flap tears are characteristic of communicating dissections. The communication of blood flow between the true lumen and the false lumen is through the entry part and the re-entry part of the tear. Figure 1 shows a schematic diagram of an aortic dissection [4].

The clinical pathological condition of an aortic dissection is classified according to three aspects: the region of dissection, blood flow in the false lumen, and the disease stage. Figure 2 shows the classifications of aortic dissections. Classifications according to the region of dissection are the Stanford [5] and DeBakey [6] classifications. The Stanford classification is divided into two types, A and B, depending on whether or not the ascending aorta is involved. The treatment methodsfor Stanford Type A (Type A) and Type B (Type B) are different based on the diagnosis of the aortic dissection. Type A requires emergency surgery, whereas Type B is generally treated by antihypertensive treatment that is regulated with medical therapy. The mortality rate for Type B is lower than that for Type A. However, one in four people with this disease die per year. The DeBakey classification is categorized as DeBakey I, II, and III. DeBakey I involves both the ascending and descending aortas, DeBakey II involves only the ascending aorta, and DeBakey III involves only the ascending aorta. In addition, aortic dissections can be classified based on blood flow in the false lumen. A dissection with patent proximal and patent distal re-entry tears in the absence of a thrombus is defined as a patent type. Dissections with a false lumen that is filled with thrombus and no longer communicates with the true lumen are defined as complete thrombosis type [7]. The complete thrombosis type is designated as intramural hematoma (IMH) in the United States and Europe [8]. Finally, the classifications according to the disease stage are categorized as acute if they occur within two weeks of the development of disease and chronic if they occur after that. As per recent trend in emergency medicine, the development of disease within 48 has been classified as a super-acute stage.

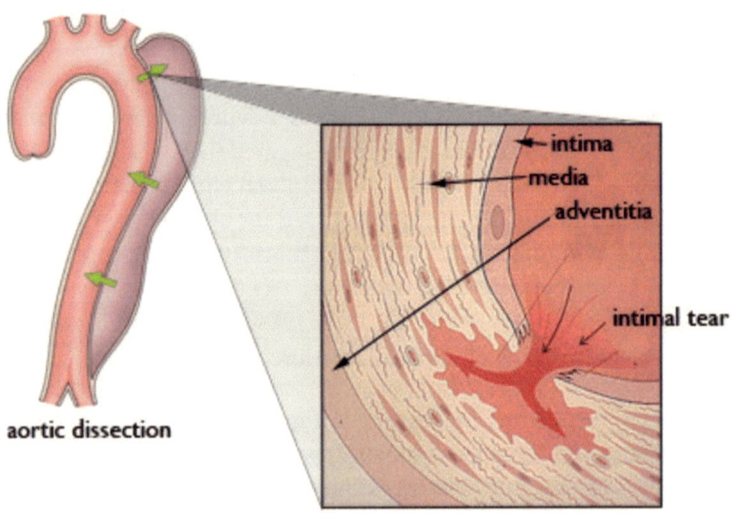

Figure 1. Schematic diagram of an aortic dissection [4].The pathogenesis of aortic dissection is an intimal tear or damage to the aortic wall.This condition is characterized by the rapid development of an intimal flap that separates the true lumen from the false lumen.

http://dx.doi.org/10.5772/52559

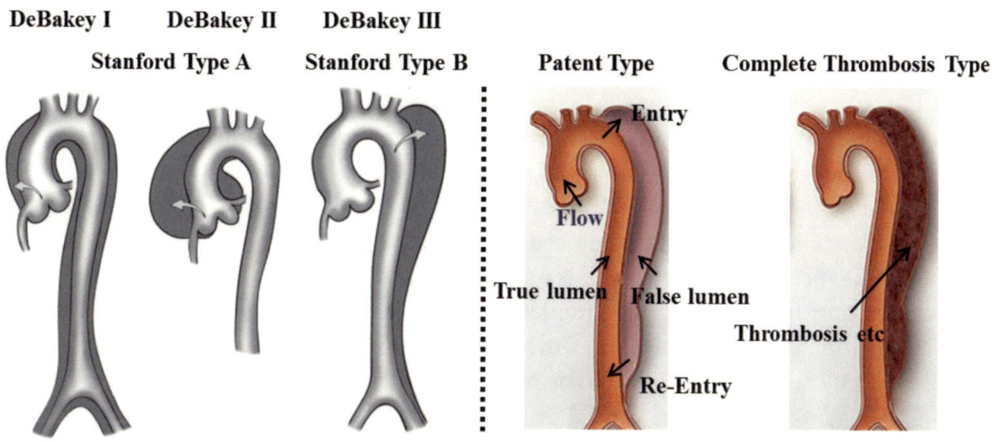

Figure 2. Classifications of aortic dissections. Based on regions of dissection: DeBakey and Stanford types (left) [9] the blood flow in the false lumen: Patent type and Complete Thrombosis type (right) [7]

1.2. Ulcer-like projection in aortic dissection

An ulcer-like projection (ULP) that occurs during the course of the complete thrombosis type [10, 11] and a penetrating atherosclerotic ulcer (PAU) due to an arteriosclerotic ulcer [12, 13] are conceptually different.ULP is an ulcerative projection image of the contrast medium that comparatively has a smooth outline and is a defect of the inner membrane continuous to the false lumen was condensed. Recently, ULP is treated as subtype (ULP type in aortic dissection) [1]. Moreover, PAU is a disease associated with bleeding and hematoma in the inner membrane. However, it is extremely difficult to clearly distinguish ULPs and PAUs in current medical diagnosis. This chapter describes ULPs.

An ULP is often detected with an improved the medical treatment imaging device such as the multi detector-row computed tomography (MDCT). A total of 170 patients admitted with acute Type B of the complete thrombosis type, 62 (36%) of these patients showed new ULP development [14]. Moreover, Kitai et al. retrospectively analyzed 38 consecutive patients who had a complete thrombosis type without an ULP. They underwent 64-row MDCT during the acute phase, and 71% of these patients were found to have intimal defects [15]. The presence of an intimal defects has been found to be a significant risk factor for evolution of IMH to an over dissection, rupture or aneurysmal dilation [16-18]. For Type A, Koshino et al. reported that ULPs developed after treatment [19]. For Type B, Tsai et al. reported that an ULP was discovered at a significant frequency for the complete thrombosis type [7]. It was clear that imaging diagnosis was an effective technique for detecting an ULP.

The survival rate of the patients who developed ULPs was higher than that of the patients who did not develop ULPs [14]. The presence or absence of ULP was a significant difference in the incidence of complications [20]. The kinds of complications were the aneurysm, aortic dissection and acute complication. Therefore, to prevent a residual ULP from forming an aneurysms and rupturing, postoperative angiography should be scheduled early after the initial surgery. In those cases when an ULP is found, surgical treatment must be done as soon as possible. For the complete thrombosis type, presence or absence of an ULP becomes a diagnostic standard. A sample CT image with an ULP reportedly has a bad prognosis [14, 16, 21]. In such cases involving an ULP, the time-dependent changes in ULPs have been discussed, which involve expansion, invariability, reduction, and disappearance [22]. The reasons for time-dependent change in an ULP are thought to be due to various factors. The parts of the aorta where the expansion tendency for an ULP is strong are the ascending aorta, the aortic arch, and the proximal descending aorta [16]. These common points are places where the influence of hemodynamics is readily applied. Moreover, an ULP can become an aneurysm during this course. The complete thrombosis type is changed to a patent type based on an ULP that might rupture. Currently, the estimation by CFD simulation for the time-dependent change is performed. The next section describes about CFD simulation.

1.3. Computed fluid dynamics simulation

It has been established using Computational Fluid Dynamics (CFD) simulations that dynamic stress is a risk factor for time-dependent changes in blood vessel configuration [23]. The recent trend in bio-fluid research is to reconstruct the blood vessel of a patient with aneurysms from the medical images and examine the distributions of several parameters, such as velocity vectors, pressures and wall shear stress (WSS) [24, 25]. Low shear has been associated with aneurysm progression [26], thrombus formation [27], and artery wall rupture [28, 29]. Karmoniket al. showed that an occlusion ofthe re-entry part increased the pressure in the false lumen in an aortic dissection [30]. Watanabe et al. reported that in the case of a partial thrombosis type,there was an increased a risk of complications [31]. In the complete thrombosis type at the systolic phase, the pressure in the false lumen is higher than that in the true lumen. In the entry part, the change in distribution indicated an effect on the intima. Shimogonya et al. performed numerical simulations to examine the formation of an aneurysm [32]. In the following sections, we will examine these factors and, in particular, concentrate on the role of hemodynamics.

2. Reconstruction shape in aortic dissection with an ULP

2.1. Observations of medical images

Imaging diagnosis using computed tomography (CT), magnetic resonance imaging (MRI), and others has significantly advanced. Thus, an accurate, prompt diagnosis is possible because of these advances. Recently, MDCT has been used. The significance of CT images has increased in the diagnosis of aortic dissections. Targeted a ULP caused by aortic dissections were all diagnosed to be saccular aneurysms. The saccular aneurysm requires a surgical adjustment because it has a tendency to rupture even when it is small.

Our study included 2 patients (sex: males; ages:Case 1, 75 years old, and Case 2, 70 years old). Both had a type B complete thrombosis aortic dissection with an ULP. The locations of their ULPs were the descending aorta. There were diagnosed by a medical doctor and ULPs showed tendencies for expansion. The period for obtaining images was approximately one month. This period included time points before the development of an ULP to immediately before the rupture of the ULP. These volunteers were treated within two weeks after an image was obtained immediately before rupture and they were recovering. Figure 3 shows the medical images of an ULP in an aortic dissection on vertical (left) and sagittal (right) views using contrast medium. By including the contrast medium, the brightness of blood flow region on the image was higher than the other parts. This ULP was caused by the aortic dissection of the complete thrombosis type. Thrombosis was present near the ULP. The format used for this image was Digital Imaging and Communications in Medicine (DICOM). DIOCM is a standard for handling, storing, printing and transmitting information for medical images. Avizo v6.3 software (Visualization Sciences Group) was used to reconstruct the aortic dissection with an ULP model based on the DICOM images of these volunteers.

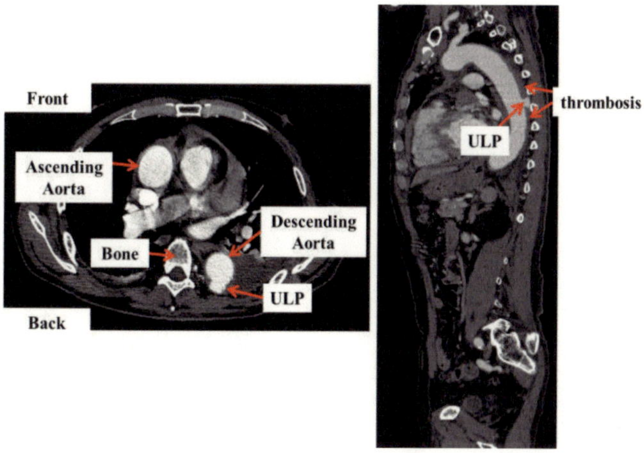

Figure 3. Ulcer-like projection in an aortic dissection of the complete thrombosis type on vertical (left) and sagittal (right) views. The location of the ULP is the descending aorta. This medical image includes a contrast medium.

2.2. Procedure of the reconstructed shape from the medical images

A realistic 3D model was reconstructed from 2D medical images using the procedure shown in figure 4. A DICOM file represents a slice of the body, as illustrated in figure3. We need to segment the blood flow region in order to generate volume data.A blood vessel region can be extracted manually by marking using Avizo v7.0.0 (VSG). The volume data are generated from the segmented part and the volume data are transferred to the stereo lithography (STL) format. STL format describes a raw, unstructured triangulated surface by a unit normal and vertices of the triangles using a 3D Cartesian coordinate system.However, the surface data that are obtained include triangle with bad aspect ratios. Thus, it is necessary to smooth the surface using Magics v9.54 (Materialize, JAPAN). A patient-specific aortic dissection with an ULP model in STL format was reconstructed from CT medical images, as illustrated in figure 4 (right).

The time-series reconstructed shape is illustrated in figure 5. The period of time-dependent change from the development of an ULP, designated Case 1A, to immediately after the rupture of the ULP, designated Case 1B, was about 1 month. In figure 5, the symbol X indicates ulceration of the artery. The symbol Y indicates that the artery is expanded, although the aneurysm was not located at this position according to the diagnosis.

A tetrahedral numerical mesh was generated using commercial software (Gambit 2.4.6, ANSYS, Inc., Canonsburg, PA).

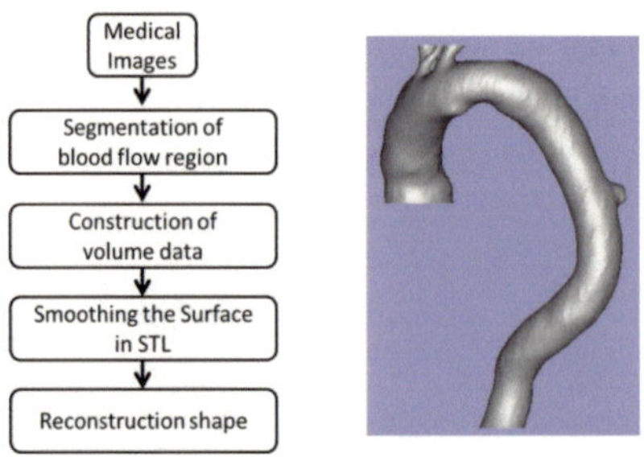

Figure 4. Procedure for reconstructing shape from medical images (left), and the reconstructed shape (right)

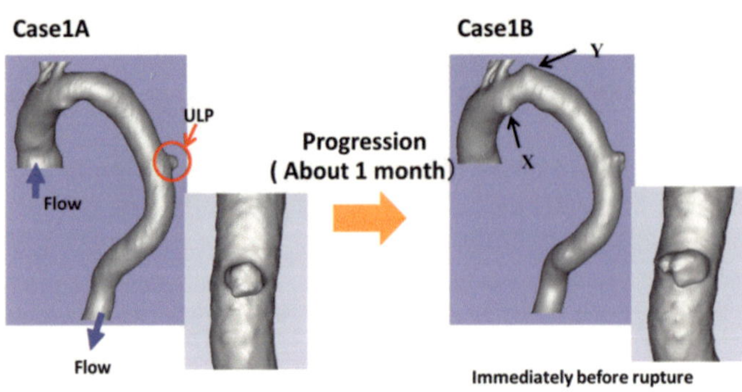

Figure 5. Time-series reconstructed shape of an aortic dissection with an ULP. The symbol X indicates ulceration of the artery and the symbol Y indicates that the artery is expanded although the aneurysm was not located at this position according to the diagnosis.

3. Numerical simulations of the time-dependent changes of an ULP in a Type B aortic dissection of the complete thrombosis type

3.1. Governing equations

This simulation calculated an unsteady-state solution. The governing equations were the following Navier-Stokes equation (1), and continuity equation (2):

$$\rho\left\{\frac{\partial \vec{u}}{\partial t}+\left(\vec{u}\cdot\nabla\right)\vec{u}\right\}=-\nabla p+\mu\nabla^2\vec{u} \qquad (1)$$

$$\nabla\cdot\vec{u}=0 \qquad (2)$$

where$\vec{u}=(u \quad v \quad w)$is a flow vector, ϱ=1.05 ×10^3 kg/m^3 is the density, p is the pressure and μ=3.5 ×10^3 N·s/m^2 is the viscosity.

We assumed the physical properties of blood. The maximum Reynolds number of the aorta at its maximum diameter in a human has been measured [33]. We assumed a Reynolds number of 6500, which is a mean value based on the literature. Blood flow was simplified as being isothermal, incompressible, and laminar Newtonian flow with a density of ϱ= 1.05 × 10^3 kg/m^{3}and a viscosity of μ= 3.5 ×10^3 N s/m^2. A k-ε model was used for turbulent flow because the flow structure of the aorta indicated that its blood flow became turbulent.

3.2. Calculation of boundary conditions

The boundary conditions used for the inlet, outlet, and blood vessel wall were as follow. The inlet boundary condition was set to the velocity profile, illustrated in figure 6 [34]. The outlet boundary condition was set to 0 Pa at the abdominal aorta. The boundary conditions for bifurcations that were at the innominate artery, the left common carotid artery, and the left subclavian artery in the upper side referred to the length from the inlet end to the outlet end and the balance of the flow rate and cross-section were set to 1:1. A no-slip condition was applied to the blood vessel wallas it was assumed to be rigid. Figure 7 illustrates the boundary conditions used in Case 1. Calculations using the finite volume method were made using a commercial solver (Fluent 6.3.26, Fluent Inc., NH). The results of similar trends were seen in Case 1 and Case 2. The results for Case 1 are shown in the following section.

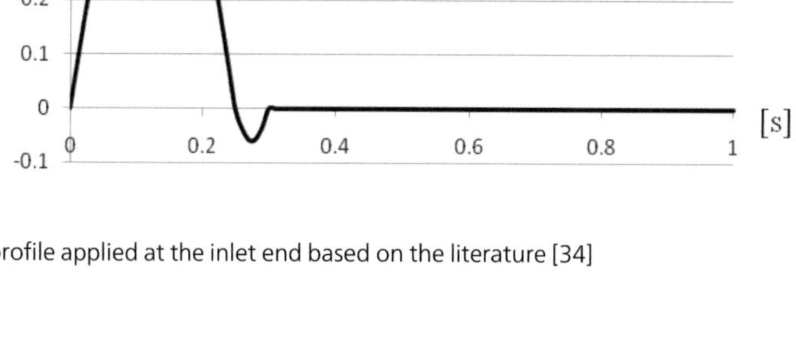

Figure 6. Velocity profile applied at the inlet end based on the literature [34]

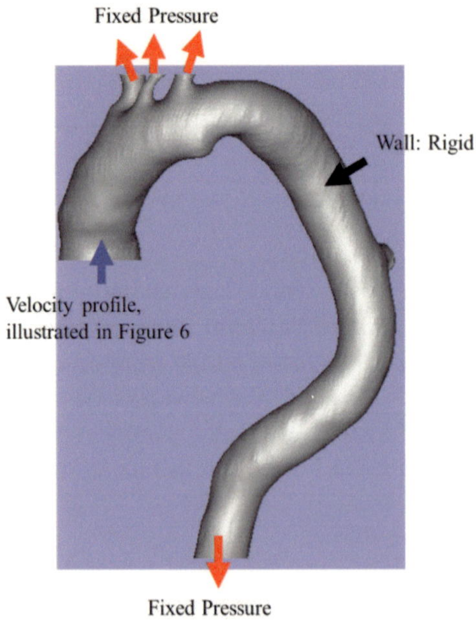

Figure 7. Boundary conditions: Inlet was set to the velocity profile in figure 6, outlet was set to a fixed pressure, and the wall was set to rigid, no-slip.

3.3. Simulation results

Figure 8 shows blood flow using the streamlines in each case at four time points (t=0.06, 0.12, 0.18, and 0.50). The flows in the aortic arch and descending aorta were faster than for Case 1B. Case 1B showed a tendency to expand and the volume of the configuration based on the time-dependent change was possibly increasing. The flow in the ULP was observed to be a vortex.

We examined the secondary flow in the ULP. During the systolic phase and excluding the adverse flow, the cross-sectional direction for the flow in the horizontal section was decided based on the flow direction in the vertical section proximal to the ULP. Figure 9 shows the secondary flow using the vectors in the ULP for Case 1A and Case 1B. The flow direction was flowing in the same direction compare to case 1A and case 1B. The flow entering from the bottom of the ULP had been outflowed from the top side after circling. In addition, the movement of the vortex core was observed using the line integral convolution (LIC) method, as illustrated in figure 10. The vortex core in the ULP moved from the outside to the inside with the passage of time. The trend for the vortex core track was consistent in each case. Therefore, there was a possibility for the ULP to expand further in Case 1B. In Case 1B, multiple vortices in the ULP were observed. Most ruptured aneurysm had complex flow patterns with multiple vortices [35, 36]. In contrast, most un-ruptured aneurysm had simple flow patterns with single vortices. Therefore, two points, which are the movements of the vortex core and multiple vortices, can be estimated for the expansion of an ULP during the movement of its vortex core.

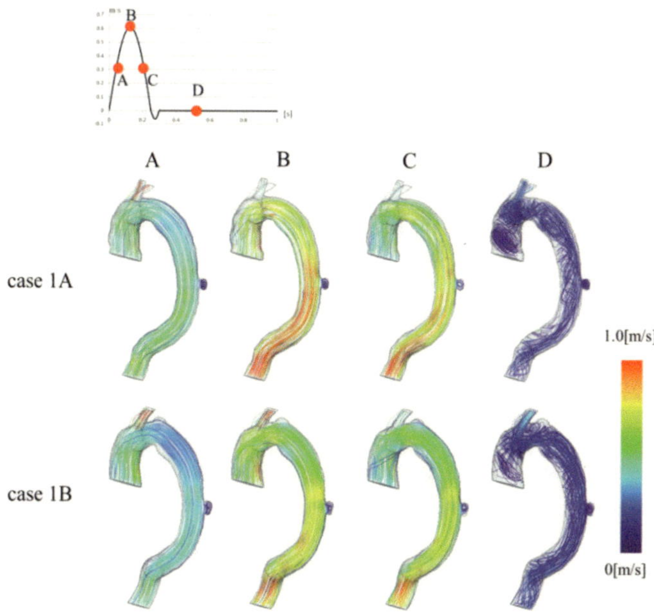

Figure 8. Flow using the streamlines in Case 1A (upper) and Case 1B (lower) at four time points (t=0.06, 0.12, 0.18, and 0.50). Blue indicates slow speed and red indicates high speed

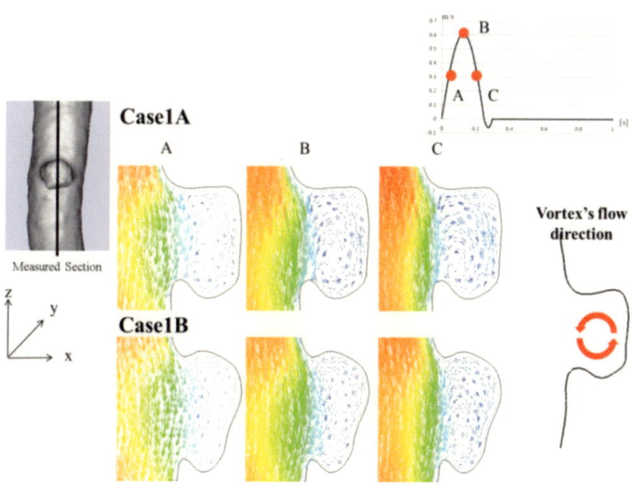

Figure 9. Secondary flow using the vectors in the horizontal sections for Case 1A (upper) and Case 1B (lower) at three time points (t=0.06, 0.12, and 0.18); the direction of the vortex flow is illustrated using the vector at the right side.

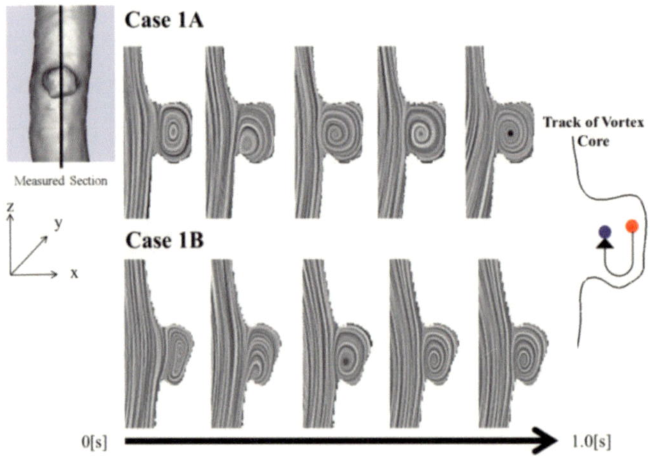

Figure 10. Movement of the vortex core using the LIC method for Case 1A (upper) and Case 1B (lower). For the track of the vortex core illustrated at the right side,the red point is the start point and the blue point is the end point.

Figure 11 shows the pressure distributions using the contours for each case at four time points. The pressure distribution values were set in the range where the ULP was emphasized. At A (t=0.06), the pressure distribution had its maximum value for the entire ULP. At the bottom side of the ULP, the pressure distribution was higher than that at other parts. Figure 12 shows the pressure distributions for each case at four time points. These four points were decided by observing the formation in Case 1B. The pressure distributions at p2, p3, and p4 were higher than at p1. When the ULP was observed in Case 1A, the progression of the configuration was observed in the high pressure region. During the progression in Case 1B, a similar trend was seen. For Case 1B, the ULP had the possibility of rupturing, which corresponded with the diagnosis made by the doctor.

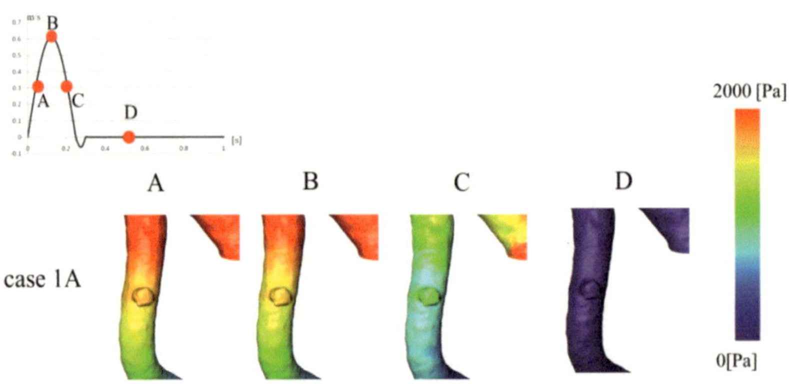

Figure 11. Pressure distributions in Case 1A at four time points. The pressure distribution values were set in the range where the ULP was emphasized.

http://dx.doi.org/10.5772/52559

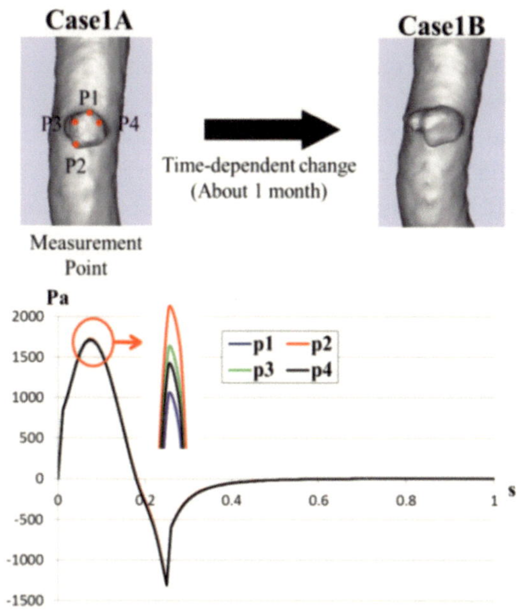

Figure 12. Pressure distributions at four time points for the ULP in Case 1A. The X axis indicatestime and the Y axis indicates the pressure distribution. Blue indicates p1 values, red indicates p2 values, green indicates p3 values, and black indicates p4 values.

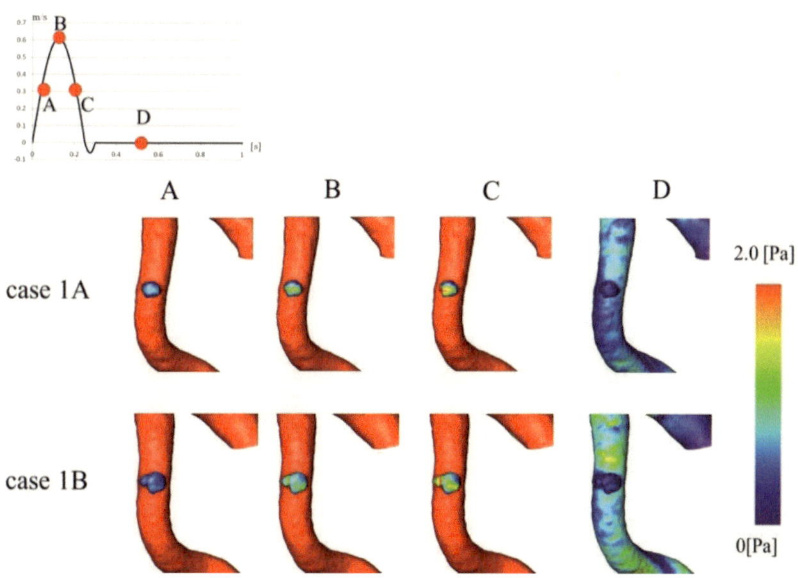

Figure 13. WSS distributionsin Case 1A and Case 1B at four time points (t=0.06, 0.12, 018, and 0.50) using their contours. The WSS distribution values were set in the range where the ULP was emphasized.

Figure 13 shows the WSS distributionsfor Case 1A and Case 1B using contours. The WSS distribution valueswere set in the range where the ULP was emphasized. At C (t=0.18), a high WSS is seen at the left side. Figure 14 shows WSS distributions in each case at four time points. The WSS distributionsat p2, p3, and p4 were lower than that at p1. When the ULP in case1A was observed, the progression of the configuration was observed in the low WSS distribution region. During the progression for Case 1B, a similar trend was seen. These results are in agreement with the results of Sheidaei [36, 37] which indicate that the region of higher expansion correlates with regions of a low WSS. Figure 15 shows the direction of WSSvectors at p2, p3, and p4. In Case 1A, the vortexes was observed at p3 and p4, and the direction of WSS vectors was separated in p2. The change in the direction of WSS vectors was seen in the area that had progressed.

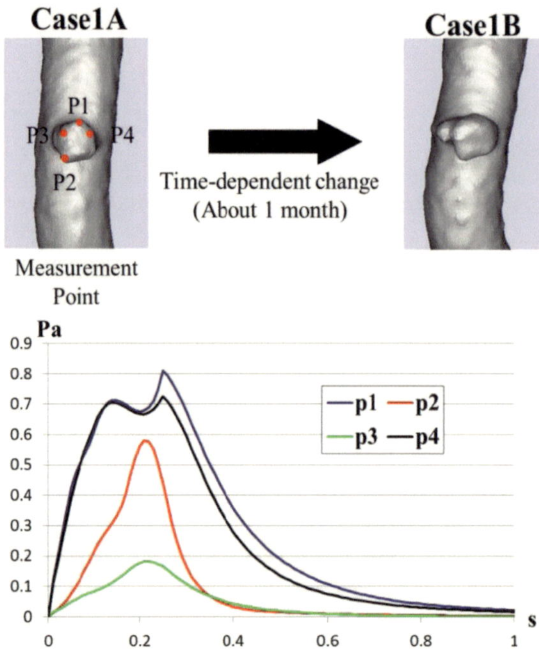

Figure 14. WSS distributions at four time points of the ULP in Case 1A. X axis indicates time and the Y axis indicates the WSS distribution. Blue indicates p1 values, red indicates p2 values, green indicates p3 values, and black indicates p4 values.

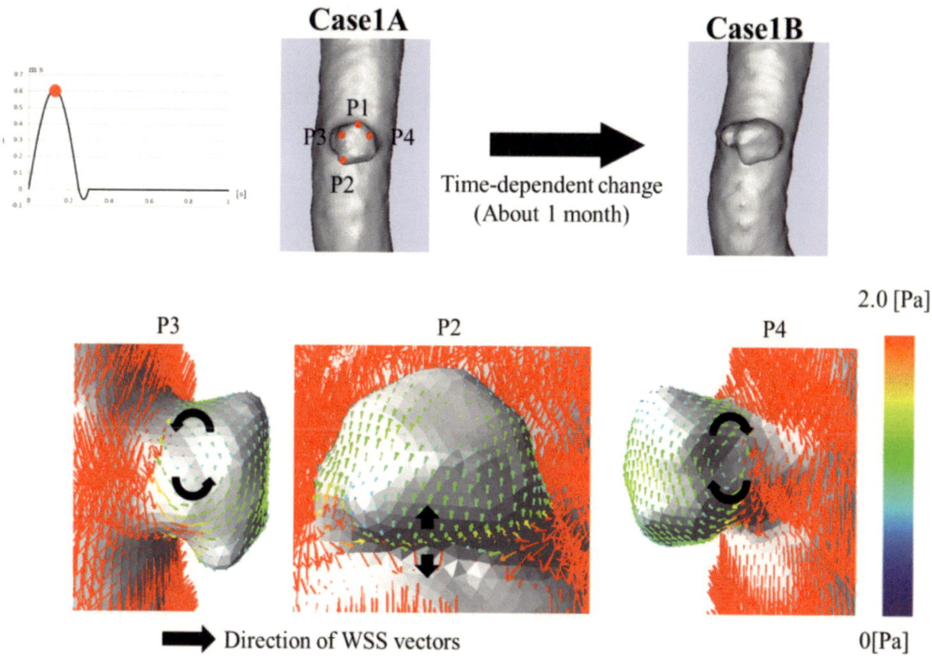

Figure 15. Direction of WSS vectors at the peak of velocity (t=0.12) using the vector. The color indicates the WSS distribution. The black arrow indicates the direction of WSS vectors. The WSS distribution values were set in the range where the ULP was emphasized.

4. Conclusions

We analyzed aortic dissections with ULPs of the complete thrombosis type using CFD simulations. In ULPs showed tendencies for expansion, the movement of the vortex cores exhibited similar tendencies. In addition, multiple vortexes were observed when a diagnosis of immediate rupture was made. Moreover, it was found that the high pressure and low WSS distribution were indictors of progression. The change in the direction of WSS vectors was seen in the area that had progressed.Thus, it is possible to predict the time-dependent change of the disease using CFD simulation.

The time-dependent change of the ULP becomes the standard of the diagnosis in aortic dissection. To examine the predictive hemodynamic factors for an ULP due to an aortic dissection of the complete thrombosis type, we reconstructed and analyzed a model blood vessel using time-series medical images. We identified the predictive hemodynamics factors. Valuable information can be obtained by combining a clinical diagnosis with fluid dynamics simulations.

Author details

Futoshi Mori[1,2,3], Hiroshi Ohtake[4], Go Watanabe[4] and Teruo Matsuzawa[5*]

*Address all correspondence to: f-mori@eri.u-tokyo.ac.jp

*Address all correspondence to: matuzawa@jaist.ac.jp

1 School of Information Science, Japan Advanced Institute of Science and Technology, Japan

2 Interfaculty Initiative in Information Studies, The University of Tokyo, Japan

3 Earthquake Research Institute, The University of Tokyo, Japan

4 Department of General and Cardiothoracic Surgery, Kanazawa University, Japan

5 Research Center for Simulation Science, Japan Advanced Institute of Science and Technology, Japan

References

[1] The Japanese Circulation Society. JCS. http://www.j-circ.or.jp/guideline/index.html/ (accessed 5August (2012).

[2] Hiratzka, L. F., Bakris, G. L., Beckman, J. A., Bersin, R. M., Carr, V. F., Casey, D. E., Jr , , Eagle, K. A., Hermann, L. K., Isselbacher, E. M., Kazerooni, E. A., Kouchoukos, N. T., Lytle, B. W., Milewicz, D. M., Reich, D. L., Sen, S., Shinn, J. A., Svensson, L. G., & Williams, D. M. 2010ACCF/AHA/AATS/ACR/ASA/SCA/SCAI/SIR/STS/SVM guidelines for the diagnosis and management of patients with thoracic aortic disease: executive summary. A report of the American College of Cardiology Foundation/ American Heart Association Task Force on Practice Guidelines, American Association for Thoracic Surgery, American College of Radiology, American Stroke Association, Society of Cardiovascular Anesthesiologists, Society for Cardiovascular Angiography and Interventions, Society of Interventional Radiology, Society of Thoracic Surgeons, and Society for Vascular Medicine. Circulation 2010;, 121, 1544-1579.

[3] Roberts WC. Aortic dissection: anatomy, consequences, and cause.American heart journal (1981). , 101, 195-214.

[4] Information for Patients from the International Registry of Acute Aortic Dissection.http://www.iradonline.org/about.htmlaccessed 5 August (2012).

[5] Daily, P. O., Trueblood, H. W., Stinson, E. B., Wuerflein, R. D., & Shumway, N. E. (1970). Management of acute aortic dissections. *The Annals of thoracic surgery*, 10, 237-247.

[6] Debakey, , Henly, W. S., Cooley, D. A., Morris, G. C., Jr , , Crawford, E. S., Beall, A. C., & Jr , . Surgical Management of Dissecting Aneurysms of the Aorta. The Journal of thoracic and cardiovascular surgery (1965). , 49, 130-149.

[7] Tsai, T. T., Evangelista, A., Nienaber, , Myrmel, T., Meinhardt, G., Cooper, J. V., Smith, D. E., Suzuki, T., Fattori, R., Llovet, A., Froehlich, J., Hutchison, S., Distante, A., Sundt, T., Beckman, J., Januzzi, J. L., Jr , , Isselbacher, E. M., & Eagle, K. A. Partial Thrombosis of the False Lumen in Patients with Acute Type B Aortic Dissection. The New England Journal of Medicine (2007). , 357, 349-359.

[8] Nienaber, , von, Kodolitsch. Y., Petersen, B., Loose, R., Helmchen, U., Haverich, A., & Spielmann, R. P. Intramural hemorrhage of the thoracic aorta. Diagnostic and therapeutic implications. Circulation (1995). , 92, 1465-1472.

[9] Aortic Dissection- Cedars-Sinai. http://www.cedars-sinai.edu/Patients/Health-Conditions/Aortic-Dissection.aspx (accessed 5August (2012).

[10] Stanson, A. W., Kazmier, F. J., Hollier, L. H., Edwards, W. D., Pairolero, P. C., Sheedy, P. F., Joyce, J. W., & Johnson, M. C. (1986). Penetrating atherosclerotic ulcers of the thoracic aorta: natural history and clinicopathologic correlations. *Annals of Vascular Surgery*, 1, 15-23.

[11] Hayashi, H., Matsuoka, Y., Sakamoto, I., Sueyoshi, E., Okimoto, T., Hayashi, K., & Matsunaga, N. Penetrating Atherosclerotic Ulcer of the Aorta: Imaging Features and Disease Concept. Radiographics (2000). , 20, 995-1005.

[12] Wu, M. T., Wang, Y. C., Huang, Y. L., Chang, R. S., Li, S. C., Yang, P., Wu, T. H., Chiou, K. R., Huang, J. S., Liang, H. L., & Pan, H. B. (2011). Intramural blood pools accompanying aortic intramural hematoma: CT appearance and natural course. *Radiology*, 258, 705-713.

[13] Park, G. M., Ahn, J. M., Kim, D. H., Kang, J. W., Song, J. M., Kang, D. H., Lim, T. H., & Song, J. K. (2011). Distal aortic intramural hematoma: clinical importance of focal contrast enhancement on CT images. *Radiology*, 259, 100-108.

[14] Kitai, T., Kaji, S., Yamamuro, A., Tani, T., Kinoshita, M., Ehara, N., Kobori, A., Kita, T., & Furukawa, Y. Impact of New Development of Ulcer-Like Projection on Clinical Outcomes in Patients With Type B Aortic Dissection With Closed and Thrombosed False Lumen. Circulation (2010). SS80., 74.

[15] Kitai, T., Kaji, S., Yamamuro, A., Tani, T., Kinoshita, M., Ehara, N., Kobori, A., Kim, K., Kita, T., & Furukawa, Y. Detection of intimal defect by 64 -row multidetector computed tomography in patients with acute aortic intramural hematoma. Circulation(2011). S174-S178.

[16] Ganaha, F., Miller, D. C., Sugimoto, K., , Y. S., Minamiguchi, H., Saito, H., Mitchell, R. S., & Dake, . Prognosis of aortic intramural hematoma with and without penetrating atherosclerotic ulcer. Circulation (2002). ; ., 106, 342-348.

[17] Sueyoshi, E., Matsuoka, Y., Sakamoto, I., Uetani, M., Kuniaki, H., & Narimatsu, M. (1997). Fate of intramural hematoma of the aorta: CT evaluation. *Journal of computer assisted tomography*, 21, 931-938.

[18] Moizumi, Y., Komatsu, T., Motoyoshi, N., & Tabayashi, K. (2004). Clinical features and long-term outcome of type A and type B intramural hematoma of the aorta. *The Journal of thoracic and cardiovascular surgery*, 127, 421-427.

[19] Enlargement of ulcer-like projections after repair of acute type A aortic dissection. The Annals of thoracic surgery; ., 68, 1860-1863.

[20] Jang, Y. M., Seo, J. B., Lee, Y. K., Chae, E. J., Park, S. H., Kang, J. W., & Lim, T. H. Newly developed ulcer-like projection (ULP) in aortic intramural haematoma on follow-up CT: is it different from the ULP seen on the initial CT?. Clinical Radiology (2008)., 63, 201-206.

[21] Kaji, S., Akasaka, T., Katayama, M., Yamabe, K., Tamita, K., Akiyama, M., Watanabe, N., Tanemoto, K., Morioka, S., & Yoshida, K. Long-term prognosis of patients with type B aortic intramural hematoma. Circulation(2003). IIII311., 307.

[22] Kawamata, H., & Kumazaki, T. Ulcerlike Projections of the Thrombosed Type Aortic Dissection- Their Incidence, Locations and Natural History-. The Journal of Japanese College of Angiology (1994)., 34, 1017-1032.

[23] Fukushima, T., Matsuzawa, T., & Homma, T. (1989). Visualization and finite element analysis of pulsatile flow in models of the abdominal aortic aneurysm. *Biorheology*, 26, 109-130.

[24] Boecher-Schwarz, H. G., Ringel, K., Kopacz, L., Heimann, A., & Kempski, O. Ex vivo study of the physical effect of coils on pressure and flow dynamics in experimental aneurysms. American Journal of Neuroradiology (2000)., 21, 1532-36.

[25] Metcalfe RW.The promise of computational fluid dynamics as a tool for delineating therapeutic options in the treatment of aneurysms. American Jounal of Neuroradiology (2003)., 24, 553-554.

[26] Boussel, L., Rayz, V., Mc Culloch, C., Martin, A., Acevedo-Bolton, G., Lawton, M., Higashida, R., Smith, W. S., Young, W. L., & Saloner, D. Aneurysm growth occurs at region of low wall shear stress patient-specificcorrelation of hemodynamics and growth in a longitudinal study. Stroke(2008)., 39, 2997-3002.

[27] Bluestein, D., Niu, L., Schoephoerster, R. T., & Dewanjee, M. K. Steady flow in ananeurysm model: correlation between fluid dynamics and blood plateletdeposition. Journal of Biomechanical Engineering-Transactions of the ASME(1996). , 118, 280-286.

[28] Shojima, M., Oshima, M., Takagi, K., Torii, R., Hayakawa, M., Katada, K., Morita, A., & Kirino, T. Magnitudeand role of wall shear stress on cerebral aneurysm-computationalfluid dynamic study of 20 middle cerebral artery aneurysms. Stroke(2004). , 35, 2500-2505.

[29] Valencia, A., Morales, H., Rivera, R., Bravo, E., & Galvez, M. Blood flow dynamicsin patient-specific cerebral aneurysm models: The relationship betweenwall shear stress and aneurysm area index. Medical Engineering & Physics(2008). , 30, 329-340.

[30] Karmonik, C., Bismuth, J., Shah, D. J., Davies, M. G., Purdy, D., & Lumsden, A. B. Computational Study of Haemodynamic Effects of Entry- and Exit-Tear Coverage in a DeBakey Type III Aortic Dissection: Technical Report. European journal of vascular and endovascular surgery (2011). , 42, 172-177.

[31] Watanabe, M., & Matsuzawa, T. (2006). Unsteady and three-dimensional simulation of blood flow in aortic dissection reconstructed from CT images. *Journal of Biomechanics*, S294 EOF.

[32] Shimogoya, Y., Ishikawa, T., Imai, Y., Matsuki, T., Yamaguchi, T. A., realistic, simulation., of, saccular., cerebral, aneurysm., formation, focusing., on, a., novel, hemodynamic., index, the., gradient, oscillatory., & number, . G. O. N. International Journal of Computational Fluid Dynamic (2009). , 8, 583-593.

[33] Stein PD., and Sabbah HN. (1976). Turbulent blood flow in the ascending aorta of humans with normal and diseased aortic valves. *Circulation research*, 39, 58-65.

[34] Fu, W., Chu, B., Chang, Yu., & Qiao, A. Construction and Analysis of Human Thoracic Aorta Based on CT Images. IFMBE Proceeding (2010). , 25, 322-325.

[35] Xiang, J., Natarajan, S. K., Tremmel, M., , D., Mocco, J., Hopkins, L. N., Siddiqui, A. H., Levy, E. L., Meng, H., & Hemodynamic, . Hemodynamic-Morphologic Discriminants for Intracranial Aneurysm Rupture. Stroke (2011). , 42, 144-152.

[36] Tremmel, M., Dhar, S., Levy, E. I., Mocco, J., & Meng, H. (2009). Influence of intracranial aneurysm-to-parent vessel size ratio on hemodynamics and implication for rupture: results from a virtual experimental study. *Neurosurgery*, 64, 622-630.

[37] Shidaei, A., Hunley, S. C., Zeinali-Davarani, S., Raguin, L. G., & Baek, S. Simulation of abdominal aortic aneurysm growth with updating hemodynamic loads using a realistic geometry. Medical Engineering & Physics (2011). , 33, 80-88.